Autoimmune Bullous Diseases

Barbara Horváth
Editor

Autoimmune Bullous Diseases

Text and Review

Second Edition

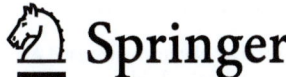

Editor
Barbara Horváth
Center for Blistering Diseases, Department of Dermatology
University Medical Center Groningen, University of Groningen
Groningen, The Netherlands

ISBN 978-3-030-91556-8   ISBN 978-3-030-91557-5   (eBook)
https://doi.org/10.1007/978-3-030-91557-5

© The Editor(s) (if applicable) and The Author(s), under exclusive license to Springer Nature Switzerland AG 2016, 2022
This work is subject to copyright. All rights are solely and exclusively licensed by the Publisher, whether the whole or part of the material is concerned, specifically the rights of translation, reprinting, reuse of illustrations, recitation, broadcasting, reproduction on microfilms or in any other physical way, and transmission or information storage and retrieval, electronic adaptation, computer software, or by similar or dissimilar methodology now known or hereafter developed.
The use of general descriptive names, registered names, trademarks, service marks, etc. in this publication does not imply, even in the absence of a specific statement, that such names are exempt from the relevant protective laws and regulations and therefore free for general use.
The publisher, the authors and the editors are safe to assume that the advice and information in this book are believed to be true and accurate at the date of publication. Neither the publisher nor the authors or the editors give a warranty, expressed or implied, with respect to the material contained herein or for any errors or omissions that may have been made. The publisher remains neutral with regard to jurisdictional claims in published maps and institutional affiliations.

This Springer imprint is published by the registered company Springer Nature Switzerland AG
The registered company address is: Gewerbestrasse 11, 6330 Cham, Switzerland

Preface to the Second Edition

Almost 5 years ago the first edition of Autoimmune Bullous Diseases study guide, edited by the late Professor Marcel Jonkman, was published. The right concept of the book was proven by its popularity, with more than 20,000 downloads of the electronic version.

However, a lot has happened in the past 5 years, both inside and outside the blistering world.

Unfortunately, Professor Marcel Jonkman passed away in 2019 due to an uncurable disease, but his legacy stayed anchored at the Center for Blistering Diseases in Groningen.

Therefore, the team in Groningen happily contributed to the second edition of this study book. We have kept the main case-based structure of the book, presenting it more as a handbook. The aim is to help clinicians in daily practice to diagnose and treat patients, rather than to provide a dry overview of the latest scientific developments. Moreover, this book became an essential resource for trainees in dermatology worldwide and for dermatologist aiming to refresh their knowledge.

Despite the fact that the basic principles of Autoimmune Bullous Diseases (AIBDs) are unchanged, we have updated the content based on current developments in diagnostics and management of AIBDs, which are still potentially life-threating diseases with an enormous impact on patients' lives. In the last decade, lots of efforts have been made by international organizations to create solid evidence in clinical trials and to publish several guidelines.

New assays, invented by our own immunodermatology laboratory, are described in the diagnostic part.

The treatment of AIBDs, especially of pemphigus, is revolutionized by the approval of rituximab for pemphigus vulgaris. Therefore, rituximab received a more pronounced place in this book (Chapter Pemphigus Vulgaris). Furthermore, with the introduction of new therapies such as novel antidiabetics or immune checkpoint inhibitors, more AIBDs are diagnosed as an adverse event in daily practice. Therefore, we adjusted the chapters on drug-induced AIBDs. Finally, two new chapters were added. First, the new chapter "Autoimmune Bullous Diseases in Childhood" aims to raise awareness for blistering cases other than epidermolysis bullosa or linear IgA disease in children. Second, we have written a chapter with the focus on "Wound care in Autoimmune Bullous Diseases" since this is crucial in the management of AIBDs but often forgotten.

I would like to thank my colleagues of the Center for Blistering Diseases and the authors for reviewing and updating the content of the first edition. I wish to thank Mrs. Katarina Ondrekova for the assistance regarding this process, and Prakash Jagannathan from Springer's office for the skillful editing. Finally, I would like to express my gratitude to all of our patients trusting in our knowledge and care and participating in our common effort to improve the management of autoimmune bullous diseases.

Groningen, The Netherlands   Barbara Horváth

Contents

1. **Basic Principles of the Immune System and Autoimmunity** 1
   Gilles F. H. Diercks and Philip M. Kluin

2. **Dermatological Examination of Bullous Diseases** 11
   Marcel F. Jonkman and Barbara Horváth

3. **How to Take a Biopsy** 29
   Gilles F. H. Diercks, Joost M. Meijer, and Marcel F. Jonkman

4. **Direct Immunofluorescence Microscopy** 35
   Gilles F. H. Diercks and Hendri H. Pas

5. **Indirect Immunofluorescence Microscopy** 43
   Gilles F. H. Diercks and Hendri H. Pas

6. **Immuno-Assays** 53
   Hendri H. Pas

7. **Structure of Desmosomes** 61
   Ena Sokol

8. **Pemphigus Vulgaris** 65
   Gerda van der Wier, Marcel F. Jonkman, and Barbara Horváth

9. **Pemphigus Foliaceus** 77
   Laura de Sena N. Maehara, Marcel F. Jonkman, and Barbara Horváth

10. **Paraneoplastic Pemphigus** 87
    Angelique M. Poot, Gilles F. H. Diercks, Hendri H. Pas, Marcel F. Jonkman, and Barbara Horváth

11. **IgA Pemphigus** 93
    Barbara Horváth and Marcel F. Jonkman

12. **Drug-Induced Pemphigus** 99
    Sylvia H. Kardaun and Laura de Sena Nogueira Maehara

13. **Structure of Hemidesmosomes and the Epidermal Basement Membrane Zone** 103
    Iana Turcan, Maria C. Bolling, and Marcel F. Jonkman

14	**Pemphigoid Diseases Affecting the Skin** 107
	Joost M. Meijer, Aniek Lamberts, and Jorrit B. Terra
15	**Mucous Membrane Pemphigoid** 121
	Joost M. Meijer, Hanan Rashid, and Jorrit B. Terra
16	**Epidermolysis Bullosa Acquisita** 131
	Joost M. Meijer and Marcel F. Jonkman
17	**Bullous Systemic Lupus Erythematosus** 137
	Marcel F. Jonkman and J. M. Meijer
18	**Linear IgA Bullous Dermatosis** 143
	Barbara Horváth and Marcel F. Jonkman
19	**Drug-Induced Pemphigoid and Linear IgA Disease** 151
	Sylvia H. Kardaun and Joost M. Meijer
20	**Dermatitis Herpetiformis** 157
	Barbara Horváth and Marcel F. Jonkman
21	**Stevens Johnson Syndrome/Toxic Epidermal Necrolysis and Erythema Exsudativum Multiforme** 165
	Sylvia H. Kardaun
22	**Porphyria Cutanea Tarda and Pseudoporphyria** 177
	Marjolein S. Bruijn and Jorrit B. Terra
23	**Bullous Dermatitis Artefacta** 181
	Marcel F. Jonkman, Wianda A. Christoffers, and Barbara Horváth
24	**Autoimmune Bullous Diseases in Childhood** 187
	Maria C. Bolling and Joost M. Meijer
25	**Wound Care in Autoimmune Bullous Diseases** 193
	Josephine C. Duipmans and Maria C. Bolling

Appendix A: Patient Support Groups and International Centers for AIBD 199

Index 203

Basic Principles of the Immune System and Autoimmunity

Gilles F. H. Diercks and Philip M. Kluin

Learning Objectives

After studying this chapter, you should know:

- The difference between the innate and adaptive immune system
- The functions of antigen presenting cells, B- and T-lymphocytes
- Causes of autoimmunity and types of hypersensitivity with emphasis on pemphigoid and pemphigus

The Immune System: A Short Introduction

Two Systems: The Innate and Adaptive System

The immune system is composed of two closely collaborative systems, an innate and an adaptive system (Fig. 1.1). *The immune system is composed of an innate and an adaptive system* These systems are activated as the first barriers of defense, mucosa and skin, are breached. The innate immune system is a constitutive present system that can act rapidly to eradicate microbes. *The innate system is a quick response system.* The primary cells of the innate immune system are macrophages, granulocytes, natural killer (NK) cells and dendritic cells, but other cells like epithelial cells can also be part of it. For instance macrophages and granulocytes are capable of phagocytosis of microorganisms by endocytosis. Pathogen-associated molecules are present on microbes and recognized by cells of the innate system by binding to toll-like receptors. In particular these cells are effective against bacteria whereas NK cells are used to fight viruses. They do this in an indirect way by recognizing and killing virally infected host cells. Besides the cellular response many proteins play an important part in the innate immune system, e.g. chemokines, interleukins, interferon and tumor necrosis factor. Binding of microbial antigens will therefore not only induce phagocytosis but also release of cytokines, which will result in an inflammatory response. Apart from these proteins the complement system constitutes an important part of the immune system. This system can be activated directly by a microorganism itself or indirectly by binding to antibodies produced by the adaptive immune system. Eventually proteins of the complement system promote phagocytosis and inflammation.

G. F. H. Diercks (✉) · P. M. Kluin
Department of Pathology, University Medical Center Groningen, University of Groningen, Groningen, The Netherlands
e-mail: g.f.h.diercks@umcg.nl

© The Author(s), under exclusive license to Springer Nature Switzerland AG 2022
B. Horváth (ed.), *Autoimmune Bullous Diseases*, https://doi.org/10.1007/978-3-030-91557-5_1

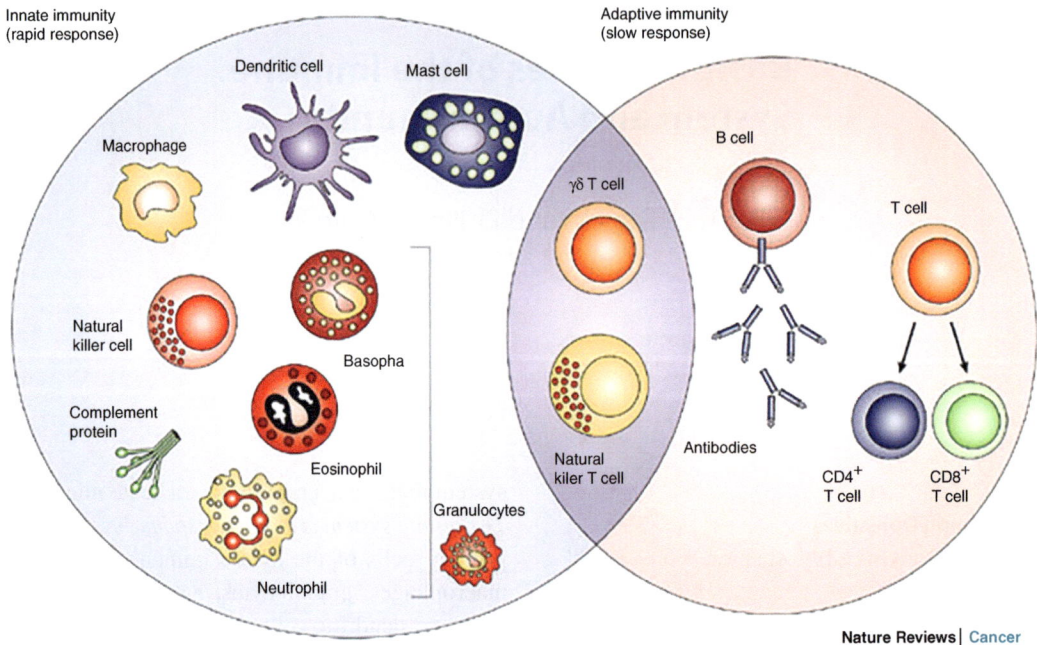

Fig. 1.1 An overview of the innate and adaptive immune system. [Reprinted by permission from Macmillan Publishers Ltd: Nature Reviews Cancer, Dranoff G. Cytokines in cancer pathogenesis and cancer therapy. 4, 11–22. Copyright 2004]

The Adaptive System in More Detail

Next to the innate system is the adaptive immunity that can be divided in a humoral and cellular system (Fig. 1.2). *The adaptive immune system is divided in a humoral and cellular system and is an antigen specific system.* By definition the adaptive immunity is a "learning" system that has to be trained. In consequence the start will be slow, but once trained, the responses will also be quite fast. In contrast to the innate system, this system is antigen specific and by that more effective. An antigen as part of a microorganism or own cells, most frequently represents a protein, but it is good to know that it also can be a carbohydrate, lipid or DNA, all being capable of inducing an antibody response.

Lymphocytes bear antigen receptors on their surface and can on basis of these receptors be divided into B-lymphocytes and T-lymphocytes. These receptors are called the B cell receptor (BCR) or cell surface immunoglobulin in B-lymphocytes and the T cell receptor (TCR) in T-lymphocytes. *B- and T-lymphocytes are the main constituents of the adaptive immune system* B-lymphocytes originate directly from and also undergo some steps of maturation with assembly of the BCR within the bone marrow, whereas T-lymphocytes start in the bone marrow but the assembly of their TCR takes place in the thymus (Fig. 1.3). After recognizing an antigen by the BCR in the peripheral lymphoid tissues such as a lymph node, B-lymphocytes are activated and altered into plasma cells and large quantities of antibody are processed and secreted by these specific B-cells. These antibodies have the same antigen-binding site as the BCR that first recognized the antigen. Antibodies can inactivate an antigen, e.g. a microorganism by complement binding or aid in phagocytosis of this microorganism, the latter called opsonization. This is entire process is thus called humoral immunity.

T-cells are part of the cellular immunity, which basically is important in eliminating intracellular microorganisms, mainly viruses. In contrast to the BCR, the T-cell receptor can only recognize

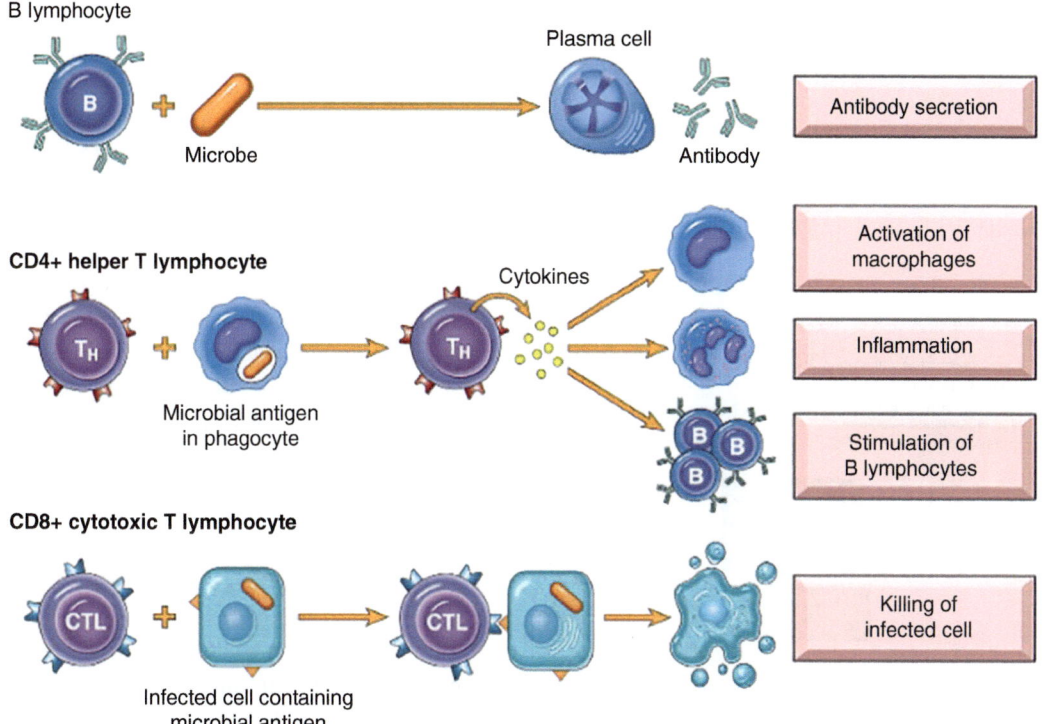

Fig. 1.2 The principle classes of lymphocytes and their functions in adaptive immunity. [Reprinted with permission from: Kumar V, Abbas AK, Fausto N, Aster J. Robbins & Cotran Pathologic Basis of Disease, 8th Edition, page 185, Copyright Elsevier 2010]

small fragments of proteins (peptide) that are presented on the surface of the infected cell by major histocompatibility complex (MHC) molecules, also called human leucocyte antigens (HLA). Thus microorganisms first have to be degraded before they can be recognized by the system. MHC molecules are divided into class-I and class-II molecules. Class-I molecules are present on all nucleated cells and platelets. Only a physical combination of an antigen-peptide within a specific MHC-I-class molecule can be recognized by the T-cell receptor. This activation transforms this particular T-cell into a cytotoxic T-cell capable of killing virally infected cells by inducing apoptosis.

MHC-II-class molecules are only expressed on certain cells of the immune system, in particular dendritic cells, macrophages and B-lymphocytes, together called antigen-presenting cells. These cells can present antigen-peptides in conjunction with MHC-II molecules to T-helper cells. These antigens are derived from degraded microorganisms that are phagocytized by the antigen-presenting cells. In addition, these T-helper cells can secrete numerous cytokines, thereby inducing activation of macrophages, stimulation of B-cells to produce antibodies but also cytotoxic T cells to do their work. T-helper cells can therefore functionally be divided into Th1 cells, stimulating a cytotoxic T-cell response, Th2 cells, involved in the humoral immune response, and different subsets of regulatory T-cells, involved in controlling these processes. *T-lymphocytes can be divided in cytotoxic T-cells and T-helper cells.* Importantly the interaction between the antigen presenting cells and the T cells with interaction between HLA molecules TCR's is helped by many other receptors and ligands on these cells, generally called "costimulatory molecules".

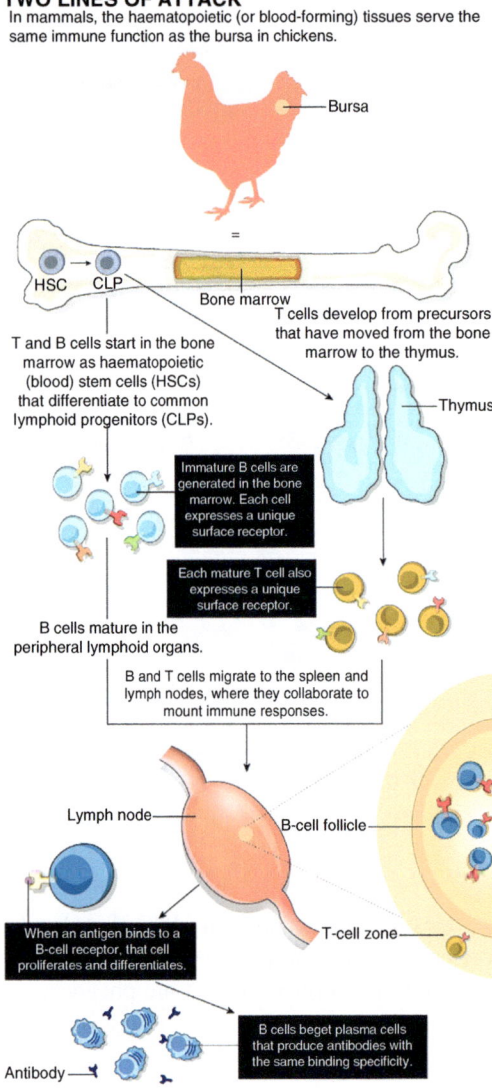

Fig. 1.3 The origin and fate of B- and T-lymphocytes. [Reprinted by permission from Macmillan Publishers Ltd: Nature, Gitlin AD, Nussenzweig MC. Fifty years of B-lymphocytes. 517, 139–141. Copyright January 2015]

Antibodies are produced by plasma cells, which are terminally differentiated B-lymphocytes (Fig. 1.4). *Antigen-specific antibodies are produced by plasma cells, which are terminally differentiated B-lymphocytes.* Each antibody is unique and produced by a single clone of plasma cells. Antibodies are composed of an antigen binding fragment (Fab) and a constant region (Fc), responsible for the effector function of the antibody. An antibody is made up of two identical heavy chains and two identical light chains. Both chains can be divided into a variable part, involved in antigen recognition, and a constant part. This constant part of the heavy chain divides the antibodies into five classes: IgM, IgA, IgG, IgE and IgD. Immature B-cells express IgM (sometimes in combination with IgD) class antibodies on the cell surface. However, under influence of cytokines B-cells can produce other classes of immunoglobulins, a process called isotype switching. This takes place in a specialized compartment of the lymph node, called the follicle or germinal center. In this compartment an additional process takes place, which is called affinity maturation and which means that binding of the BCR of individual B-cells to the antigen is further improved. B-cells with these improved receptors will more efficiently recognize the antigen after rechalllenge and therefore provide a better and faster immune response, which is the idea behind the effect of boost vaccinations in all vaccination programs. While B-cells that did not encounter an antigen before are called naive B-cells, these improved B-cells are called memory B-cells.

As already mentioned, the function of free antibodies is twofold: microorganisms loaded with antibodies are phagocytized more easily because phagocytizing cells are capable of binding the Fc part of the antibodies. Besides that, once fixed to an antigen, antibodies are capable of stimulating the complement system. *Antibodies aid in phagocytosis of microbes and stimulate the complement system.*

All cells of the immune system originate from the bone marrow. The myeloid stem cells mature into granulocytes, macrophages, erythrocytes and thrombocytes, while lymphoid stem cells differentiate to precursor B- and T-cells (and natural killer cells not discussed here). Maturation of B-cells occurs in the bone marrow with formation of unique antigen receptors on the cell surface. In contrast, maturation of T-cells takes place in a specialized organ, called the thymus. It is important that B- and T-cells do not react against

Fig. 1.4 Basic structure of an antibody. [Adapted from Y_tambe: Wikipedia under a Creative Commons Attribution-Share Alike 3.0 License.]

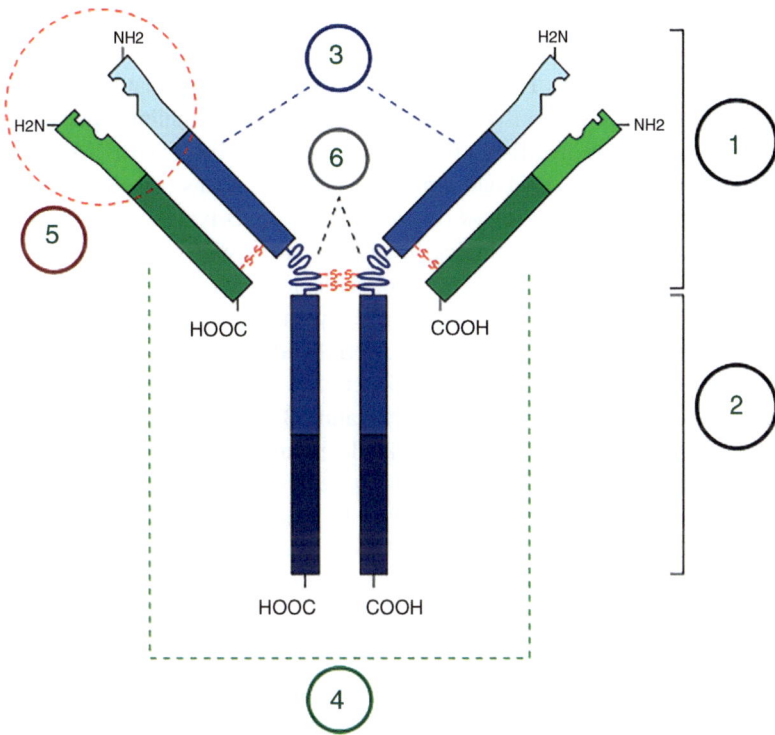

self-antigens, since this might result in autoimmunity. Normally, these potentially auto-reactive and therefore dangerous cells go into apoptosis, a process called negative selection or clonal deletion. After maturation in the bone marrow and thymus the lymphoid cells migrate to secondary lymphoid organs, e.g. lymph nodes, spleen and mucosa associated lymphoid tissues.

Whereas intact microorganisms can be transported directly to be presented to the B-cells in these tissues, for interaction with T-cells transport of antigens is mostly done by dendritic cells. In these peripheral lymphoid organs both the already mentioned naïve and faster and more efficient memory B- and T-cells reside, which can directly be activated.

A Closer Look at the Skin

Besides having a barrier function, the skin itself is also an important immunogenic organ. *The skin functions in the innate as well as in the adaptive immune system*. The skin possesses an innate immune response, characterized by synthesis and release of antimicrobial peptides like defensins and substance P. Next to the innate immunity, the adaptive immunity is provided by Langerhans cells, a population of dendritic cells that reside in the epidermis. These Langerhans cells can phagocytize antigens, migrate to regional lymph nodes (sometimes called veiled cells), and present the antigen to a T-lymphocyte, which can result in a cellular or humoral immune response, the latter only if the antigen is also presented to B-cells. Moreover, circulating macrophages, T-cells and dendritic cells, present in the dermis, provide continuous immunological surveillance.

Autoimmunity

Cells of the innate immune system recognize so-called pathogen associated molecules on microorganisms. Human cells lack these patterns on their surface, thereby preventing auto-reactivity.

The adaptive immune system avoids auto-reactivity by the aforementioned clonal deletion or negative selection. This result is also called immunological tolerance. When this tolerance is breached, auto-reactive B- and T-cells might be formed, a process called autoimmunity. *Auto-reactive B- and T-lymphocytes can induce autoimmune diseases.* Immunological tolerance can be achieved by central tolerance, i.e. clonal deletion of B- and T-cells in bone marrow and thymus respectively, and peripheral tolerance. Peripheral tolerance is achieved by functional inactivation and active suppression of auto-reactive mature B- and T-cells that have escaped clonal deletion. *Central and peripheral tolerance prevents autoimmunity.* For complete activation of B- and T-cells, besides antigen-antibody binding, the already mentioned co-stimulatory signals are also necessary. These co-stimulatory signals are mostly present on cells of the innate system, i.e. macrophages and dendritic cells. Absence of these signals, e.g. in case of auto-reactivity, will result in functional inactivation of the immune response. This is called anergy. Regulatory T-cells (Tregs) play an important role in active suppression of the immune response by inhibitory effects on T-cells, macrophages and dendritic cells. In addition to stimulation, some of these costimulatory molecules have an opposite effect by dampening the immune interaction, a physiological process necessary to stop an immune reaction. One of these molecules is CTLA4. Interestingly, some recently developed drugs interact with these costimulatory interactions, for instance Ipilimumab, which blocks CTLA4, is presently used to improve the immune reaction against metastatic melanoma.

Unfortunately these mechanisms are not perfect and auto-reactivity can still occur and might eventually result in autoimmune diseases. Several mechanisms can be responsible for breaching immunological tolerance. First, certain microorganisms can bind to the constant part of membranous IgM on the cell surface of B-lymphocytes, thereby avoiding the need of co-stimulatory signals of T-helper cells. This is called a superantigen stimulated polyclonal lymphocytic activation. In addition, the Epstein-Barr-virus (EBV), after internalization, stimulates B-cell proliferation and inhibits apoptosis by producing certain proteins, like EBNA-2 and EBNA-LP. These mechanisms result in an uncontrolled polyclonal B-lymphocyte response that might produce self-reactive antibodies. Second, antigens of microorganisms might have a strong resemblance to self-antigens. This might result in a cross reaction of B- and T-cells against auto-antigens, a process called molecular mimicry. Finally, exposure of the immune system to normally shielded antigens (eye, testis, brain) or exposure to newly formed antigens (neoepitopes) can result in an immune response to a self-antigen that has not previously been recognized as such. An example of a neoepitope in blistering diseases is the shed ectodomain of collagen XVII that might serve as a self-antigen.

Important modulating factors in autoimmunity are sex hormones, explaining the predominance of autoimmune diseases in women, and genetic background. *Sex hormones and genetic background are important factors for developing autoimmune diseases.* In particular MHC genes are an important factor in developing autoimmune diseases. Associations have been found between certain MHC haplotypes and autoimmune diseases. For instance, HLA-DQβ1*0301 has been associated with various variants of pemphigoid, whereas several studies have demonstrated an association between HLA-DRB1 and pemphigus vulgaris.

Various pathophysiological mechanisms in autoimmune diseases are eventually responsible for the clinical manifestations. These hypersensitivity reactions are classified after the proposal of Gell and Coombs. In Type II reactions autoantibodies are directed against cell or matrix components. Pemphigoid and pemphigus are the result of type II hypersensitivity. *Autoimmune blistering diseases are the result of type II hypersensitivity, whereas systemic lupus erythematosus results from a type III hypersensitivity reaction.* A Type III reaction is the result of deposition of antigen-antibody immune complexes in various organs, eventually resulting in tissue destruction. An example of a type III hypersensitivity reaction is systemic lupus erythematosus (SLE). Typically, SLE is more prominent in women and genetic factors contribute to the disease. SLE is characterized by the formation of IgG antibodies against nuclear antigens (ANA), in particular against double stranded DNA (dsDNA). These circulating IgG-dsDNA complexes deposit in various organs, especially in kidneys (glomerulonephritis), skin (facial erythema) and joints (synovitis). These immune complexes are the mediators of tissue injury, mainly by activating the complement system. As shown in Fig. 1.5, these complexes can directly be visualized by immunofluorescent techniques in a skin biopsy of the patient. Such a pattern is also called a lupus band. In fact, complement consumption and low levels of circulating complement factors C3 and C4 characterize disease activity.

Type IV hypersensitivity or delayed type hypersensitivity is the result of stimulation of Th1-lymphocytes, that can induce tissue damage by secretion of certain cytokines. Eczema is an example of a type IV reaction.

As stated above pemphigoid and pemphigus are the result of a type II hypersensitivity reaction. In bullous pemphigoid autoantibodies are directed against collagen XVII (BP180) and/or BP230, important components of the hemidesmosome, responsible for attachment of the epidermis to the dermis. *Pemphigoid diseases are characterized by antibodies against hemidesmosomal components.* These antibodies are mainly of the IgG class, although often in conjunction with IgA. These circulating autoantibodies react with these hemidesmosomal antigens, giving rise to a cascade of events. Binding of IgG to BP180 results in complement activation, attraction of inflammatory cells to the dermis and release of proteases by granulocytes that ultimately induce dermal-epidermal splitting [1] (Fig. 1.6). Besides this inflammatory response another mechanism has been proposed responsible for detachment of the epidermis from the dermis. Adhesion of antibodies to BP180 can result in internalization and endocytosis of this protein, thereby weakening the hemidesmosome (Fig. 1.7) [2]. In this case an inflammatory response is not necessary for subepidermal blistering and explains the existence of pemphigoid blisters without an inflammatory infiltrate.

Also pemphigus is caused by autoreactive antibodies, in this case directed against desmoglein 1 and 3. *Pemphigus is characterized by antibodies against desmosomal proteins, mainly desmogleins.* Desmogleins are components of the desmosome, responsible for the attachment between keratinocytes. The exact mechanism by which these antibodies are responsible for acantholysis and subsequent intraepidermal blistering is not completely clear. In contrast to pemphigoid an inflammatory response seems not to be primarily responsible. Several alternative theories have been proposed. First is the steric hindrance theory, which is based on the idea that direct interference of IgG with the extracellular domain of desmoglein results in acantholysis [3]. The second theory implies that deranged cell signaling, i.e. activation of p38 MAPK [4], RhoA [5] and plakoglobin [6], interferes with desmosomal function. Finally, pemphigus IgG might influence desmosome assembly and disassembly. Binding of IgG to desmoglein could result in internalization of desmoglein by endocytosis, eventually reducing the adhesion strength between keratinocytes [7].

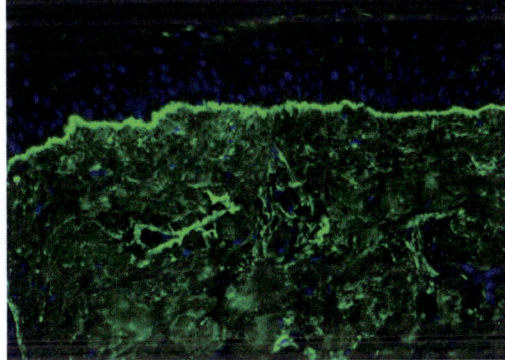

Fig. 1.5 The lupus band: deposition of immunoglobulins along the basement membrane zone

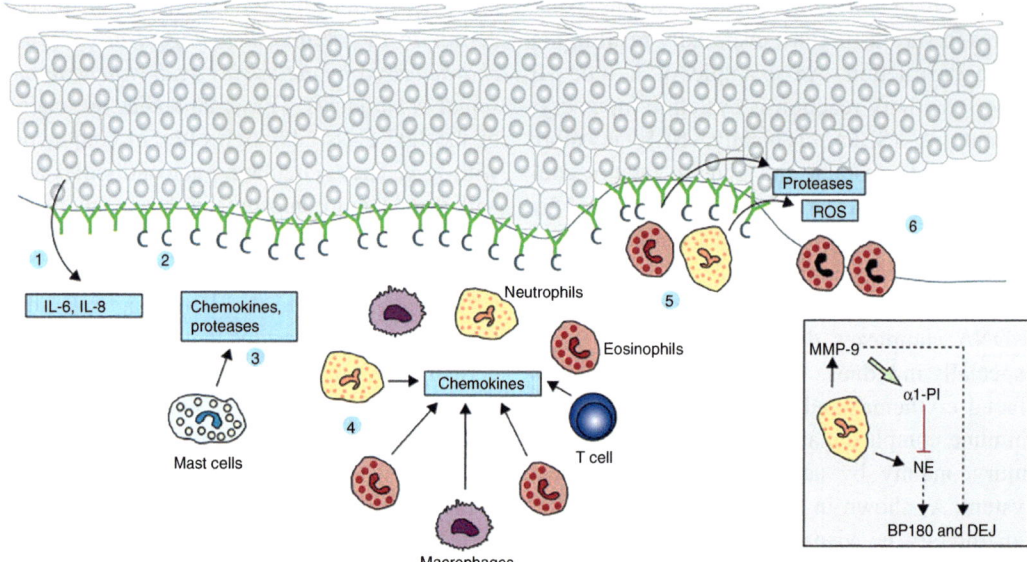

Fig. 1.6 Hypothetical sequence of events leading to blister formation in bullous pemphigoid. Binding of autoantibodies to BP180 initiates Fc receptor-independent events leading to the release of interleukin 6 (IL-6) and IL-8 from basal keratinocytes (1). Complement is activated (2) at the dermal–epidermal junction (DEJ) and mast cells degranulate (3). Complement activation and chemokine gradients result in the infiltration of inflammatory cells into the upper dermis (4). Secretion of inflammatory mediators further increases the inflammatory reaction before granulocytes at the DEJ release proteases (insert) and reactive oxygen species (ROS) (5) that ultimately induce dermal–epidermal splitting (6). As shown in the neonatal mouse model of bullous pemphigoid, matrix metalloproteinase 9 (MMP-9) secreted from neutrophils cleaves (green arrow) α1-proteinase inhibitor (α1-PI) to remove neutrophil elastase inhibition (red bar). Both MMP-9 and NE also directly degrade proteins of the DEJ including BP180 (insert). [Reprinted from The Lancet, 381, Schmidt N, Zillikens D, Pemphigoid diseases 320–332, with permission from Elsevier.]

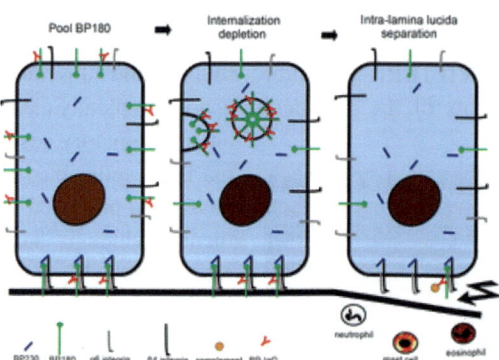

Fig. 1.7 Potential mechanisms of blistering in BP. Hemidesmosomal proteins are distributed homogeneously on the plasma membrane, and some of them compose HD at the ventral side of basal cells (left). HD seemed to be constantly remodelled, assembly and disassembly. Initially, autoantibodies bind to BP180, which is distributed on the plasma membrane of basal cells, and lead to internalization of BP180 and depleting BP180 from the plasma membrane (middle). The depletion of BP180 by anti-BP180 autoantibodies may disturb the supply of BP180 and impair HD formation. Insufficient HD lacking BP180 may not have enough adhesional strength to basement membrane. Finally, intra-lamina lucida separations may be caused by mechanical stress or inflammation, such as fixation of complement and FcgR-dependent activation of neutrophils, induced via Fc fragment of pathogenic IgG (right). [Reprinted from: Iwata H, KitajimaY. Bullous pemphigoid: role of complement and mechanisms for blister formaation within the lamina lucida. Exp Derm 2013; 22:381–385. With permission from Wiley.]

Review Questions

1. The innate immune system
   a. Is an antigen-specific system
   b. Is a quick response system
   c. Is made up of mainly lymphocytes
2. B-lymphocytes
   a. Are efficient in killing viruses
   b. Mature in the thymus
   c. Differentiate into plasma cells, which produce antibodies
3. Autoimmune blistering diseases
   a. Can be the result of a disturbed peripheral tolerance
   b. Are an example of type III hypersensitivity
   c. Both answers are true

   Answers

1. b
2. c
3. a

References

1. Schmidt E, Zillikens D. Pemphigoid diseases. Lancet. 2013;38:320–32.
2. Iwata H, Kitajima Y. Bullous pemphigoid: role of complement and mechanisms for blister formation within the lamina lucida. Exp Dermatol. 2013;22:381–5.
3. Heupel WM, Zillikens D, Drenckhahn D, Waschke J. Pemphigus vulgaris IgG directly inhibit desmoglein 3-mediated transinteraction. J Immunol. 2008;181:1825–34.
4. Berkowitz P, Hu P, Warren S, Liu Z, Diaz LA, Rubenstein DS. p38MAPK inhibition prevents disease in pemphigus vulgaris mice. Proc Natl Acad Sci U S A. 2006;103:12855–60.
5. Waschke J, Spindler V, Bruggeman P, Zillikens D, Schmidt G, Drenckhahn D. Inhibition of Rho A activity causes pemphigus skin blistering. J Cell Biol. 2006;175:721–7.
6. Caldelari R, de Bruin A, Baumann D, Suter MM, Bierkamp C, Balmer V, Müller E. A central role for the armadillo protein plakoglobin in the autoimmune disease pemphigus vulgaris. J Cell Biol. 2001;153:823–34.
7. Aoyama Y, Kitajima Y. Pemphigus vulgaris-IgG causes a rapid depletion of desmoglein 3 (Dsg3) from the Triton X-100 soluble pools, leading to the formation of Dsg3-depleted desmosomes in a human squamous carcinoma cell line, DJM-1 cells. J Invest Dermatol. 1999;112:67–71.

Suggested Further Reading

Robbins and Cotran. Pathologic basis of disease. Saunders, 9th edition.
Abbas and Lichtman. Cellular and Molecular Immunology. Saunders 8th edition.

Dermatological Examination of Bullous Diseases

2

Marcel F. Jonkman and Barbara Horváth

Introduction & AIMS

Short Definition in Layman Terms

The vesicle or blister is the top efflorescence in the clinical reasoning chain for dermatological diagnosis. Finding only one single blister on the skin is sufficient to make the diagnosis bullous disease. The notion that a skin disease might be autoimmune emerges after a blister is found by physical examination. However, autoimmune bullous diseases not always present with blisters. In this chapter the skills and knowledge is outlined of the dermatological examination.

Autoimmune bullous diseases not always present with blisters.

Learning Objectives

After reading this chapter you know the algorithm and definitions for the physical examination of skin and mucous membranes for bullous diseases.

Case Study: Part 1

A 61-year-old male presented with a widespread bullous eruption of 3 months duration. Clinically, he had numerous flaccid blisters, and a few tense bullae on both inflamed and non-erythematous skin involving primarily the scalp, face, neck, and breast. Examination of the oral mucosa revealed extensive desquamative gingivitis and three erosions on hard palate and buccal measuring up to 2 cm in diameter. Perilesional skin of an erosion exhibited a positive marginal Nikolsky's sign, the base of which was moist and exudative.

A biopsy for histopathology of the left arm revealed suprabasal blister formation with acantholysis. A biopsy for direct immunofluorescence revealed immunoglobulin G (IgG) and C5 deposition throughout the epidermis in a pattern along the cell surface. Indirect IF on monkey esophagus circulating anti-cell surface antibodies were detected. The ELISA indices of autoantibodies for desmoglein 1 was 57 and for desmoglein 3 was >150.

M. F. Jonkman (Deceased) · B. Horváth (✉)
Center for Blistering Diseases, Department of Dermatology, University Medical Center Groningen,
University of Groningen,
Groningen, The Netherlands
e-mail: b.horvath@umcg.nl

Didactical Questions; Cross Section of Questions to Prime the Readers Interest

Meticulous skin examination is needed when a vesiculo-bullous disorder is suspected, since finding one vesicle is sufficient for making the diagnosis. However the absence of a vesicle does not exclude bullous disease, since several may come with only erythema, wheals, papules, nodules, erosions, or crusts. Vesicles are hard to identify on the mucous membranes. For instance, erosions on the gingiva may look like bright red erythema (enanthema), but the glistening surface betrays the lack of epithelium. How can the disease activity be scored?

Facts & Figures

Definitions and Classification

The efflorescences of vesiculo-bullous diseases as defined by the International League of Dermatological Societies are:

- Vesicle (vesicula): A circumscribed elevation ≤1 cm in diameter that contains liquid (clear, serous or hemorrhagic).
- Blister (bulla): A circumscribed elevation >1 cm in diameter that contains liquid (clear, serous or hemorrhagic).
- Pustule (pustula): A circumscribed lesion that contains purulent material.
- Crust (crusta): Dried serum, blood or pus on the surface of the skin.
- Erosion: Loss of either a portion of or the entire epidermis.

The nomenclature of efflorescences are defined by the International League of Dermatological Societies.

The distribution of vesicles may be solitary, grouped (herpetiform), or arch-like (circinate). The content of vesicles or bullae may be clear (transudate), opaque (serous), red-blue (hemorrhagic). If the blister cavity is hollow (air-filled) within the corneal layer, than in sensu strictu it does not fulfill the definition of a bulla, and might be called exfoliation or skin peeling. If the content is yellow (pustular) but yet also serous than the transitional word vesiculo-pustule is used.

Symptoms

Burning and pain are almost invariable features of blisters; pruritus is particularly associated with pemphigoid diseases, and dermatitis herpetiformis. Bullous diseases may start with erythematous lesions that can be macular, papular, urticarial, or nodular before a vesicle or blister erupts. Serous vesicles may become pustular with time as secondary efflorescence. Tense bullae are characteristic of blistering diseases with subepidermal split level such as pemphigoid, whereas slack bullae that break easily are seen in bullous diseases with intra-epidermal split, such as pemphigus. When the roof of the blister is lost, an erosion develops. When the liquid in the blister cavity is released it dries out into a crust. The color of the crust depends on the nature of the blister liquid (light yellow = exudate, blue-black = blood, gold = pus). If the blister does not have an underlying erythema, it is called monomorphic (monomorphic pemphigoid, pseudoporphyria).

Bullous diseases may come with itch, that evokes scratching, which results in excoriations. The lifetime of a vesicle may be extremely short by immediate scratching such as in dermatitis herpetiformis. Milia (horny pearls in the upper dermis) and scarring appear when the basement membrane is interrupted, such as in epidermolysis bullosa acquisita.

The distribution pattern of the lesions may by solitary (solitary bullous mastocytosis), grouped 'en bouquet'/herpetiform (herpes simplex), circinate (linear IgA bullous disease), linear (phytophotodermatitis) or randomly (bullous pemphigoid).

Lesions may be distributed over de whole body such as in bullous pemphigoid, present in a circumscriptive area such as to head and neck in pemphigus, segmental in herpes zoster, or confined to skin folds such as in pemphigus vegetans.

The mucous membranes of body openings (eyes, nose, mouth, genitals) might be involved. Examine the eye for erythema of upper and lower conjunctiva, synechiae of conjunctival sac (symblepharon), and corneal abnormalities (pannus), inverted eyelashes (trichiasis). In the nose (blood) crusts or erosions can be found on the septum in the nasal vestibule. White patches in the mouth cavity may consist of blister roof of thickening of epithelium (leukoplakia). Other efflorescences are erosions, and intact vesicles or blisters. Erosions are intense red and differ from red epithelium by their glistering. Patients with bullous disease of the mucous membranes complain of pain or burnings sensations of the sensitive mucosa. Ask your patient for photophobia, nasal cleaning, hoarseness, dysphagia, dysuria and dyspareunia.

Signs

The physician may evoke sign's to disclose epidermal dislodgement with the (hand gloved!) fingers. The most commonly used is the Nikolsky sign, however there are several other physical signs of blistering diseases. Since the broad availability of modern immunodiagnostics their relevance in the daily practice is limited (see box).

Physical Signs of Blistering Diseases

- *Nikolsky or Nikolsky's sign I* (normal or direct Nikolsky sign): ability to split the epidermis on skin areas distant from the lesions of normal appearing skin by a lateral pressure with a finger (Fig. 2.1).
- *Nikolsky or Nikolsky's sign II* (marginal or indirect Nikolsky sign): ability to split the epidermis of the skin far beyond the preexisting erosion, extending to a great distance on the normal-appearing skin, by pulling the remnant of a ruptured blister or rubbing at the periphery of existing lesions [1].
- *Pear sign*: old blisters become flaccid and acquire a pear-like shape due to weight of the exudate, resembling a rubber sack filled with fluid.
- *Sheklakov's sign* (perifocal subepidermal separation): ability to extend to a limited distance a lesion in direction of the periphery by pulling the remnant of a ruptured blister, producing erosions that are limited in size, do not have a tendency to subsequent spontaneous extension, heal fast, and may show a drop of blood.
- *Pseudo-Nikolsky sign* (epidermal peeling): ability to peel off the entire epidermis by a lateral pressure (rubbing) only on the erythematous skin areas (Fig. 2.2).
- *Asboe-Hansen's or Lutz' sign* (blister spread): ability to enlarge a blister in direction of the periphery by applying mechanical pressure on the roof of intact blister (Fig. 2.3).

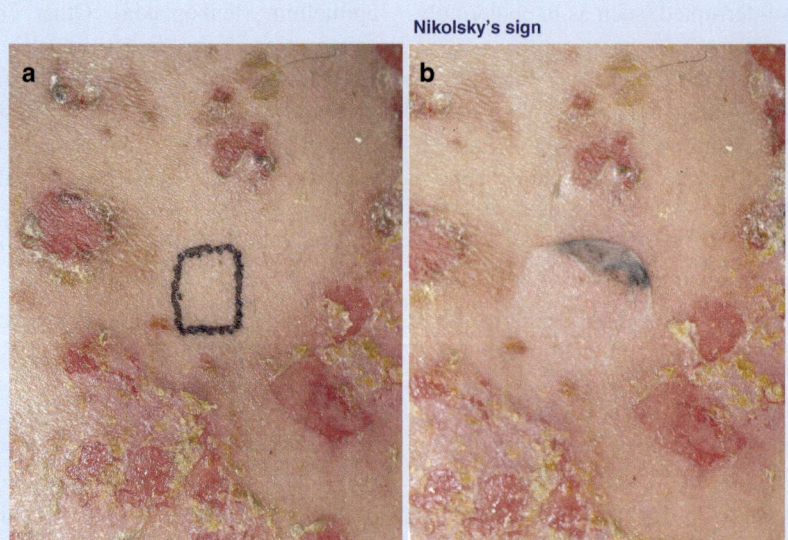

Fig. 2.1 Nikolsky sign type I procedure in pemphigus vulgaris (**a**) before and (**b**) after pressure with a finger

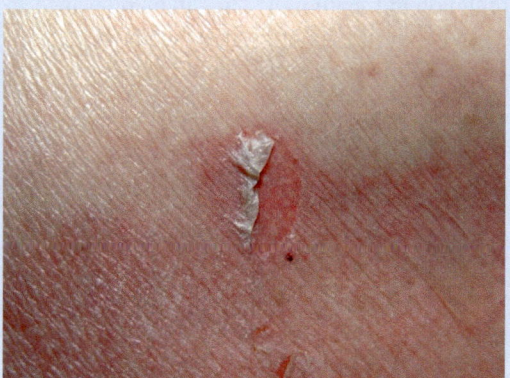

Fig. 2.2 Pseudo-Nikolsky sign in toxic epidermal necrolysis

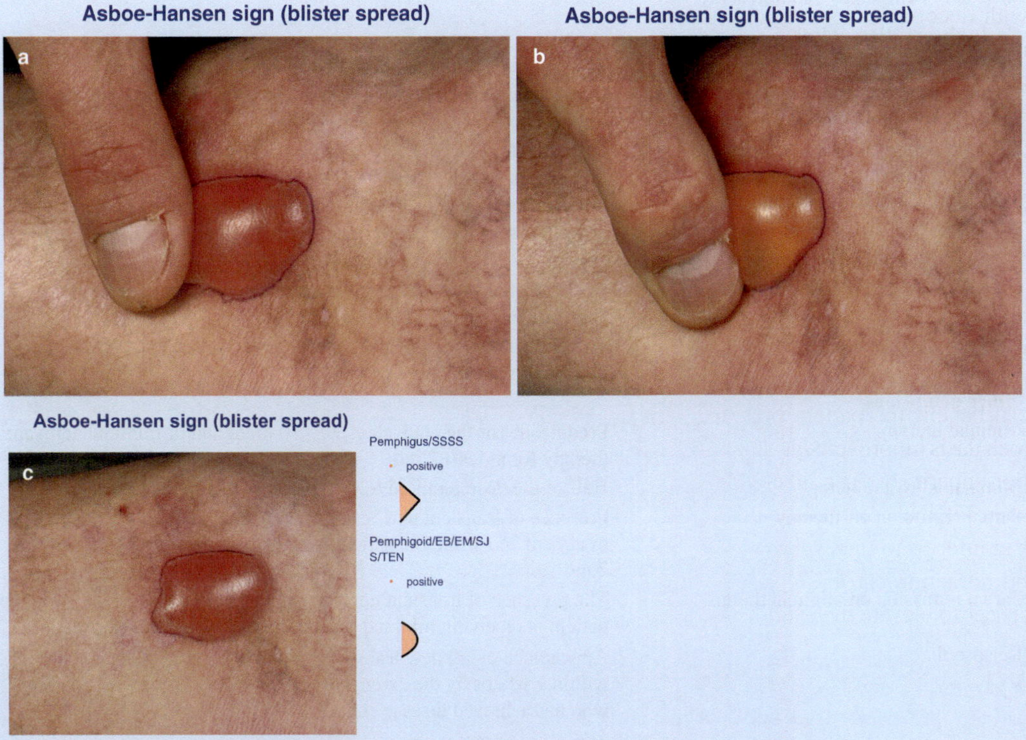

Fig. 2.3 Asboe-Hansen's (or blister spread) sign. (**a**) Draw line around the blister edge, and (**b**) press with thumb on blister. (**c**) Asboe-Hansen's sign is positive if the blister has spread beyond the line

The Nikolsky sign is positive in epidermal acantholysis such as in all forms of pemphigus and in staphylococcal scaled skin syndrome (SSSS) [2].

The pseudo-Nikolsky sign is positive in Erythema exsudativum multiforme (EEM), Stevens-Johnson syndrome (SJS) and Toxic epidermal necrolysis (TEN). Asboe-Hansen sign is positive in all bullous diseases.

Definitions and Activity Scores

Pemphigus

Definitions
The consensus definitions of the clinical milestones for pemphigus are listed [3] (Table 2.1).

Pemphigus Disease Area Index (PDAI)
The activity, extent and damage of skin and mucous membranes pemphigus can scored with PDAI [4] (Fig. 2.4 and Table 2.2).

Bullous Pemphigoid

The consensus definitions of the clinical milestones for pemphigoid are listed [5] (Fig. 2.5 and Table 2.3).

Bullous Pemphigoid Area Index (BPDAI)

The activity, extent and damage of skin and mucous membranes pemphigus can scored with BPDAI [5] (Fig. 2.6 and Table 2.4).

Table 2.1 Pemphigus definitions [3]

Early observation points	
Baseline	The day that therapy is started by a physician
Control of disease activity (disease control; beginning of consolidation phase)	The time at which new lesions cease to form and established lesions begin to heal
Time to disease control	The time interval between baseline and control
End of the consolidation phase	The time at which no new lesions have developed for a minimum of 2 wks, approximately 80% of lesions have healed, and when most clinicians start to taper steroids
Late observation end points	
Complete remission off therapy	Absence of new or established lesions while the patient is off all systemic therapy for at least 2 mo
Complete remission on therapy	The absence of new or established lesions while the patient is receiving minimal therapy
Other definitions	
Minimal therapy	Prednisone (or the equivalent) at ≤10 mg/d and/or minimal adjuvant therapy for at least 2 mo
Minimal adjuvant therapy	Half of the dose required to be defined as treatment failure
Partial remission off therapy	Presence of transient new lesions that heal within 1 wk without treatment and while the patient is off all systemic therapy for at least 2 mo
Partial remission on minimal therapy	The presence of transient new lesions that heal within 1 wk while the patient is receiving minimal therapy, including topical steroids
Relapse/flare	Appearance of ≥3 new lesions/mo that do not heal spontaneously within 1 wk, or by the extension of established lesions, in a patient who has achieved disease control

[Reprinted from: Murrell DF, Dick S, Ahmed AR, Amagai M, Barnadas MA, Borradori L, et al. Consensus statement on definitions of disease, end points, and therapeutic response for pemphigus. Journal of the American Academy of Dermatology 2008;58:1043-6, with permission from Elsevier.]

Case Study: Part 2

The patient was diagnosed with pemphigus vulgaris. At the start of therapy the PDAI score was 23 on skin and 12 on mucous membranes.

He was successfully treated with prednisone 1 mg/kg daily tapered in 4 months, and in addition 2× 1000 mg rituximab. During the induction phase, non-inflamed skin exhibited a positive direct Nikolsky's sign, beneath which was a non-exudative blister base. After 2 weeks control of disease was reached where no new lesions anymore developed. The skin improved quicker than the mouth with a PDAI at the end of the consolidation phase of 0 and 5 respectively.

Mucous Membrane Pemphigoid Area Index (MMPDAI)

The consensus definitions of the clinical milestones for mucous membrane pemphigoid are listed [6] (Table 2.5).

The activity, extent and damage of skin and mucous membranes pemphigus can scored with MMPDAI [6] (Fig. 2.7 and Table 2.6).

Case Study: Part 3

Patient reached complete remission while off therapy by 6 months that sustained during the total follow up period of 18 months. The PDAI dropped to 0.

2 Dermatological Examination of Bullous Diseases

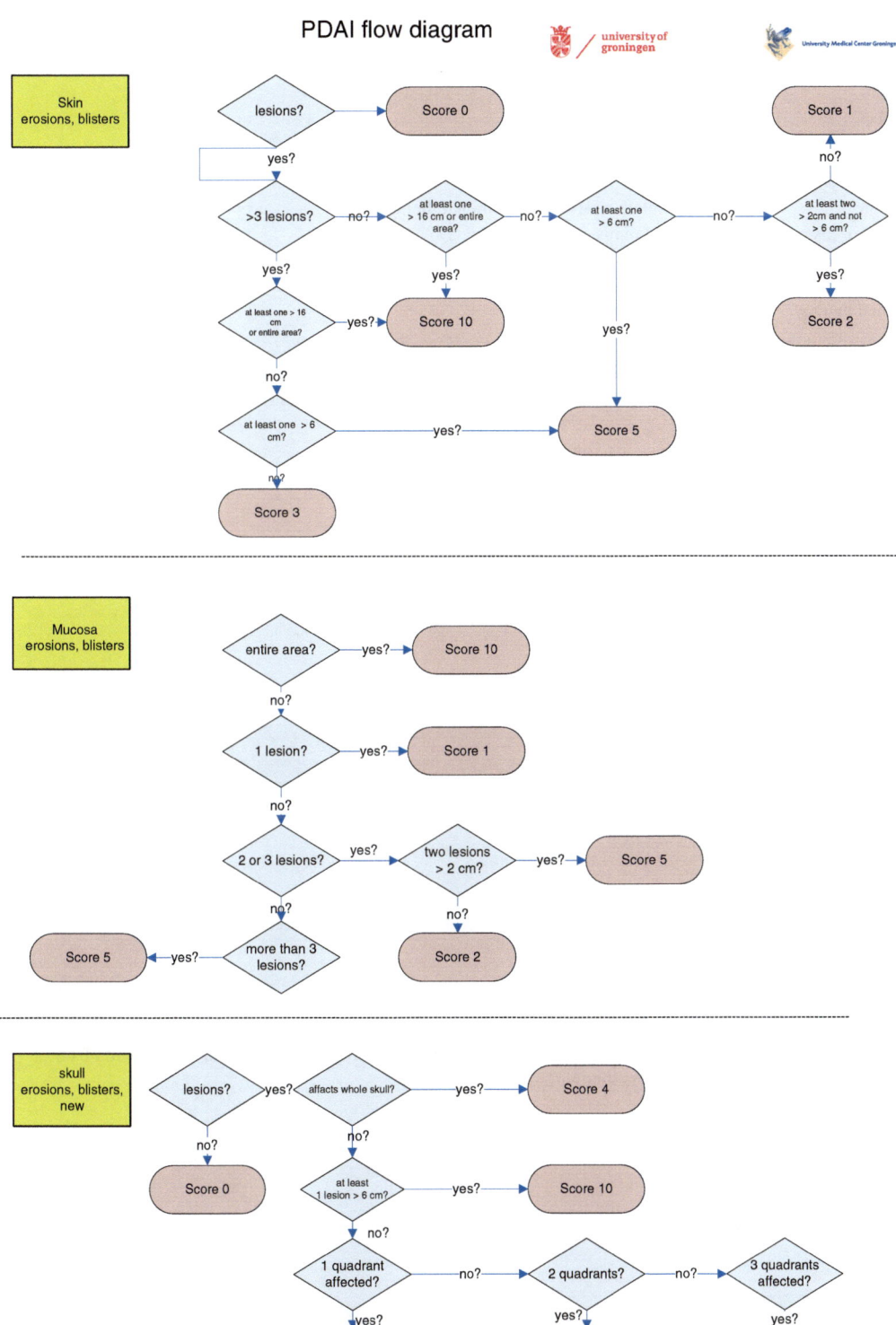

Fig. 2.4 Pemphigus Disease Area Index (PDAI) flow diagram

Table 2.2 Pemphigus Disease Area Index

PDAI			
Name:			
DOB:			
Number:			
Date:			

Treatment phase	
Baseline	Complete remission on minimal therapy
Control of disease	Partial remission off therapy
Consolidation phase	Complete remission off therapy
Partial remission on minimal therapy	Flare

Skin	Activiity		Damage
Anatomical location	Erosions/Blisters or new erythema		Post-inflammatory hyperpigmentation or erythema from resolving lesion
	0	absent	0 absent
	1	1-3 lesions, up to one lesion >2 cm in any diameter; none > 6 cm	1 present
	2	2-3 lesions, at least two lesions > 2cm; none > 6 cm	
	3	> 3 lesions, none > 6 cm	
	5	>3 lesions; and/or at least one lesion > 6 cm	
	10	>3 lesions; and/or at least one > 16 cm or entire area	
Ears			
Nose			
Rest of the face			
Neck			
Chest			
Abdomen			
Back, buttocks			
Arms			
Hands			
Legs			
Feet			
Genitals			
Total skin scores	/120		/12

Scalp	Erosions/Blisters or new erythema		Post-inflammatory hyperpigmentation or erythema from resolving lesion
	0	absent	0 absent
	1	in 1 quadrant	1 present
	2	in 2 quadrants	
	3	in 3 quadrants	
	4	affects whole skull	
	10	at least 1 lesion > 6 cm	
Total scalp scores	/10		/1
Total score of damage skin and scalp			/13

(continued)

Table 2.2 (continued)

Mucous membranes	
Anatomical location	**Erosions/Blisters**
	0 absent
	1 1 lesion
	2 2-3 lesions
	5 >3 lesions of 2 lesions > 2 cm
	10 entire area
Eyes	
Nose	
Buccal mucosa	
Hard palate	
Soft palate	
Upper gingiva	
Lower gingiva	
Tongue	
Floor of mouth	
Labial mucosa	
Posterior pharynx	
Anogenital	
Total Mucosa Score	/120
Total Activity Score Skin+Scalp+Mucosa	/250
Total Damage Score Skin+Scalp	/13

[Reprinted from: Murrell DF, Dick S, Ahmed AR, Amagai M, Barnadas MA, Borradori L, et al. Consensus statement on definitions of disease, end points, and therapeutic response for pemphigus. Journal of the American Academy of Dermatology 2008;58:1043-6, with permission from Elsevier.]

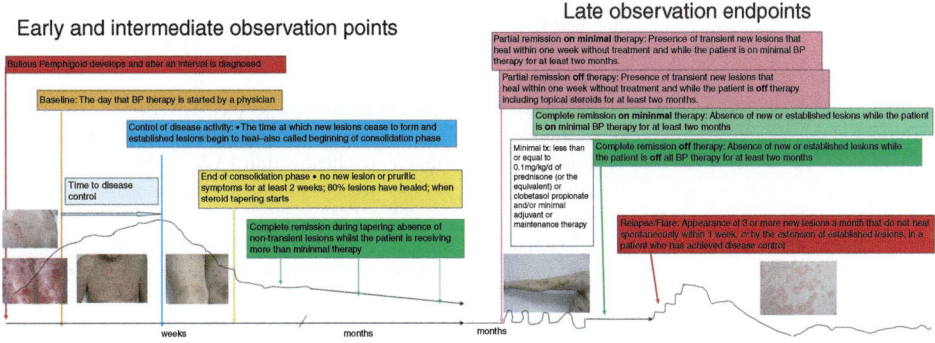

Fig. 2.5 Pictorial depiction of end points in bullous pemphigoid

Table 2.3 Definitions for Bullous Pemphigoid

Early observation points	
Baseline	Day that BP therapy is started by physician
Control of disease activity	Time at which new lesions cease to form and established lesions begin to heal or pruritic symptoms start to abate
Time to control of disease activity (disease control; beginning of consolidation phase)	The time interval between baseline and control of disease activity
End of the consolidation phase	Time at which no new lesions have developed for minimum of 2 wk and approximately 80% of lesions have healed and pruritic symptoms are minimal
Intermediate observation end points	
Transient lesions	New lesions that heal within 1 wk or pruritus lasting <1 wk and clearing without treatment
Nontransient lesions	New lesions that do not heal within 1 wk or pruritus continuing >1 wk with or without treatment
Complete remission during tapering	Absence of nontransient lesions while patient is receiving more than minimal therapy
Late observation end points	
Minimal therapy	≤0.1 mg/kg/d of prednisone (or equivalent) or 20 g/wk of clobetasol propionate and/or minimal adjuvant or maintenance therapy
Minimal adjuvant therapy and/or maintenance therapy	Following doses or less: methotrexate 5 mg/wk; azathioprine 0.7 mg/kg/d (with normal thiopurine s-methyltransferase level); mycophenolate mofetil 500 mg/d; mycophenolic acid 360 mg/d; or dapsone 50 mg/d
Partial remission on minimal therapy	Presence of transient new lesions that heal within 1 wk while patient is receiving minimal therapy for at least 2 mo
Complete remission on minimal therapy	Absence of new or established lesions or pruritus while patient is receiving minimal therapy for at least 2 mo
Partial remission off therapy	Presence of transient new lesions that heal within 1 wk without treatment while patient is off all BP therapy for at least 2 mo
Complete remission off therapy	Absence of new or established lesions or pruritus while patient is off all BP therapy for at least 2 mo
Mild new activity	<3 Lesions/mo (blisters, eczematous lesions, or urticarial plaques) that do not heal within 1 wk, or extension of established lesions or pruritus once/wk but less than daily in patient who has achieved disease control; these lesions have to heal within 2 wk
Relapse/flare	Appearance of ≥ 3 new lesions/mo (blisters, eczematous lesions, or urticarial plaques) or at least one large ([10 cm diameter) eczematous lesion or urticarial plaques that do not heal within 1 wk, or extension of established lesions or daily pruritus in patient who has achieved disease control
Failure of therapy for initial control	Development of new nontransient lesions or continued extension of old lesions, or failure of established lesions to begin to heal or continued pruritus despite: Clobetasol propionate 40 g/d for 4 wk; or Prednisone 0.75 mg/kg/d equivalent for minimum of 3 wk with or without drugs used for maintenance therapy; or A tetracycline on full dosing for 4 wk; or Dapsone 1.5 mg/kg/d for 4 wk; or Methotrexate 15 mg/wk (if [60 kg and no major renal impairment) for 4 wk; or Azathioprine 2.5 mg/kg/d for 4 wk (if thiopurine s-methyltransferase level is normal); or Mycophenolate mofetil 40 mg/kg/d (if normal renal function, otherwise according to age/creatinine clearance) for 4 wk

[Reprinted from: Murrell DF, Daniel BS, Joly P, Borradori L, Amagai M, Hashimoto T, et al. Definitions and outcome measures for bullous pemphigoid: recommendations by an international panel of experts. J Am Acad Dermatol 2012;66:479–485, with permission from Elsevier.]

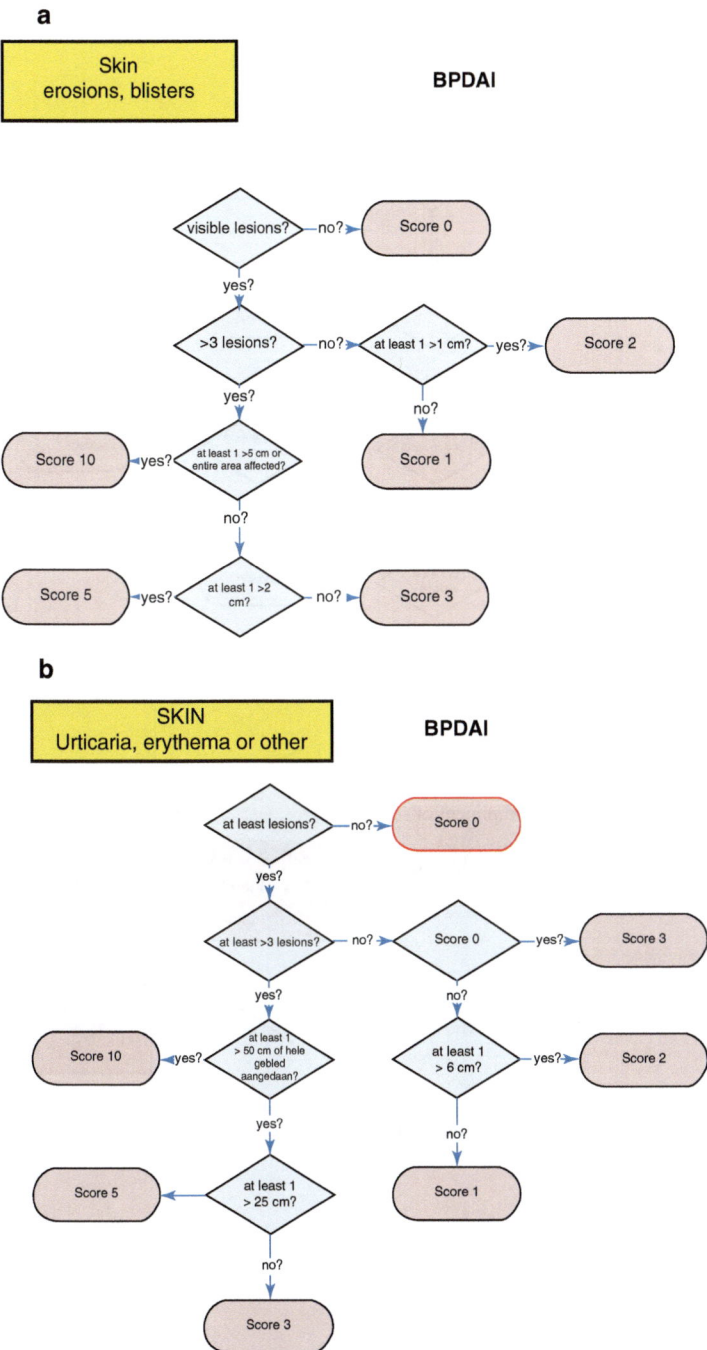

Fig. 2.6 Bullous Pemphigoid Area Index (BPDAI) flow diagram for assessment of (**a**) skin blistesr and erosions, (**b**) skin erythema and other lesions, (**c**) mucous membrane blisters and erosions

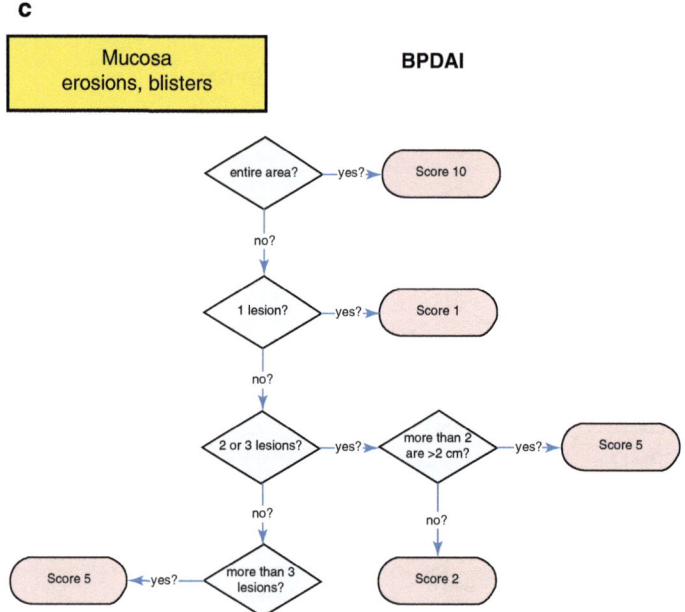

Fig. 2.6 (continued)

Fig. 2.7 Eye quadrants for Mucous Membrane Pemphigoid Area Index (MMPDAI). Diagram to illustrate how erythema is to be scored in different quadrants of each eye for the mucosal component of the Mucous Membrane Pemphigoid Disease Area Index. The degree of pinkness represents how high to score this parameter

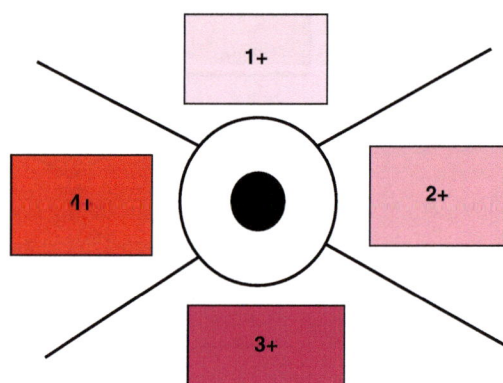

Table 2.4 Bullous Pemphigoid Disease Area Index (BPDAI)

Name:	
DOB:	
#:	
Date:	
Diagnosis:	
Treatment phase:	
Number of weeks after baseline:	
Current medication:	
Baseline	Complete remission on minimal therapy
Control of disease	Partial remission off therapy
Consolidation phase	Complete remission off therapy
Partial remission on minimal therapy	Flare

[Reprinted from: Murrell DF, Daniel BS, Joly P, Borradori L, Amagai M, Hashimoto T, et al. Definitions and outcome measures for bullous pemphigoid: recommendations by an international panel of experts. J Am Acad Dermatol 2012;66:479-485, with permission from Elsevier.]

BPDAI skin Anatomical location	Activity Erosions/Blisters		Activity Urticaria/Erythema/Other		Damage Pigmentation/Other
	0	absent	0	absent	0 absent
	1	1-3 lesions; none > 1 cm	1	1-3 lesions; none > 6 cm	1 present
	2	1-3 lesions, at least 1 lesion >1 cm	2	1-3 lesions, at least 1 lesion > 6 cm	
	3	>3 lesions, none >2 cm	3	>3 lesions, at least 1 lesion > 10 cm	
	5	>3 lesions, and at least 1 lesion >2 cm	5	>3 lesions, at least 1 lesion > 25 cm	
	10	>3 lesions, and at least 1 lesion >5 cm or entire area	10	>3 lesions, at least 1 lesion > 50 cm or entire area	
Head					
Neck					
Chest					
Left arm					
Right arm					
Hands					
Abdomen					
Genitals					
Back/Buttocks					
Left leg					
Right leg					
Feet					
Total skin score	/120		/120		/12
MUCOSA	Erosions/Blisters				0
	0 Absent				
	2 2-3 lesions				
	5 3>lesions, of 2 > 2 cm				
	10 Entire area				
Eyes					
Nose					
Buccal mucosa					
Hard palate					
Soft palate					
Upper gingiva					
Lower gingiva					
Tongue					
Floor of mouth					
Labial mucosa					
Posterior pharynx					
Anogenitaal					
Total score mucosa	/120				
Total activity score skin (blist./urtic.) + mucosa	/360		**Total damage score skin**	/12	

Table 2.5 Definitions for Mucous Membrane Pemphigoid

Early observation points	
Baseline	The day that MMP therapy is started by a physician
Control of disease	The time at which new inflammatory lesions cease to form and established lesions begin to heal
Time to control disease activity (disease control; beginning of consolidation phase)	The time interval from baseline to the control of disease activity
Control of scarring	The time needed to control scarring progression
End of the consolidation phase	The time at which no new lesions have developed for minimum of 4 wk, and approximately 80% of inflammatory lesions have healed
Intermediate observation end points	
Transient lesions	New lesions that heal within 1 wk or clear without treatment
Nontransient lesions	New lesions that do not heal within 1 wk
Complete remission during tapering	The absence of nontransient lesions while the patient is receiving more than minimal therapy
Minimal therapy	Dapsone ≤ 1.0 mg/kg/d; ≤ 0.1 mg/kg/d of prednisone (or the equivalent); minocycline ≤ 100 mg/d; doxycycline 100 mg/d; lymecycline 300 mg/d; topical corticosteroids once a day including fluticasone propionate suspension 400 g/once a day; colchicine 500 g/d; Salazopyrin 1 g/d; sulfapyridine 500 mg/d; sulfamethoxypyridazine 500 mg/d; nicotinamide 500 mg/d
Minimal adjuvant therapy (and/or maintenance therapy)	The following doses or less: azathioprine (1 mg/kg/d) with normal thiopurine S-methyltransferase level; mycophenolate mofetil 500 mg/d; mycophenolic acid 360 mg/d; methotrexate 5 mg/wk; cyclosporine 1 mg/kg/d
Long-term biological therapy	Refers to therapies given intermittently, for example, when rituximab is used for MMP, or IVIG monthly
Late observation end points	
Partial remission on minimal therapy	Presence of transient new lesions that heal without scarring within 1 wk while patient is receiving minimal therapy for at least 2 mo
Complete remission on minimal therapy	The absence of new or established lesions or pruritus while patient is receiving minimal therapy for at least 2 mo
Partial remission off therapy	Presence of transient new lesions that heal within 1 wk without treatment while patient is off all MMP therapy for at least 2 mo
Complete remission off therapy	Absence of new or established lesions or pruritus while patient is off all MMP therapy for at least 2 mo
Relapse/flare	Appearance of ≥ 3 new lesions a month (blisters, erosions) that do not heal within 1 wk, or extension of established lesions in patient who has achieved disease control

IVIG Intravenous immunoglobulin, *MMP* mucous membrane pemphigoid
[Reprinted from: Murrell DF, Marinovic B, Caux F, Prost C, Ahmed R, Wozniak K, et al. Definitions and outcome measures for mucous membrane pemphigoid: Recommendations of an international panel of experts. J Am Acad Dermatol 2015;72:168–174., with permission from Elsevier.]

Table 2.6 Mucous Membrane Pemphigoid Disease Area Index (MMPDAI)

Name:
DOB:
:
Date:

Treatment phase	
Baseline	Complete remission on minimal therapy
Control of disease	Partial remission off therapy
Consolidation phase	Complete remission off therapy
Partial remission on minimal therapy	Flare

[Reprinted from: Murrell DF, Marinovic B, Caux F, Prost C, Ahmed R, Wozniak K, et al. Definitions and outcome measures for mucous membrane pemphigoid: Recommendations of an international panel of experts. J Am Acad Dermatol 2015;72:168-174., with permission from Elsevier.]

Skin	Activity		Damage
Anatomical location	Erosions/Blisters or new erythema		Post-inflammatory hyperpigmentation or erythema from resolving lesion or scarring
	0	absent	0 absent
	1	1-3 lesions, up to one >2 cm in any diameter, none > 6 cm	1 present
	2	2-3 lesions, at least two > 2 cm diameter, none > 6cm	
	3	>3 lesions, none > 6 cm diameter	
	5	>3 lesions, and/or at least one >6 cm	
	10	>3 lesions, and/or at least one lesion >16 cm diameter or entire area	
Ears			
Forehead			
Rest of the face			
Neck			
Chest			
Abdomen			
Shoulders, Back			
Buttocks			
Arms & hands			
Legs & feet			
Anal			
Genitals			
Total skin scores	/120		/12

Scalp	Erosion/Blisters/active erythema		Post-inflammatory hyperpigmentation or erythema from resolving lesion or scarring
	0	absent	0 absent
	1	in 1 quadrant	1 present
	2	in 2 quadrants	
	3	in 3 quadrants	
	4	affects whole scalp	
	10	at least 1 lesion > 6 cm	
Total scalp	/10		/1

Mucous membranes	Activity	Damage
Anatomical location	Erosion/Blisters/active erythema	Post-inflammatory hyperpigmentation or erythema from resolving lesion or scarring

Mucous membranes	Activity		Damage
Eyes (quadrants upper, lower, medial and lateral)	0	No erythema	0 absent
	1	Light pink	1 present
	2	Moderate pink	
	3	Dark pink	
	4	Bright red	
	add up quadrants		
Left eye (0-16) × 0.625			
Right eye (0-16) × 0.625			
	0	absent	0 absent
	1	1 lesion, or 1 quadrant eye	1 present
	2	2-3 lesions, or 2 quadrants eye	
	5	> 3 lesions or two lesions > 2 cm, or three quadrants eye	
	10	entire area, or four quadrants eye	
Nose			
Buccal mucosa			
Palate			
Upper gingiva			
Lower gingiva			
Tongue/Floor of mouth			
Labia			
Posterior pharynx			
Anus			
Genitals			
Total mucosa scores	/120		/12
Total scores skin + scalp + mucosa	/250		/25

Review Questions

1. A vesicle is a circumscribed elevation
   a. ≥ 1 cm in diameter that contains clear liquid
   b. ≤ 1 cm in diameter that contains serous liquid
   c. ≥ 1 cm in diameter that contains purulent material
   d. Is a bulla
2. The liquid contents of a serous vesicle is
   a. Transparent
   b. Opaque
   c. Purulent
   d. Leaking
3. The Nikolsky sign is positive, except
   a. Pemphigus vulgaris
   b. Staphylococcal scaled skin syndrome (SSSS)
   c. Pemphigus foliaceus
   d. Bullous pemphigoid
4. Which is NOT an severity scores in autoimmune blistering diseases?
   a. PASI
   b. BPDAI
   c. PDAI
   d. MMPDAI
5. The beginning of the consolidation phase in BP is the moment when reached
   a. Control of disease activity
   b. Partial remission on minimal therapy
   c. Partial remission off therapy
   d. Complete remission on minimal therapy

Answers

1. b
2. b
3. d
4. a
5. a

On the web

International Pemphigus and Pemphigoid Foundation www.pemphigus.org

Supplement 2.1 ILDS – Nomenclature for description of cutaneous lesions (attached)

References

1. Grando SA, Grando AA, Glukhenky BT, Doguzov V, Nguyen VT, Holubar K. History and clinical significance of mechanical symptoms in blistering dermatoses: a reappraisal. J Am Acad Dermatol. 2003;48:86–92.
2. Mignogna MD, Fortuna G, Leuci S, Ruoppo E, Marasca F, Matarasso S. Nikolsky's sign on the gingival mucosa: a clinical tool for oral health practitioners. J Periodontol. 2008;79:2241–6.
3. Murrell DF, Dick S, Ahmed AR, Amagai M, Barnadas MA, Borradori L, et al. Consensus statement on definitions of disease, end points, and therapeutic response for pemphigus. J Am Acad Dermatol. 2008;58:1043–6.
4. Rosenbach M, Murrell DF, Bystryn JC, Dulay S, Dick S, Fakharzadeh S, et al. Reliability and convergent validity of two outcome instruments for pemphigus. J Invest Dermatol. 2009;129:2404–10.
5. Murrell DF, Daniel BS, Joly P, Borradori L, Amagai M, Hashimoto T, et al. Definitions and outcome measures for bullous pemphigoid: recommendations by an international panel of experts. J Am Acad Dermatol. 2012;66:479–85.
6. Murrell DF, Marinovic B, Caux F, Prost C, Ahmed R, Wozniak K, et al. Definitions and outcome measures for mucous membrane pemphigoid: Recommendations of an international panel of experts. J Am Acad Dermatol. 2015;72:168–74.

Additional Reading

Powell AM, Black M. A stepwise approach to the diagnosis of blisters in the clinic. Clin Dermatol. 2001;19:598–606.

How to Take a Biopsy

Gilles F. H. Diercks, Joost M. Meijer, and Marcel F. Jonkman

Introduction & AIMS

Short Definition in Layman Terms

A skin biopsy is a technique in which a skin sample is taken for microscopic examination by a pathologist. For autoimmune bullous diseases, different types of punch biopsies may give clues for a diagnosis. The level of the blistering in the skin is different in pemphigus and pemphigoid. A skin biopsy for immunofluorescence microscopy visualizes the autoimmune reaction in the skin and is an important diagnostic test for autoimmune bullous diseases. Biopsies can also be taken of mucous membranes, such as the oral mucosa or the conjunctiva.

G. F. H. Diercks (✉)
Center for Blistering Diseases, Departments of Dermatology, University Medical Center Groningen, University of Groningen,
Groningen, The Netherlands

Center for Blistering Diseases, Department of Dermatology and Pathology, University Medical Center Groningen, University of Groningen,
Groningen, The Netherlands
e-mail: g.f.h.diercks@umcg.nl

J. M. Meijer · M. F. Jonkman (Deceased)
Center for Blistering Diseases, Departments of Dermatology, University Medical Center Groningen, University of Groningen,
Groningen, The Netherlands
e-mail: j.m.meijer@umcg.nl

Learning Objectives
- Procedure of the biopsy
- Where to take a skin or mucosal biopsy in a patient suspected of an autoimmune blistering disease
- How to transport and handle a biopsy

Didactical Questions; Cross Section of Questions to Prime the Readers Interest

What is a perilesional biopsy? What is the preferred location to biopsy for DIF in nonbullous pemphigoid? How is the DIF biopsy transported?

Histopathology

Procedure of the Punch Biopsy

There is no rational for AIBD diagnosis to take larger samples by oval excision, than by punch biopsy. For histopathology, the punch biopsy sample should measure at least 3 to 4 mm in diameter to minimize sampling error and to provide sufficient tissue for any special staining that may be required. The procedure for performing the biopsy is explained on video [1]. Ideally, a biopsy of a very recent lesion should be sent in formalin to the histopathology laboratory. Older lesions may yield confusing information, because there may be regeneration changes or secondary infection.

Biopsy Site

The biopsy should include two-third blister cavity and one-third peribullous skin. One may draw a line that touches the blister (tangent) for orientation before giving local anesthesia, and biopsy perpendicular to the tangent (Fig. 3.1).

Transport and Handling of Biopsies

For histopathology the biopsy is submersed in a tube with 4% formaldehyde fixative and sent at room temperature to the histopathology laboratory.

Direct Immunofluorescence

Procedure of the Biopsy

Skin
For direct immunofluorescence (DIF) microscopy of the skin, the punch biopsy sample should measure at least 4 mm in diameter. The wound is sutured at the end of the procedure.

Buccal Mucosa
For DIF of the oral mucosa, the punch biopsy sample should measure at least 3 mm in diameter. A perilesional biopsy location is preferred, but when not feasible also healthy buccal mucosa is suitable. The recommended location is one third of the distance from the mouth corner to the last molar to avoid the parotid duct. The wound is not sutured at the end of the procedure. The use of a resorbable suture has no additional benefit unless hemostasis is not reached without one.

Conjunctiva
For the diagnosis of ocular AIBD DIF of the conjunctiva is the reference standard. The front of the eye is anesthetized by two droplets of oxybuprocaine 0.4% in the conjunctival sac. The eye is closed; required anesthesia is reached after 15 seconds. An eye spreader is placed below the upper and lower eyelids (Fig. 3.2a, b). The conjunctiva above the ocular bulbus is picked up with micro forceps, and an oval peace of mucous membrane with 3 mm in length is cut with a micro scissors (Fig. 3.2b). The tissue sample is place on a piece of polystyrene (from a coffee cup), and pierced at the tip with small needle tips (bend 90 °) (Fig. 3.2c). The needles are turned to each other and the whole fits into an aluminum container (Fig. 3.2d). After screwing the cup on the container, the whole is immersed in liquid nitrogen until the boiling stops. The specimen would be lost, or would curl up if it was not pinned down.

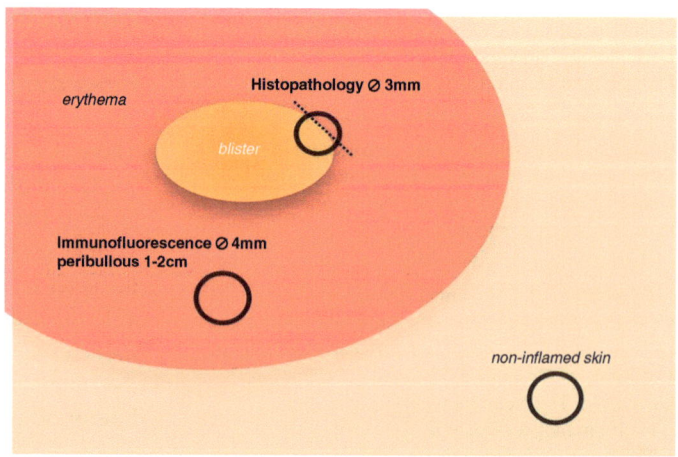

Fig. 3.1 Preferred locations of biopsies for histopathology and direct immunofluorescence microscopy is 2/3 in bulla and perilesional erythema adjacent to a vesicle or blister, respectively

3 How to Take a Biopsy

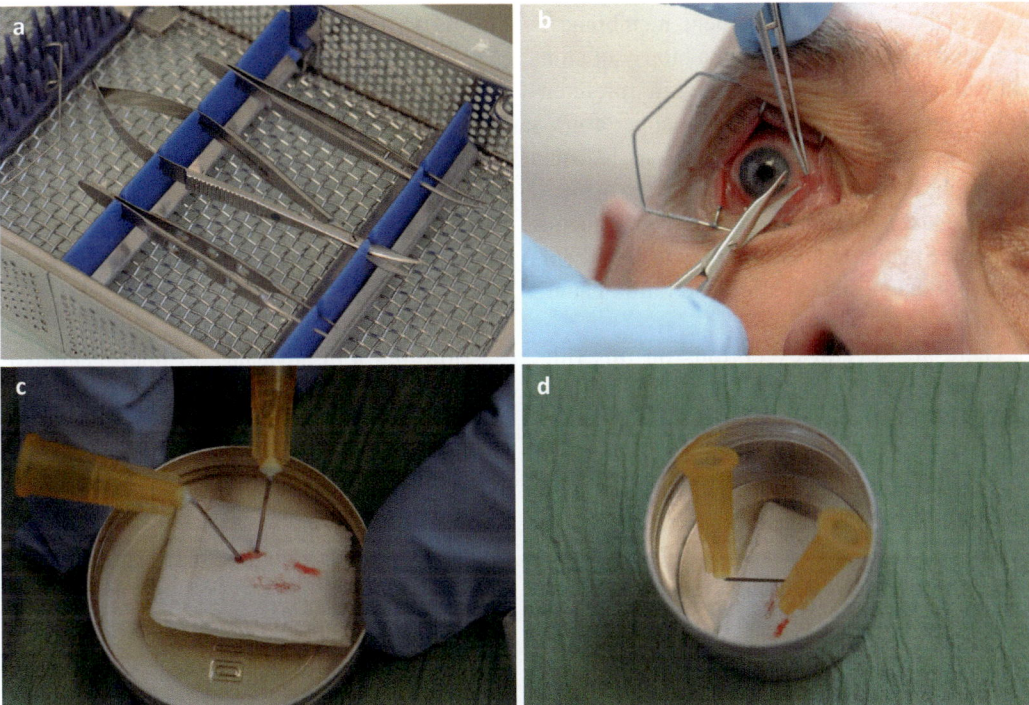

Fig. 3.2 Immunofluorescence biopsy of conjunctiva. (**a**) micro eye tweezer, micro eye Castroviejo curved scissors, two 25 Gauge 5/8th inch orange needles bend 90 °, and aluminum container with screwed top, (**b**) cutting of small oval piece of conjunctiva with micro scissors, (**c**) conjunctiva specimen pinned to polystyrene, (**d**) pinned specimen placed in container

Table 3.1 Recommendation of immunofluorescence biopsy sites in autoimmune blistering diseases

	Perilesional	Uninvolved skin	Lesional
In general	✓	(inner aspect upper arm)	
Exceptions			
Bullous SLE	✓	dorsal site wrist	✓
Lichen planus pemphigoides	✓		✓
Dermatitis herpetiformis	✓	extensor site elbow	
Nonbullous pemphigoid		✓	✓
Mucous membrane pemphigoid	✓	✓ (optional)	

Include 2/3rd of bulla in punch biopsy for histopathology.

Biopsy Sites (Table 3.1)

For direct immunofluorescence microscopy it is important to take an adequate skin or mucosal biopsy in order to avoid false negative results. A *perilesional* biopsy is recommended in general. The definition of a perilesional biopsy is of erythematous skin 1 to 2 centimeters adjacent to a vesicle or bulla (*lesional peribullous biopsy*).

A perilesional biopsy will increase the possibility of a positive result and one avoids a false negative result by taking a lesional biopsy with secondary changes, e.g. erosion or ulceration of the epidermis. Moreover, lesional biopsies in pemphigoid often yield negative findings because the epidermal basement membrane is destroyed. Although in general a biopsy of clinically uninvolved non-inflamed skin (preferentially from the inner aspect of the upper arm) is not necessary for diagnostic purposes [2], this still might be considered for diagnosis of pemphigoid, since especially in cases of mucous membrane pemphigoid a skin biopsy can be sufficient for diagnosis and allows serration pattern analysis (see below).

There are several exceptions on this rule. In bullous systemic lupus erythematosus (SLE) apart from taking a perilesional biopsy, it is also recommended to take a biopsy of lesional skin in order to find a lupus band. In addition, it has been demonstrated that a biopsy of non-sun exposed skin of the wrist with a positive lupus band has a predictive value of possible renal involvement. In lichen planus pemphigoides one can decide to take a lesional and a perilesional biopsy. The lesional biopsy will typically show a lichenoid infiltrate and deposition of fibrin along the basement membrane (see below). The preferred biopsy site of clinically uninvolved skin in dermatitis herpetiformis is the extensor side of the elbow, since this is a predilection site. Finally, in nonbullous pemphigoid it is recommended to take a lesional biopsy to increase sensitivity [2].

Taking a perilesional biopsy for DIF is recommended in general.

Transport and Handling of Biopsies

Several options exist for handling biopsy specimens. The most widely used method is snap-frozen in liquid nitrogen. Alternatively, Michel's solution [3], which contains ammonium sulfate, N-ethyl-maleimide, potassium citrate buffer, magnesium sulfate, and distilled water, can be used and facilitates transport of biopsies from referral hospitals.

However, a disadvantage of both methods is the high dermal background fluorescence due to undesired specific (dermal IgG) and non-specific staining. This lowers the signal to noise ratio, which yields false negative cases, especially in cases of pemphigoid with a weak linear staining of the basement membrane zone (Fig. 3.3a).

Alternatively, transport and overnight storage in normal saline can be used. Saline stored biopsies result in a decreased background staining and an increased signal to noise ratio, eventually leading to a higher diagnostic yield [4] (Fig. 3.3b). This due to wash out of nonspecific bound dermal IgG.

When feasible, transport an IF biopsy in 0.9% saline.

However, there are several drawbacks to this method. First, the biopsies shouldn't be kept longer than 36–48 h in saline. Longer than 48 hours might washout desired immunoreactants. Second disadvantage might be the loss of epidermal *in vivo* anti-nuclear antibodies. Therefore, in cases

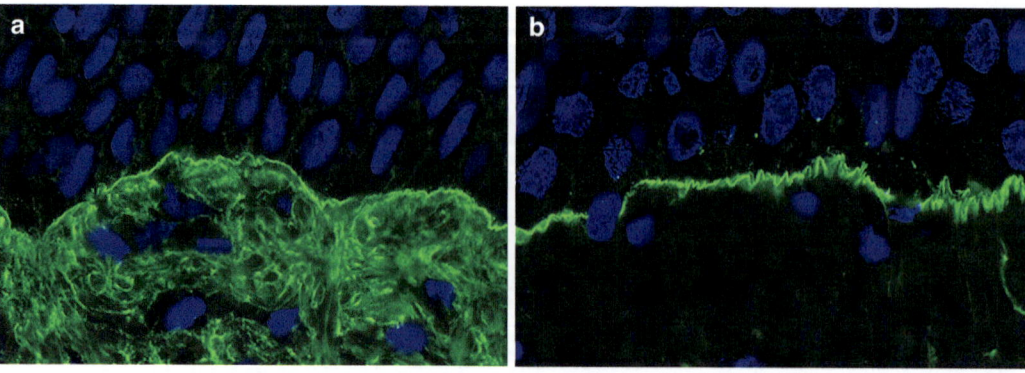

Fig. 3.3 A biopsy stored in normal saline (**b**) yields a higher signal to noise ratio than a biopsy stored in liquid nitrogen (**a**)

of suspected subacute cutaneous lupus erythematosus a snap-frozen biopsy is advisable.

After overnight storage in saline the biopsy is snap frozen and can be stored in a -80 C freezer or processed further for immunofluorescence microscopy. Serration pattern analysis is possible in a biopsy stored in either 0.9% saline or Michel's medium [5].

Review Questions

1. A skin biopsy for direct immunofluorescence should preferably be taken from
   a. Lesional bullous skin
   b. Perilesional erythematous skin
   c. Perilesional noninflamed skin
2. A skin biopsy for direct immunofluorescence is preferably transported in
   a. liquid nitrogen
   b. Michel's medium
   c. 0.9% saline
   d. 4% formaldehyde
3. A skin biopsy for direct immunofluorescence for the diagnosis of subacute lupus erythematosus is preferably transported in
   a. liquid nitrogen
   b. Michel's medium
   c. saline
   d. 4% formaldehyde

Answers

1. b
2. c
3. a

On the Web

Levitt J, Bernardo S, Whang T (2013) Videos in clinical medicine. How to perform a punch biopsy of the skin. N Eng J Med 369:e13 http://www.nejm.org/doi/full/10.1056/NEJMvcm1105849

References

1. Levitt J, Bernardo S, Whang T. Videos in clinical medicine. How to perform a punch biopsy of the skin. N Eng J Med. 2013;369:e13.
2. Meijer JM, Diercks GFH, de Lang EWG, Pas HH, Jonkman MF. Assessment of diagnostic strategy for early recognition of bullous and nonbullous variants of pemphigoid. JAMA Dermatol. 2019;155(2):158–65.
3. Michel B, Milner Y, David K. Preservation of tissue-fixed immoglobulins in skin biopsies of patients with lupus erythematosus and bullous diseases-Preliminary report. J Invest Dermatol. 2003;59:449–52.
4. Vodegel RM, de Jong MCJM, Meijer HJ, Weytingh MB, Pas HH, Jonkman MF. Enhanced diagnostic immunofluorescence using biopsies transported in saline. BMC Dermatol. 2004;4:10.
5. Meijer JM, Ingeborg Atefi GFH, Diercks AV, Zuiderveen J, Meijer HJ, Pas HH, Zillikens D, Schmidt E, Jonkman MF. Serration pattern analysis for differentiating epidermolysis bullosa acquisita from other pemphigoid diseases. J Am Acad Dermatol. 2018;78(4):754–759.e6.

Additional Reading

Powell AM, Black M. A stepwise approach to the diagnosis of blisters in the clinic. Clin Dermatol. 2001;19:598–606.

Direct Immunofluorescence Microscopy

4

Gilles F. H. Diercks and Hendri H. Pas

Learning Objectives

After studying this chapter, you should know:

- The various cutaneous immunodeposition patterns in pemphigus, pemphigoid, dermatitis herpetiformis and porphyria
- The difference between an n-serrated and u-serrated pattern in pemphigoids

Introduction & Aims

Ever since the discovery of the presence of autoantibodies in pemphigus in 1964 by Beutner and Jordon [1], immunofluorescence microscopy has become an essential part in the diagnostics of blistering diseases. Both serum and biopsy specimens can be examined by this method. The next chapter will describe the technique of direct immunofluorescence microscopy, i.e. visualization of *in vivo* bound autoantibodies. After reading this chapter the reader knows the different patterns that can be recognized in various blistering diseases.

G. F. H. Diercks (✉) · H. H. Pas
Center for Blistering Diseases, Department of Dermatology and Pathology, University Medical Center Groningen, University of Groningen, Groningen, The Netherlands
e-mail: g.f.h.diercks@umcg.nl; h.h.pas@umcg.nl

Laboratory Preparation

The purpose of direct immunofluorescence microscopy is to detect *in vivo* antibodies. This is done by adding a fluorescent labeled antibody against a human antigen, e.g. a goat antibody directed against human IgG, on a frozen section. To prepare a skin or mucosa biopsy for immunofluorescence microscopy the following steps are recommended (Groningen protocol):

- Cut frozen sections at a thickness of 4 um.
- Blow dry the sections with a cold dryer for 15 min
- Rinse the slides with PBS (NaCl 8.75 g/l, Na2HPO4 1.14 g/l, KH2PO4 0.27 g/l) for a minimum of 5 seconds. Wipe off excess PBS.
- Place fluorescent isothiocyanate (FITC)-conjugated antibody on the slides and incubate in a moist chamber for 30–40 min. See Table 4.1 for used antibodies.
- Rinse the slides with PBS and wash the slides subsequently for 30 min in PBS.
- Wipe off excess PBS.
- Place bisbenzimide (Hoechst 33258), which binds to double stranded DNA and therefore provides a nuclear staining, on the slides and incubate for 5–10 min on room temperature.
- Rinse the slides with PBS and wash the slides subsequently for 30 min in PBS.
- Place a drop of PBS/glycerin (1:1) on each section and top with a cover slip.

Table 4.1 Recommended FITC conjugated antibodies

Antibodies	Manufacturer
FITC-conjugated Goat F(ab)2 anti-human IgG	Protos 311, Protos immunoresearch, Burlingame, CA, US
FITC-conjugated Goat F(ab)2 anti-human IgA	Protos 312, Protos immunoresearch, Burlingame, CA, US
FITC-conjugated Goat F(ab)2 anti- human IgM	Protos 313, Protos immunoresearch, Burlingame, CA, US
FITC-conjugated Rabbit anti-human fibrinogen	Dako F111, Dako, Glostrup, Denmark
FITC-conjugated Rabbit anti-human C3c complement	Dako F201, Dako, Glostrup, Denmark

Immunofluorescence Patterns

Pemphigus

Pemphigus is caused by autoantibodies directed against desmosomal antigens, in particular desmoglein 1 (pemphigus foliaceus) or desmoglein 3 (mucosal pemphigus vulgaris) or desmoglein 1 and 3 (mucocutaneous pemphigus vulgaris) [2], although cases have been described with antibodies against desmocollin 1 or 3. Whatever the nature of the antibodies or the pemphigus variant, direct immunofluorescence of pemphigus shows depositions of immunoglobulins and/or complement on the epithelial cell surface (ECS) in virtually all patients [3]. This ECS deposition is in most cases throughout the entire epidermis and mucosal epithelium, therefore a subclassification can not be made. In the majority of textbooks this is described as a smooth pattern throughout the epidermis (Fig. 4.1a). However, in many biopsies a fine or coarse granular pattern can be observed (Fig. 4.1b, c). *Pemphigus is characterized by ECS deposition of immunoglobulins and complement in a smooth or granular pattern* These clusters seem to be the result of clustering of IgG, Dsg3 and plakoglobin, but no other desmosomal components are involved [4]. Due to its bivalency, IgG crosslinks non-junctional Dsg molecules and these crosslinked molecules then concentrate in dots. In addition to deposits throughout the epidermis, immunoglobulins can in many cases also be observed in adnexal structures, e.g. hair follicles and sweat glands. False positive ECS deposition can be observed in biopsies of eczema lesions. In these cases a "tram rails" pattern between the keratinocytes can be observed in contrast to the smooth or granular patterns in pemphigus (Fig. 4.2).

On top of ECS deposition, in some cases also a granular deposition of autoantibodies and complement can be found along the dermal-epidermal junction, especially in pemphigus erythematosus, now considered to be a localized form of pemphigus foliaceus (Fig. 4.3). It seems that these granules consist of IgG directed against the ectodomain of desmoglein 1, which is shed along the epidermal basement membrane.

In most cases of pemphigus the ECS deposition consists of IgG with or without complement binding, although in some cases also IgA is present. However, in rare cases only IgA depositions can be found, a so-called IgA pemphigus (see Chap. 11). In general two variants of IgA pemphigus are considered, the subcorneal pustulosis type and the intraepidermal neutrophilic type. Direct immunofluorescence of the subcorneal pustulosis type shows deposits of IgA only in the upper part of the epidermis, while in the intraepidermal neutrophilic type IgA is present on the ECS throughout the entire epidermis.

Paraneoplastic pemphigus is a severe autoimmune multiorgan disease different from pemphigus vulgaris [5]. It is characterized clinically by painful stomatitis and polymorphous cutaneous manifestations in patients with underlying neoplasia. PNP comprises many antibodies; the most characteristic are periplakin and envoplakin next to desmoglein. *Paraneoplastic pemphigus is a severe multiorgan disease with in almost all cases antibodies against envoplakin and periplakin.* Direct immunofluorescence shows ECS deposits of IgG and complement throughout the epidermis consistent with other variants of pemphigus. In addition, in some cases a linear deposition of IgG and complement can be seen, which can be attributed to additional antibodies against hemidesmosomal components (Fig. 4.4).

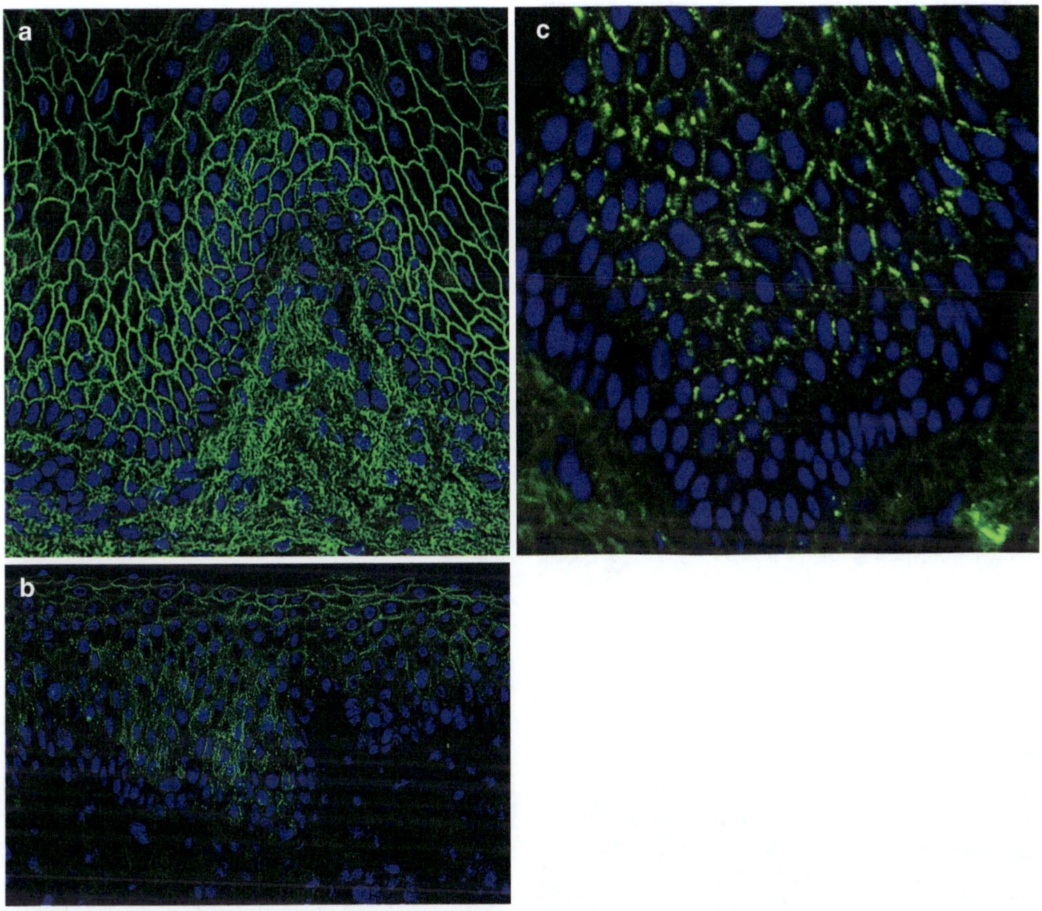

Fig. 4.1 Patterns of epithelial cell surface (ECS) staining in pemphigus: (**a**) smooth pattern, (**b**) fine granular pattern, (**c**) coarse granular pattern

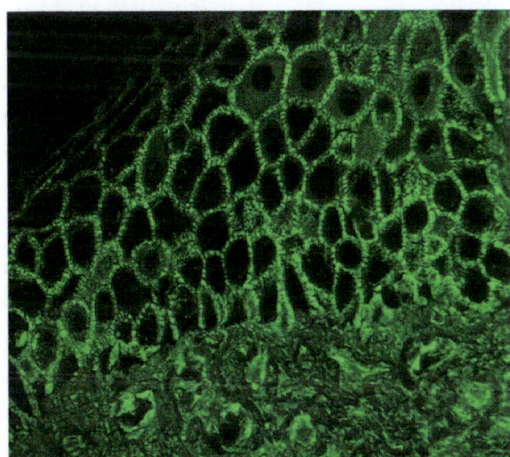

Fig. 4.2 Fals-positive pseudo-epithelial cell surface (ECS) staining of IgG in a tram rail pattern in eczema due to spongiotic edema

However, in these cases the diagnosis of paraneoplastic pemphigus has to be confirmed by serology, since rare cases of coexisting pemphigus and pemphigoid are described in literature.

Pemphigoid

All variants of are characterized by a linear deposition of immunoglobulins and/or complement along the epidermal basement membrane zone [6] (Fig. 4.5a). *Pemphigoid is characterized by a linear deposition of immunoreactants along the basement membrane* These antibodies are directed against various hemidesmosomal components and connecting molecules; (1) type XVII collagen (BP180) in

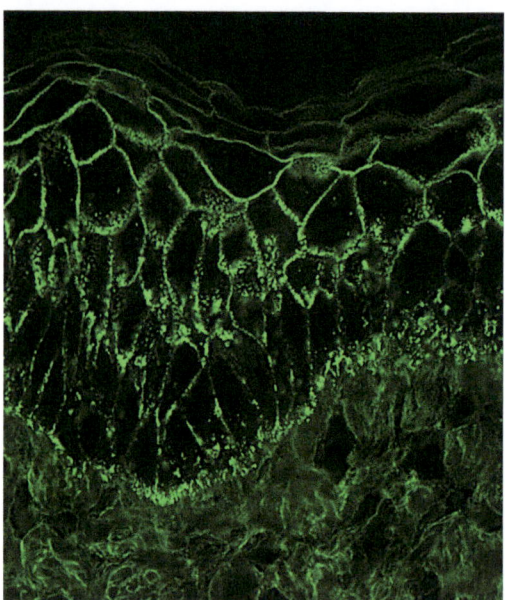

Fig. 4.3 Pemphigus erythematosus with IgG in a smooth/granular ECS deposition, and additionally a granular deposition along the epidermal basement membrane zone

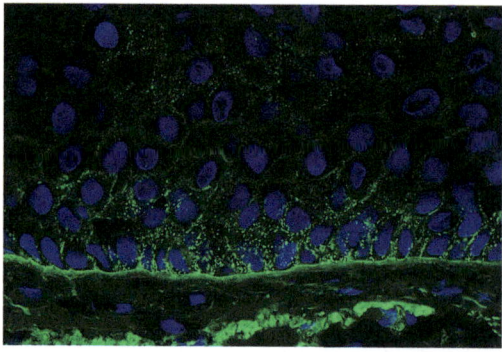

Fig. 4.4 Paraneoplastic pemphigus with IgG in a granular ECS deposition and additionally a linear deposition along the epidermal basement membrane zone

bullous pemphigoid (BP), mucous membrane pemphigoid (MMP), pemphigoid gestationis (PG), lichen planus pemphigoides (LPP), and linear IgA disease (LAD), (2) BP230 in BP, (3) laminin 332 in anti-laminin 332 pemphigoid, (4) integrin beta4 in ocular mucous membrane pemphigoid, and (5) p200 in anti-p200 pemphigoid. Moreover, in epidermolysis bullosa acquisita (EBA) and bullous SLE, antibodies against type VII collagen, present in the sublamina densa, also give rise to a linear deposition pattern.

In case a linear deposition is observed it is important to determine the nature of the deposits. In most variants of BP and in EBA the deposits consist of IgG and complement. Mixed IgG/IgA depositions are commonly encountered, especially in mucosal dominant cases of pemphigoid. In addition, in some cases only IgA is present, leading to a diagnosis of LAD or IgA EBA [7, 8]. However, in mucosal dominant pemphigoid with mixed IgA/IgG depositions, the IgG component might be very weak, which might result in a misdiagnosis of linear IgA disease. PG shows in virtually all cases a strong linear deposition of complement along the basement membrane with a weaker staining for IgG. Strikingly, in many cases of PG interruptions in this linear deposition can be seen, caused by the presence of melanocytes (Fig. 4.5b). This can also been seen in other cases of pemphigoid, but is usually less obvious. Although in a number of cases linear IgM deposition might be present in adjunct to IgG and complement, cases have been described with only linear IgM deposition. Whether these cases should be considered a variant of pemphigoid or merely a coincident finding is unknown.

In LPP, clinically characterized by blisters next to typical lichen planus lesions, in addition to a linear IgG deposition, shaggy deposition of fibrin and lichenoid infiltrate is often found (Fig. 4.5c). Furthermore, colloid bodies, ovoid or round structures consisting of keratin filaments and covered with immunoglobulins, can be found in the underlying dermis.

Bullous SLE is characterized by antibodies to type VII collagen in a patient fulfilling the ARA criteria for systemic lupus erythematosus. In bullous SLE, next to or superimposed on a linear IgG deposition, a biopsy might show a lupusband, characterized by granular deposition of immunoglobulins and complement, and the presence of epidermal *in vivo* anti-nuclear antibodies.

In most cases of pemphigoid a linear-serrated pattern can be discerned. This serration pattern can be separated in an n-serrated pattern and a u-serrated pattern [9] (Fig. 4.6a, b). *Bullous pemphigoid shows an n-serrated pattern,*

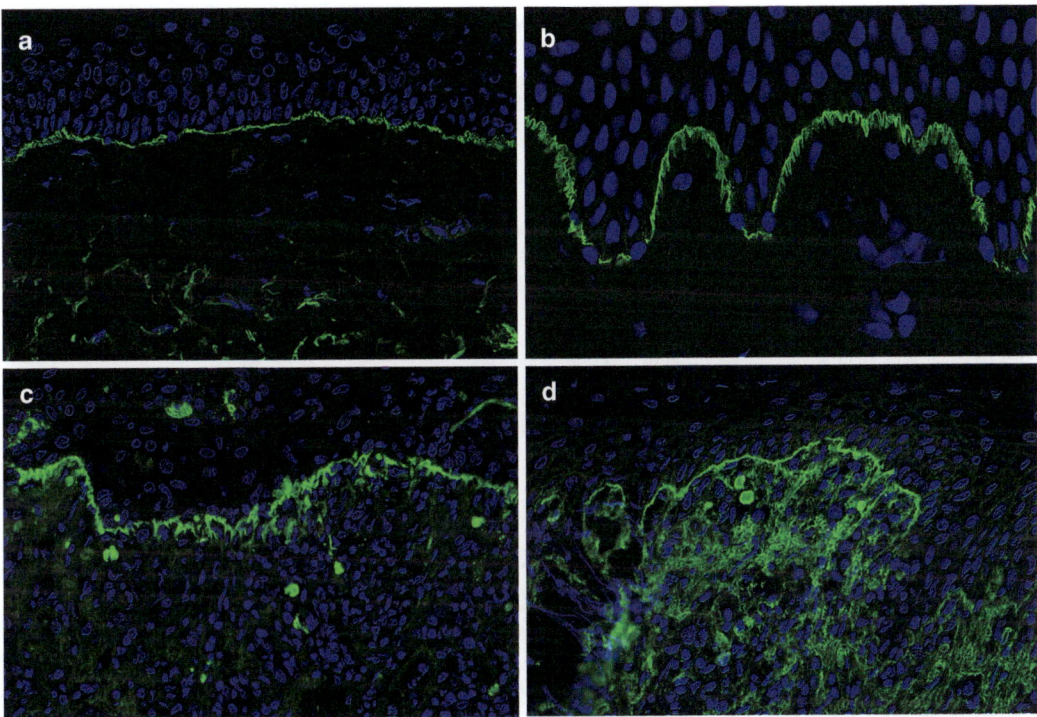

Fig. 4.5 (a) Linear deposition of IgG along the basement membrane in bullous pemphigoid. (b) Linear deposition of complement with marked gaps due to the presence of melanocytes in pemphigoid gestationis. Shaggy deposition of fibrin (c) and a linear deposition of IgG (d) along the epidermal BMZ in lichen planus pemphigoides

whereas epidermolysis bullosa acquisita shows a u-serrated pattern. The recognition of these serration patterns makes it possible to differentiate between (1) sublamina densa binding diseases caused by autoantibodies against type VII collagen, e.g. EBA and bullous SLE and (2) blistering diseases with binding above the lamina densa with antibodies against hemidesmosomal components, e.g. BP, PG, MMP, anti-p200 pemphigoid, and anti-laminin 332 pemphigoid. This differentiation can be explained by the fact that in cases with antibodies against type VII collagen the immunodeposits are located between the rootlets of the basal keratinocytes, leading to a u-serrated pattern (Fig. 4.6c). On the other hand, depositions above the lamina densa follow the plasma membrane in the basal cell rootlets, resulting in an n-serrated pattern (Fig. 4.6d). In some cases it is not possible to determine the serration pattern, especially in mucosal biopsies. In these cases it is wise to cut thinner sections or to take a biopsy of clinically uninvolved skin.

However, a few cases remain in which it is impossible to differentiate between an n-serrated and an u-serrated pattern. In these cases the level of the deposition of the antibodies can be determined by fluorescent overlay antigen mapping (FOAM). FOAM is a technique based on the possibility to visualize a targeted antigen relative to a topographic marker. For instance, in Fig. 4.6 red staining is used for type VII collagen, as topographic reference marker and a green staining for IgG deposits. In case of BP separate patterns of IgG deposits (green) and type VII collagen (red) can be seen with red staining on the dermal side. In contrast, EBA skin shows a pattern with overlap of green IgG deposits and red type VII collagen staining, resulting in a yellow-orange fluorescence and lacking red staining on the dermal side. FOAM can be done using a standard immunofluorescence microscope, providing appropriate software is available. However, better results are accomplished using confocal microscopy.

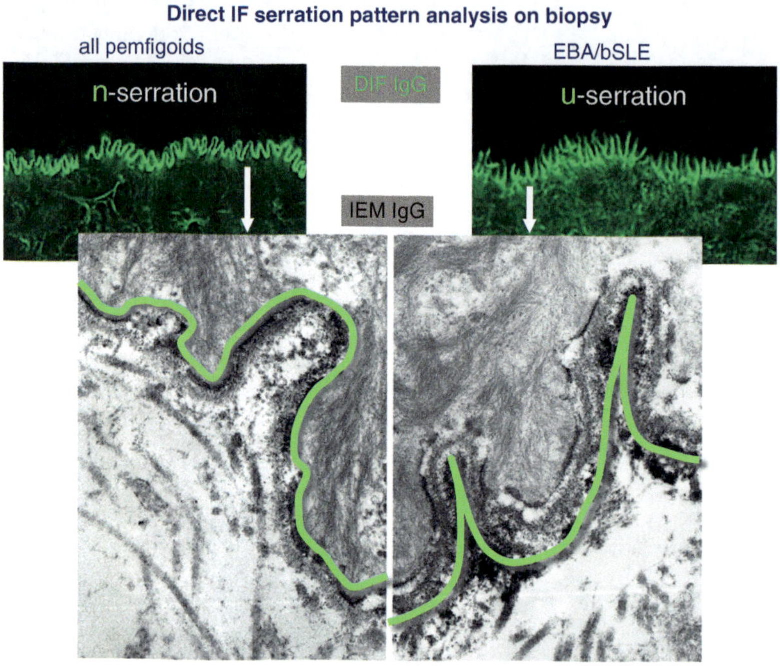

Fig. 4.6 (**a**) n-serrated pattern in bullous pemphigoid, (**b**) u-serrated pattern in epidermolysis bullosa acquisita, (**c–d**) immunoelectron microscopy of peroxidase labeled IgG of perilesional skin from a patient with bullous pemphigoid (**c**) and epidermolysis bullosa acquisita (**d**). The n-serrated pattern follows the undulations of the plasma membrane, whereas the u-serrated pattern is the result of staining of anchoring fibrils between the rootlets. [Reprinted from: Vodegel, R. M., Jonkman, M. F., Pas, H. H. & de Jong, M. C. J. M. U-serrated immunodeposition pattern differentiates type VII collagen targeting bullous diseases from other subepidermal bullous autoimmune diseases. Br. J. Dermatol. 151, 112–118 (2004), with permission from Wiley]

Dermatitis Herpetiformis

Dermatitis herpetiformis (DH) is characterized by IgA antibodies against tissue transglutaminase and although it has typical pruritic blisters on predilection sites, the clinical picture might resemble various variants of pemphigoid. However, direct immunofluorescence can make a clear distinction between these entities. Direct immunofluorescence of DH shows a granular deposition of IgA along the dermal-epidermal junction [10]. *Dermatitis herpetiformis is characterized by a granular deposition of IgA along the dermal-epidermal junction.* Typically, these depositions are concentrated in the dermal papillae, although in many cases a linear granular is present (Fig. 4.7). This deposition is most probably the result of the precipitation of IgA antibodies against epidermal transglutaminase (TG3). These IgA-TG3 immune complexes can also be detected in small vessels in the papillary dermis.

Porphyria Cutanea Tarda and Pseudoporphyria

Porphyria cutanea tarda (PCT) is characterized by cell poor blisters mostly present on the dorsal sites of hand and feet, induced by photosensitization of endogenous (porphyrins) or exogenous (e.g. NSAID's) agents. Although this disease shows a typical clinical presentation and has a characteristic histology, the differentiation from mechanobullous EBA can be difficult. Fortunately, both entities have different immunofluorescent patterns. As described above EBA is characterized by u-serrated linear deposition of IgG and complement along the basement membrane. PCT, on the other hand,

4 Direct Immunofluorescence Microscopy

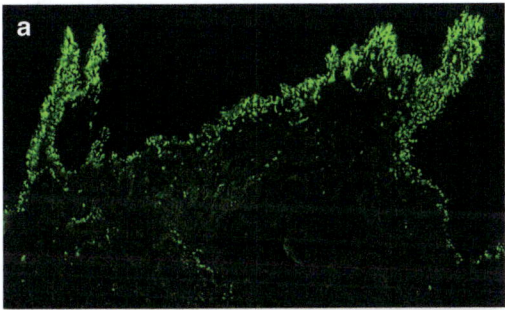

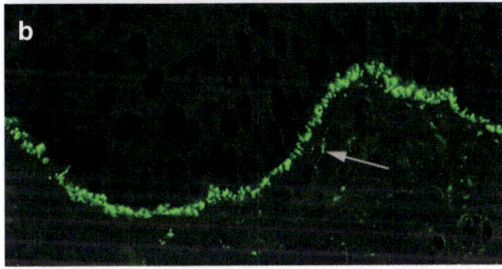

Fig. 4.7 (**a**) The granular IgA depositions in dermatitis herpetiformis are located in the dermal papillae, or (**b**) more along the dermal-epidermal junction and in superficial vessel walls (arrows)

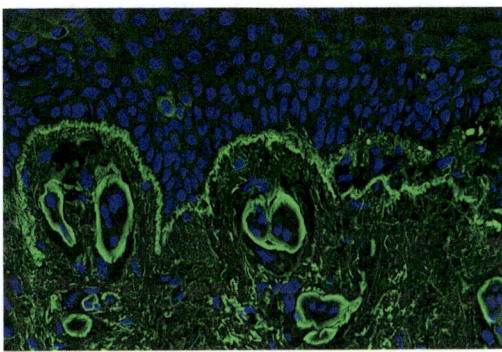

Fig. 4.8 Homogeneous deposition of IgG along the dermal-epidermal junction and in vessel walls is the hallmark of (pseudo)porphyria

shows a homogeneous deposition of immunoglobulins, preferably IgG, in vessel walls and in most instances a homogeneous deposition along the dermal-epidermal junction (Fig. 4.8), although also granular and fibrillar depositions have been described. *A homogeneous deposition of particularly IgG along the dermal-epidermal junction and in vessel walls is typical in porphyria* It has been hypothesized that the depositions in the vessel walls might reflect a reaction between physiological autoantibodies and damaged vascular endothelium. The formation of separation at the lamina lucida is a secondary event caused by the release of proteolytic enzymes and destruction of laminin and type IV collagen.

Review Questions

1. Pemphigus is characterized by
   a. A smooth epithelial surface staining
   b. A granular epithelial surface staining
   c. Both patterns can be observed

2. An u-serrated linear staining along the basal membrane zone can be observed in
   a. Bullous pemphigoid
   b. Epidermolysis bullosa acquisita
   c. Anti-p200 pemphigoid

Answers

1. c
2. b

Acknowledgements Dr M.C. de Jong is acknowledged for providing some of the IF pictures.

References

1. Beutner EH, Jordon RE. Demonstration of skin antibodies in sera of pemphigus vulgaris patients by indirect immunofluorescent staining. Proc Soc Exp Biol Med. 1964;117:505–10.
2. Mahoney MG, et al. Explanations for the clinical and microscopic localization of lesions in pemphigus foliaceus and vulgaris. J Clin Invest. 1999;103:461–8.
3. Beutner EH, Lever WF, Witebsky E, Jordon R, Chertock B. Autoantibodies in pemphigus vulgaris: response to an intercellular substance of epidermis. JAMA. 1965;192:682–8.
4. Oktarina DAM, van der Wier G, Diercks GFH, Jonkman MF, Pas HH. IgG-induced clustering of desmogleins 1 and 3 in skin of patients with pemphigus fits with the desmoglein non-assembly depletion hypothesis. Br J Dermatol. 2011;165:552–62.

5. Anhalt GJ, Kim SC, Stanley JR, Korman NJ, Jabs DA, Kory M, Izumi H, Ratrie H 3rd, Mutasim D, Ariss-Abdo L, et al. Paraneoplastic pemphigus. An autoimmunemucocutaneous disease associated with neoplasia. N Engl J Med. 1990;20:1729–35.
6. Jordon RE, et al. Basement zone antibodies in bullous pemphigoid. JAMA. 1967;200:751–6.
7. Wilson BD, Beutner EH, Kumar V, Chorzelski TP, Jablonska S. Linear IgA bullous dermatosis. An immunologically defined disease. Int J Dermatol. 1985;24:569–74.
8. Vodegel RM, de Jong MCJM, Pas HH, Jonkman MF. IgA-mediated epidermolysis bullosa acquisita: two cases and review of the literature. J Am Acad Dermatol. 2002;47:919–25.
9. Vodegel RM, Jonkman MF, Pas HH, de Jong MCJM. U-serrated immunodeposition pattern differentiates type VII collagen targeting bullous diseases from other subepidermal bullous autoimmune diseases. Br J Dermatol. 2004;151:112–8.
10. van der Meer JB. Granular deposits of immunoglobulins in the skin of patients with dermatitis herpetiformis. An immunofluorescent study. Br J Dermatol. 1969;81:493–503.

Indirect Immunofluorescence Microscopy

5

Gilles F. H. Diercks and Hendri H. Pas

Learning Objectives

After studying this chapter, you should know:

- The various substrates used in indirect immunofluorescence microscopy in auto-immune blistering diseases
- The binding patterns of autoantibodies to monkey esophagus in pemphigus, pemphigoid and dermatitis herpetiformis
- The principle of salt split skin and the difference between epidermal and dermal staining
- The use of rat bladder for the diagnosis of paraneoplastic pemphigus

Introduction

Indirect immunofluorescence microscopy is used to detect circulating antibodies in patient's serum. For this purpose an adequate substrate is necessary to visualize these antibodies. In this chapter various substrates and techniques are described to (sub)type the different variants of autoimmune blistering diseases. A summary of intraepidermal and subepidermal autoimmune blistering diseases with associated antigens and immunofluorescence patterns is described in Table 5.1.

Indirect immunofluorescence is used to detect circulating antibodies.

Technique

To detect circulating autoantibodies with immunofluorescence microscopy the following steps are recommended (Groningen protocol):

- Collect 5–10 ml of blood without anticoagulants.
- Dilute patient's serum: for testing on monkey esophagus a dilution of 1:40 is recommended, for human salt split skin 1:8 and for endomysium antibodies 1:4.
- Apply diluted serum onto a substrate for 30–40 min.
- Rinse the slides with PBS (NaCl 8.75 g/l, Na2HPO4 1.14 g/l, KH2PO4 0.27 g/l) for a minimum of 5 seconds. Wipe off excess PBS.
- Apply fluorescein isothiocyanate (FITC)-conjugated antibodies for 30–40 min (see Chap. 3 for the recommended IgG and IgA antibodies).
- Rinse the slides with PBS. Wipe off excess PBS.
- Rinse the slides now for 15–20 min with PBS.
- Place a drop of PBS/glycerin (1:1) on each section and top with a cover slip.

G. F. H. Diercks (✉) · H. H. Pas
Center for Blistering Diseases, Department of Dermatology and Pathology, University Medical Center Groningen, University of Groningen, Groningen, The Netherlands
e-mail: g.f.h.diercks@umcg.nl; h.h.pas@umcg.nl

Table 5.1 Laboratory diagnosis of autoimmune blistering diseases by direct and indirect immunofluorescence microscopy

Bullous disease	Antigen	Direct IF skin/mucosa		Indirect IF serum		Salt split skin	
				Esophagus	Anti-BMZ	Anti-BMZ	
		ECS	BMZ	Anti-ECS		Epidermal	Dermal
Intraepidermal							
Pemphigus vulgaris	Desmoglein 3±1	IgG±A, C	–	IgG	–	–	–
Pemphigus foliaceus	Desmoglein 1	IgG±A, C	–	IgG	–	–	–
Paraneoplastic pemphigus	Plakines, desmoglein 3±1, BP230, plectin, a2ML1	IgG±A, C	IgG±A, C	IgG	(IgG)	(IgG)	–
IgA-pemphigus	Desmocollin	IgA	–	IgA	–	–	–
Subepidermal					Anti-BMZ		
Bullous pemhigoid	BP230/BP180/LAD/plectin	–	IgG±A, C n-serrated	–	IgG±A	IgG±A	–
Pemphigoid gestationis	BP180	–	C, (IgG) n-serrated	–	(IgG)	(IgG)	–
Mucous membrane pemphigoid	BP230/BP180/LAD/Integrinα6β4	–	IgG±A, C n-serrated	–	IgG±A	IgG±A	–
Lichen planus pemphigoides	BP180	–	IgG, C n-serrated	–	IgG	IgG	–
Linear IgA disease	BP180/LAD/plectin	–	IgA n-serrated	–	IgA	IgA	–
Anti-laminin 332 pemphigoid	Laminin 332	–	IgG, C n-serrated	–	–	–	IgG±A
Anti-p200 pemphigoid	P200	–	IgG, C n-serrated	–	–	–	IgG±A
Epidermolysis bullosa acquisita	Collagen type VII	–	IgG, IgA, C u-serrated	–	–	–	IgG±A, IgA
Dermatitis herpetiformis	Transglutaminase	–	IgA granular	EMA IgA	–	–	–

IF immunofluorescence, *ECS* epithelial cell surface, *BMZ* basement membrane zone, *EMA* endomysium antibodies, *C* complement

Monkey Esophagus

Monkey esophagus was the first substrate used for detecting of circulating autoantibodies in patients with autoimmune blistering diseases [1]. Other substrates that have been used are guinea pig lip, guinea pig esophagus or monkey tongue. However, monkey esophagus seems to yield the best results [2]. Studies have shown that using two substrates, e.g. monkey esophagus and guinea pig esophagus or human skin yields a higher sensitivity for the diagnosis of pemphigus. Moreover, due to different staining patterns on various substrates, one might differentiate pemphigus vulgaris from foliaceus. However, in daily practice it might not be feasible to use two substrates. With commercially distributed monkey esophagus widely available, this seems to be the substrate of choice. Moreover, a reliable differentiation between pemphigus vulgaris and foliaceus is available by the introduction of specific ELISA kits for desmoglein 1 and 3.

Although studies have proposed human skin as the substrate of choice, many specimens have to be tested to find a reactive one. Moreover, sera with pemphigus autoantibodies might react with patient's own skin, but not with normal skin of other individuals, yielding false negative results.

Monkey esophagus is normally tested with FITC-conjugated anti-human IgG (Fig. 5.1a). In addition one can also detect IgA, however these results have to be carefully interpreted, since anti-IgA is known to give false *positive* results.

In practice two main patterns can be discerned. In all variants of true pemphigus IgG class antibodies show an epithelial cell surface (ECS) pattern (Fig. 5.1b), resulting from present autoantibodies against the desmosomal transmembrane adhesion molecules desmoglein 1 and/or 3. The ECS pattern is also called chicken wire or honeycomb pattern. The old term intercellular substance (ICS) pattern is abandoned since the immunoglobulin binding is not to a 'substance' between the cells, but to the cell surface. In pemphigoid a linear deposition along the epithelial basement membrane can be observed, caused by autoantibodies against hemidesmosomes or their connecting proteins underneath (Fig. 5.1c).

Monkey esophagus can detect circulating antibodies against desmosomal and basal membrane zone molecules.

Indirect immunofluorescence on monkey esophagus always shows a smooth ECS pattern (Fig. 5.1b), in contrast to the more granular pattern observed with direct immunofluorescence microscopy on skin biopsies. The sensitivity of this test for active pemphigus is up to 90%, whereas results might be negative in quiescent cases or cases in remission. One should be aware that false positive sera could be encountered. An important reason is the existence of blood group AB antigens on monkey epithelial cells, which might react with anti-A or anti-B antibodies present in patient's blood. This gives rise to a pseudo- ECS pattern, which at close examination reveals a coarse "barbed wire" pattern (Fig. 5.1d), instead of the sharply defined smooth pattern seen with pemphigus sera (Fig. 5.1b). Moreover, sera with pseudo-ECS pattern tend not to bind to the basal epithelial layer [3]. Absorption of A and B antibodies might resolve this problem. In addition, various other conditions might give a false positive ECS staining, among which burn wound victims seem to be the most important.

Early studies have shown that indirect immunofluorescence microscopy on monkey esophagus has a sensitivity for bullous pemphigoid of around 60-80% with a high specificity [4]. In this respect it is important to notice that active disease activity is more likely to give a positive result, while inactive cases are mostly negative. Although numbers vary, most studies on mucous membrane pemphigoid show a much lower sensitivity, as low as 10–20% [5] probably due to lower concentration of circulating antibodies. The sensitivity of indirect immunofluorescence is also low in epidermolysis bullosa acquisita (EBA) [6].

In addition to the pemphigus and pemphigoid staining patterns, other binding patterns can be encountered. Cytoplasmic staining of epithelial basal cells has been associated with drug-induced skin reactions (Fig. 5.2). However, sensitivity and specificity seem to be low. These antibodies might

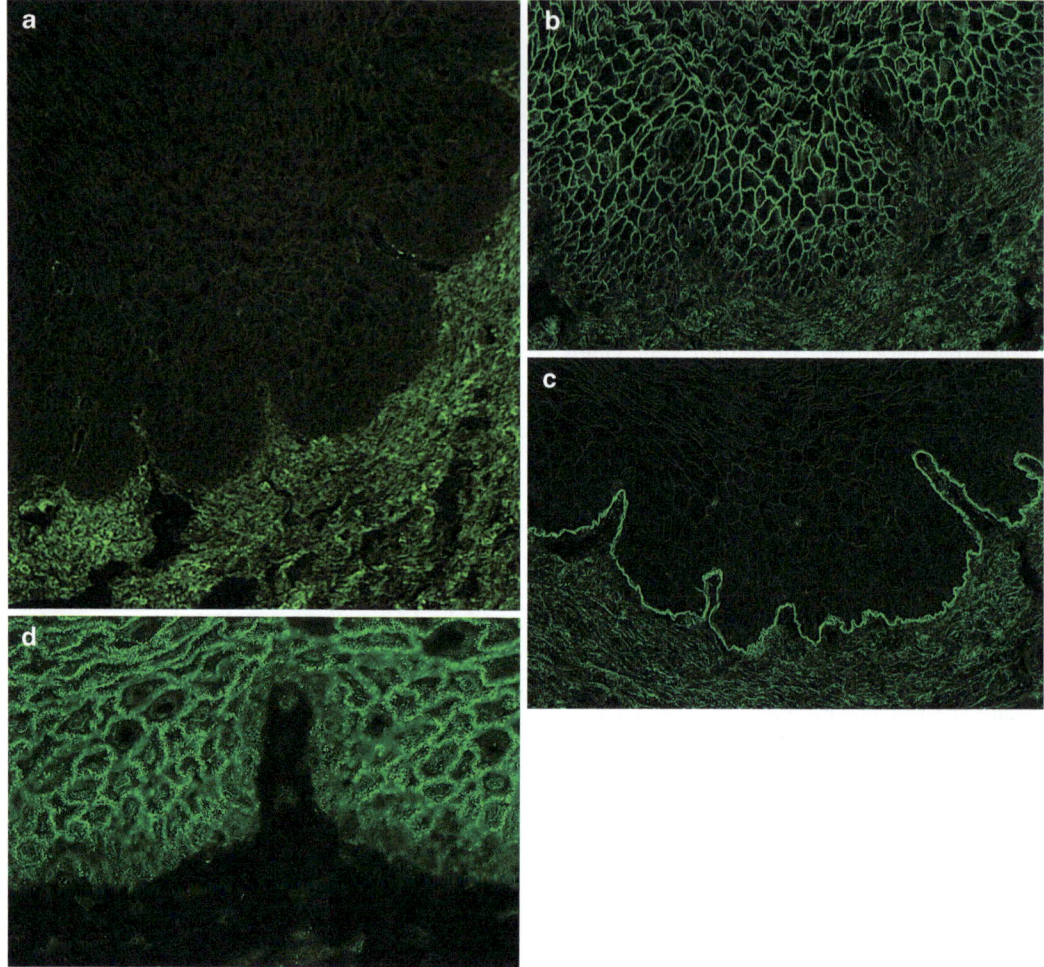

Fig. 5.1 Indirect immunofluorescence on monkey esophagus. (**a**) Control serum with negative binding, (**b**) pemphigus serum IgG binds in a smooth epithelial cell surface (ECS) pattern, (**c**) pemphigoid serum IgG binds in a linear pattern along the epithelial basement membrane membrane zone, and (**d**) false positive ECS binding

amongst others also be demonstrated in burn victims and after bone marrow transplantation, but also in pemphigus and pemphigoid patients. Antinuclear antibodies can be observed in monkey esophagus, although monkey esophagus is not the substrate of choice for assessing antinuclear antibodies. One pattern that might be of some importance is a stratified epithelium-specific antinuclear antibody that is directed against a 70-kd antigen and is characterized by a fine speckled nuclear staining. This antibody can be found in chronic ulcerative stomatitis, a condition closely related to erosive lichen planus [7].

An important use of monkey esophagus is detection of IgA anti-endomysium antibody in patients with celiac disease or dermatitis herpetiformis and will detect IgA antibodies directed against the endomysium, a connective tissue layer that surrounds individual muscle fibers (Fig. 5.3). This layer contains transglutaminase, the primary autoantigen in celiac disease and dermatitis herpetiformis [8].

IgA binding to the endomysium of smooth muscle cells is indicative of celiac disease and dermatitis herpetiformis

Human Salt Split Skin

In the 80s the first studies using human salt split skin for the diagnosis of subepidermal autoimmune blistering diseases were performed [9] and this technique proved to be a valuable asset to monkey esophagus. *salt split skin is the substrate of choice for detecting antibodies in pemphigoid disease* Normal human skin is incubated for 48–72 h in 1.0 mol sodium chloride, which produces a reproducible split in the lamina lucida, separating epidermal and dermal located pemphigoid antigens. Important antigens in the roof of salt split skin are type XVII collagen (BP180) and BP230, whereas laminin 332, p200 and type IV collagen are situated in the floor of the blister (Fig. 5.4a). This implies that bullous pemphigoid, mucous membrane pemphigoid, pemphigoid gestationis, and lichen planus pemphigoides show staining of IgG on the epidermal side of the blister (Fig. 5.4b). On the other hand anti-laminin 332 pemphigoid, anti-p200 pemphigoid, epidermolysis bullosa acquisita, and bullous SLE show staining on the dermal side (Fig. 5.4c). *Bullous pemphigoid shows an epidermal staining on salt split skin, whereas EBA shows a dermal staining* In various cases also expression of IgA in addition to IgG can be demonstrated. Solely IgA deposition can be seen in linear IgA disease and IgA epidermolysis bullosa acquisita on the epidermal and dermal side respectively.

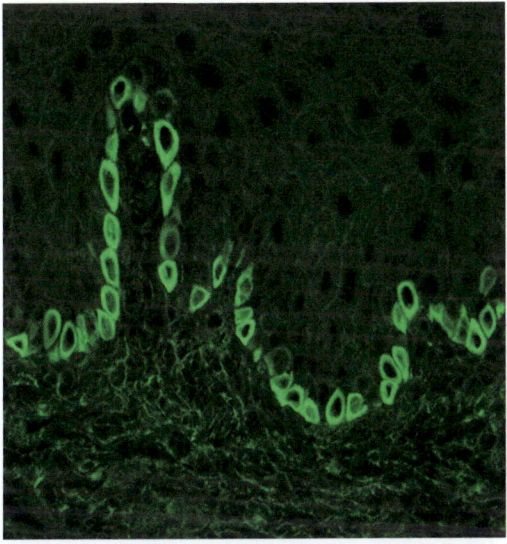

Fig. 5.2 Basal cell cytoplasmic staining by indirect immunofluorescence on monkey esophagus

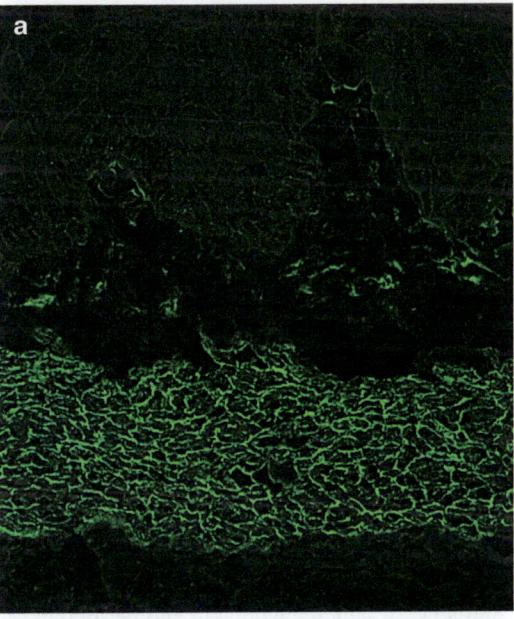

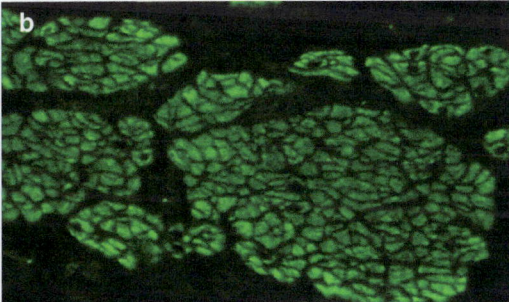

Fig. 5.3 IgA antibodies directed against (**a**) the endomysium of smooth muscle fibers in dermatitis herpetiformis and (**b**) a negative control

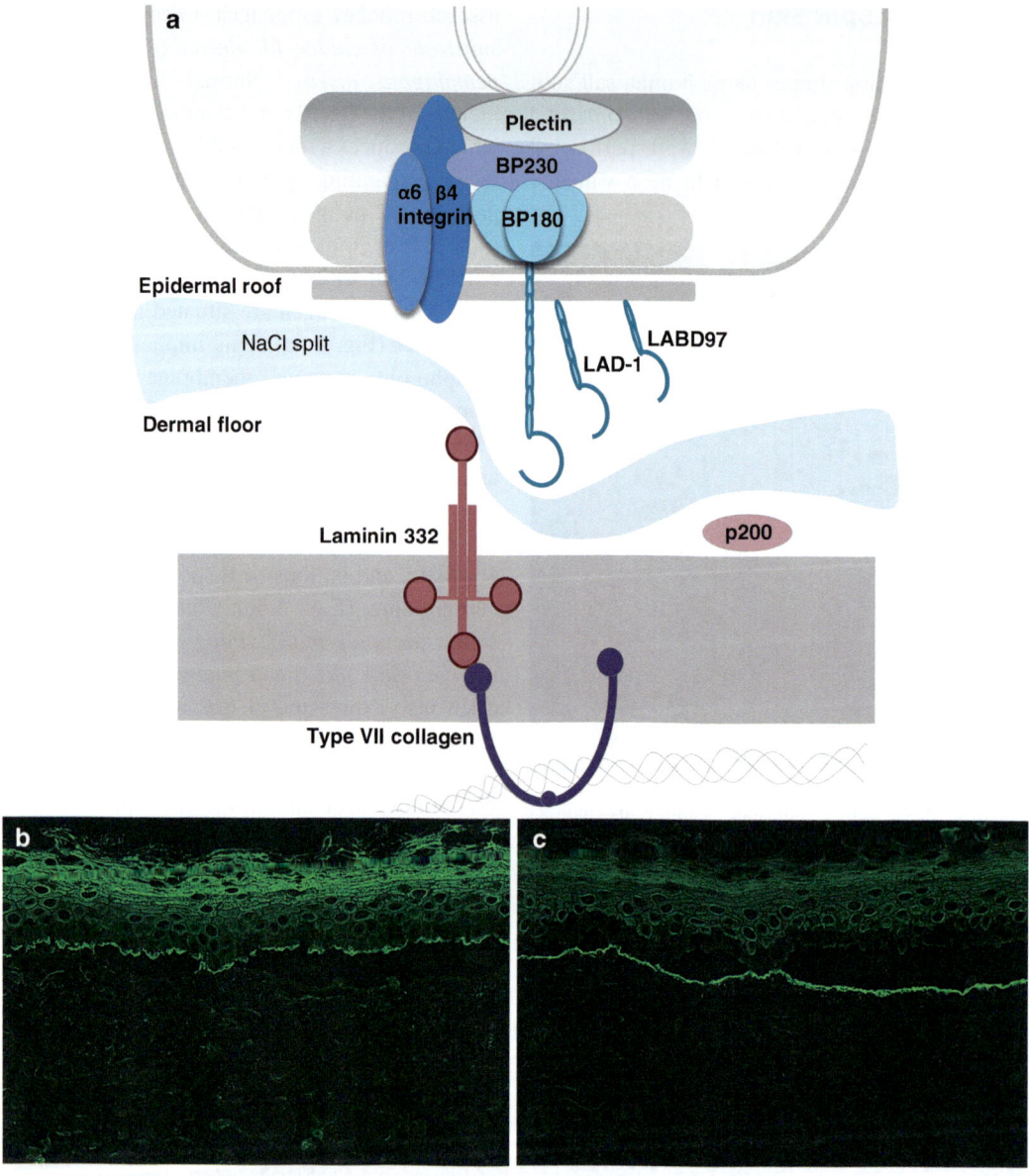

Fig. 5.4 (**a**) Diagram of basement membrane zone in salt split skin. Indirect IF in bullous pemhigoid with antibodies to BP180 shows (**b**) an epidermal staining, epidermolysis bullosa acquisita with antibodies against type VII collagen shows a (**c**) dermal staining

The sensitivity of salt split skin in comparison with monkey esophagus for pemphigoid sera is comparable to that of monkey oesophagus with a sensitivity between 70 and 80%. For EBA the sensitivity is around 40–50% [6]. Specificity of salt split skin is high for all types of autoimmune blistering diseases, and ranges between 97 and 100%.

Rat bladder

Paraneoplastic pemphigus is an autoimmune blistering disease associated with an underlying neoplasm and with antibodies directed against various antigens, of which envoplakin and periplakin are considered the most important, but also includes desmoglein 1 and 3, desmoplakins and plectin.

5 Indirect Immunofluorescence Microscopy

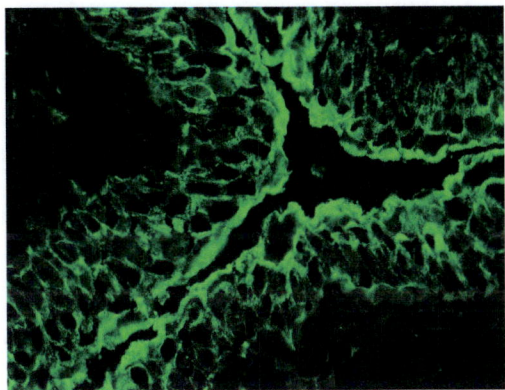

Fig. 5.5 Positive indirect IF on rat bladder with IgG staining in ECS pattern in paraneoplastic pemphigus

Indirect immunofluorescence on monkey esophagus might show a smooth ECS pattern and therefore does not differentiate between pemphigus and paraneoplastic pemphigus. However, the transitional epithelium of rat bladder is rich in envoplakin and periplakin, but is devoid of desmoglein 1 and 3. In case of paraneoplastic pemphigus rat bladder shows an ECS staining, whereas pemphigus will be negative (Fig. 5.5).

Rat bladder testing for paraneoplastic pemphigus has a sensitivity of about 74%, but a high specificity [10]. With respect to the low sensitivity additional testing using immunoblot or immunoprecipitation raises the sensitivity to 100%.

Knock-Out Skin

In addition to the above-mentioned more or less routine techniques for serological detection of autoantibodies, more advanced immunofluorescence techniques can be used to further characterize present autoantibodies.

One of these techniques is using knock-out skin, i.e. skin of patients with inherited forms of epidermolysis bullosa (EB) completely lacking certain molecules at the dermoepidermal junction [11]. Patients with severe recessive dystrophic EB are devoid of type VII collagen, whereas patients with junctional EB, Herlitz type lack laminin 332. Using skin of these patients as a substrate makes it possible to differentiate between EBA and anti-laminin 332 pemphigoid, diseases that both are characterized by dermal staining on salt split skin. EBA will show absence of staining on type VII collagen-deficient skin, but in contrast will show a linear staining along the BMZ in laminin 332-deficient skin (Fig. 5.6). Anti-laminin 332 pemphigoid will show opposite results. A dermal staining on salt split skin and a positive staining on both deficient-skin substrates suggests an anti-p200 pemphigoid.

A major disadvantage of this technique is the need of a sufficient concentration of circulating antibodies, which might be low, particularly in EBA. In these cases one needs a skin biopsy to determine the serration pattern or eventual use fluorescent overlay antigen mapping by direct immunofluorescence (see previous chapter) to differentiate between these diseases.

Review Questions

1. Using monkey esophagus as a substrate, pemphigus is characterized by
   a. A linear pattern along the basement membrane
   b. A epithelial cell surface staining in a chicken wire pattern
   c. Both patterns can be observed
2. A dermal staining in salt split skin can be observed in
   a. Anti-laminin 332 pemphigoid
   b. Anti-p200 pemphigoid
   c. Epidermolysis bullosa acquisita
   d. All of the above mentioned variants
3. The substrate of choice for testing for paraneoplastic pemphigus is
   a. Monkey esophagus
   b. Rat bladder
   c. Salt split skin

Answers

1. b
2. d
3. b

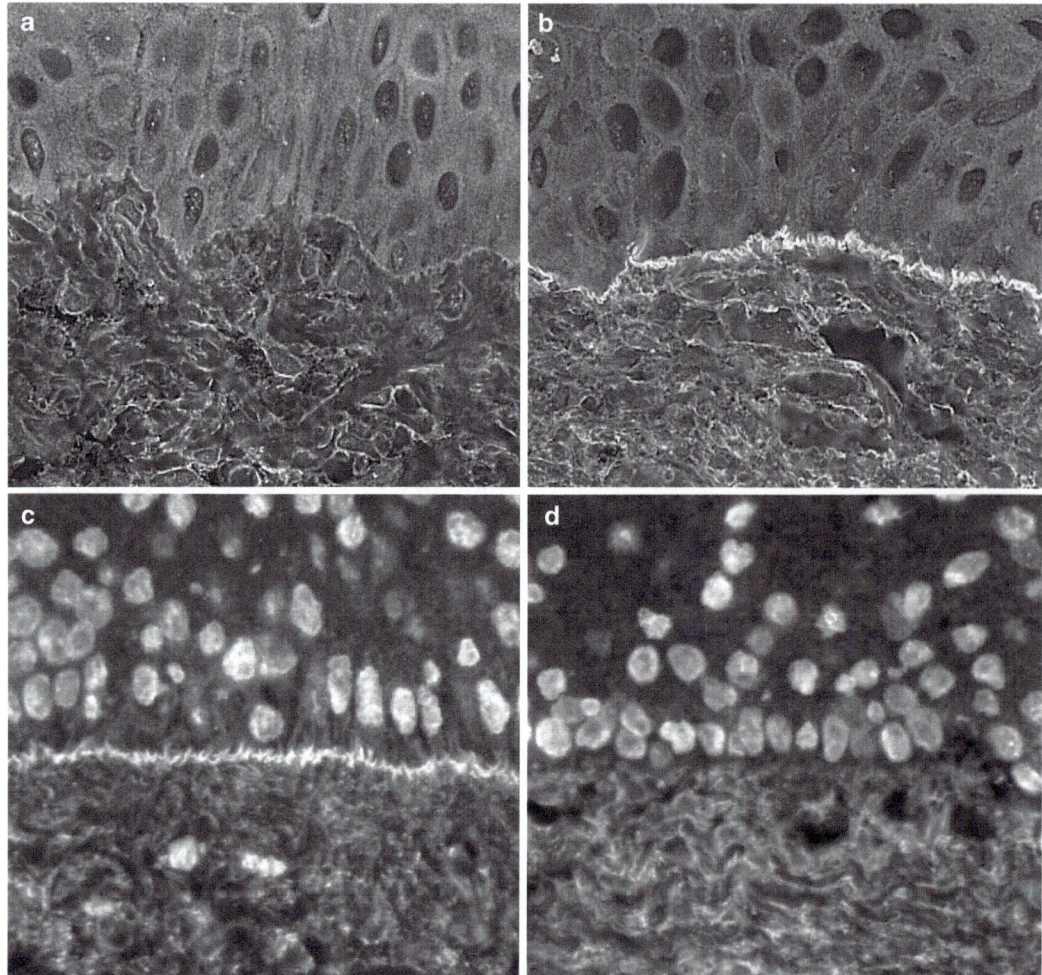

Fig. 5.6 Staining for serum IgG on knockout skin substrates lacking either (**a** and **c**) laminin 332 or (**b** and **d**) type VII collagen. Anti-laminin 332 pemphigoid shows absent IgG binding in (**a**) laminin 332 deficient-skin, while a positive binding in (**b**) type VII collagen-deficient skin. EBA shows a reverse binding pattern (**c** and **d**). [Reprinted from J Am Acad Dermatol, 48, Vodegal RM, de Jong MCJM, Pas HH, Yancey KB, Jonkman MF, Anti-epiligrin cicatricial pemphigoid and epidermolysis bullosa acquisita: Differentiation by use of indirect immunofluorescence microscopy, 542-7, copyright 2003, with permission from Elsevier]

Acknowledgements Dr M.C. de Jong is acknowledged for providing some of the IF pictures.

References

1. Beutner EH, Jordon RE. Demonstration of skin antibodies in sera of pemphigus vulgaris patients by indirect immunofluorescent staining. Proc Soc Exp Biol Med. 1964 Nov;117:505–10.
2. Feibelman C, Stolzner G, Provost TT, Pemphigus vulgaris. Superior sensitivity of monkey esophagus in the determination of pemphigus antibody. Arch Dermatol. 1981 Sep;117(9):561–2.
3. Goldblatt F, Gordon TP. Antibodies to blood group antigens mimic pemphigus staining patterns: a useful reminder. Autoimmunity. 2002 Mar;35(2):93–6.
4. Jordon RE, Beutner EH, Witebsky E, Blumental G, Hale WL, Lever WF. Basement zone antibodies in bullous pemphigoid. JAMA. 1967 May 29;200(9):751–6.
5. Bean SF. Cicatricial pemphigoid. Immunofluorescent studies. Arch Dermatol. 1974 Oct;110(4):552–5.
6. Terra JB, Jonkman MF, Diercks GF, Pas HH. Low sensitivity of type VII collagen enzyme-linked

immunosorbent assay in epidermolysis bullosa acquisita: serration pattern analysis on skin biopsy is required for diagnosis. Br J Dermatol. 2013 Jul;169(1):164–7.
7. Jaremko WM, Beutner EH, Kumar V, Kipping H, Condry P, Zeid MY, Kauffmann CL, Tatakis DN, Chorzelski TP. Chronic ulcerative stomatitis associated with a specific immunologic marker. J Am Acad Dermatol. 1990 Feb;22(2 Pt 1):215–20.
8. Chorzelski TP, Beutner EH, Sulej J, Tchorzewska H, Jablonska S, Kumar V, Kapuscinska A. IgA anti-endomysium antibody. A new immunological marker of dermatitis herpetiformis and coeliac disease. Br J Dermatol. 1984 Oct;111(4):395–402.
9. Woodley D, Sauder D, Talley MJ, Silver M, Grotendorst G, Qwarnstrom E. Localization of basement membrane components after dermal-epidermal junction separation. J Invest Dermatol. 1983 Aug;81(2):149–53.
10. Poot AM, Diercks GF, Kramer D, Schepens I, Klunder G, Hashimoto T, Borradori L, Jonkman MF, Pas HH. Laboratory diagnosis of paraneoplastic pemphigus. Br J Dermatol. 2013 Nov;169(5):1016–24.
11. Vodegel RM, de Jong MC, Pas HH, Yancey KB, Jonkman MF. Anti-epiligrin cicatricial pemphigoid and epidermolysis bullosa acquisita: differentiation by use of indirect immunofluorescence microscopy. J Am Acad Dermatol. 2003 Apr;48(4):542–7.

Immuno-Assays

Hendri H. Pas

Introduction & AIMS

Pemphigus and pemphigoid are autoimmune bullous diseases that are characterized by autoantibodies to epithelial proteins. Immunoblot, immunoprecipitation and ELISA are laboratory techniques that can visualize to which epithelial protein(s) the autoantibodies are directed. ELISA furthermore can quantify the autoantibody titer. Furthermore we will discuss the keratinocyte binding assay and the keratinocyte footprint assay. In this chapter we will briefly outline how these techniques work and how results should be interpreted.

> **Learning Objectives**
>
> After reading this chapter you should be able to:
>
> - Understand the principle of immuno-assays
> - Interpret the results of immunoassays
> - Decide if immuno-assays could be helpful in managing your patient
> - Choose which immuno-assays to perform for individual patients

Immunoblotting

Immunoblotting is a qualitative test to identify which autoantigen(s) are involved a particular AIBD patient. Briefly, denatured skin proteins are separated and sorted on molecular mass by polyacrylamide gel electrophoresis (PAGE) and then transferred onto membrane filters to facilitate further incubation and washing steps. The filters are overlaid with patient serum and after washing bound IgG is stained. The antigens then become visible as purple bands and are identified by apparent molecular weight (Fig. 6.1) [1]. Skin proteins are obtained by extracting cultured human keratinocytes or human skin with the harsh soap sodium dodecyl sulphate (SDS). SDS

H. H. Pas (✉)
Center for Blistering Diseases, Departments of Dermatology, University Medical Center Groningen, University of Groningen, Groningen, The Netherlands
e-mail: h.h.pas@umcg.nl

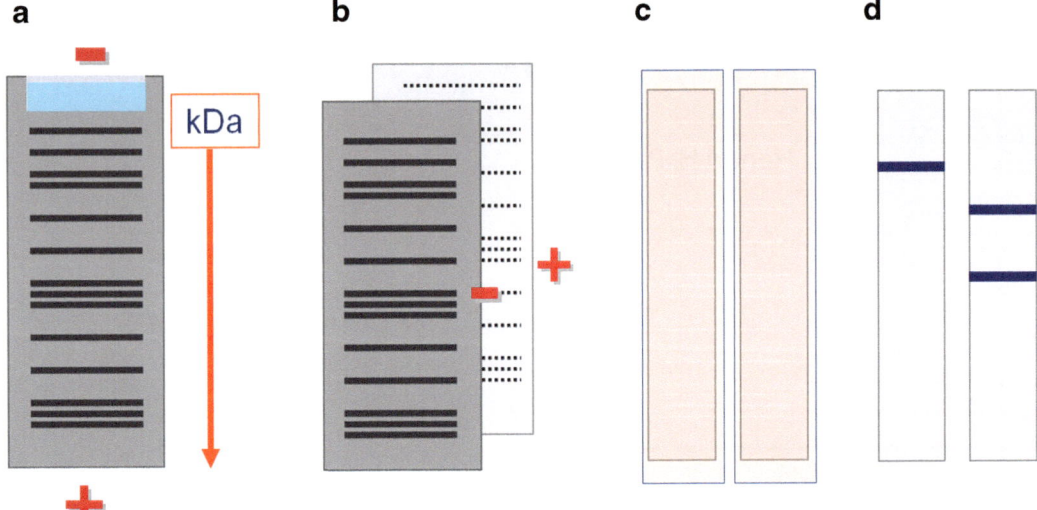

Fig. 6.1 Principle of immunoblotting. (**a**) Molecules in a skin protein extract are separated by gel electrophoresis. (**b**) The protein pattern is electrophoretically transferred to a membrane filter what facilitates further handling. (**c**) The filter is immersed in diluted patient serum. (**d**) Bound IgG is visualized by staining

has the ability to completely dissolve protein complexes including large structures as hemidesmosomes and desmosomes that contain major pemphigus and pemphigoid autoantigens. SDS is a negatively charged molecule and binds to proteins in an assumed SDS:protein ratio of 1.4. This destroys the native conformation of proteins that enroll and take on a linear shape. As all proteins become negatively charged with an even distribution of charge per unit mass they are fractionized according to size during electrophoresis.

Immunoblotting is a qualitative test to identify the targeted autoantigen.

SDS also has a disadvantage as it destroys conformational epitopes. An epitope is the part of the antigen that is recognized by the antibody and they have an average size of around 15 amino acids [2]. Epitopes are divided in two categories: linear epitopes that consist of a continuous stretch of amino acids and are thus determined by the primary structure and conformational epitopes formed by separate stretches of amino acids that lie close together in the native conformation of the protein and which are thus determined by the tertiary structure (Fig. 6.2). It is this last category of epitopes that is destroyed by the SDS and is missed in immunoblotting. For this reason immunoblotting is not suited for diagnosing pemphigus vulgaris (PV) or pemphigus foliaceus (PF) as the pathogenic epitopes of the autoantigens desmoglein 1 and 3 are largely conformational epitopes. In case of paraneoplastic pemphigus (PNP) however it is a good option as here immunoblotting has a reported 89% sensitivity and 100% specificity for detecting the simultaneous presence of antibodies to envoplakin and periplakin that is specific for PNP [3]. For identification of autoantibodies to pemphigoid antigens immunoblotting has a varying sensitivity and is not first choice when alternatives are available. For type VII collagen and BP230 ELISA's can now be commercially obtained. Diagnosis of anti-p200 pemphigoid seems to have high sensitivity but the quality of the dermal extract, which requires a sophisticated extraction procedure, is important and the assay is therefore only performed in a few highly specialized laboratories. Although plectin antibodies were found by immunoblotting in 4% of all pemphigoid patients the sensitivity is not known. Immunoblotting has additional value for detecting antibodies to BP180 which is the dominant antigen of the pemphigoid group. An ELISA for BP180 is available but can only detect antibodies to a small stretch of BP180 named NC16A that is

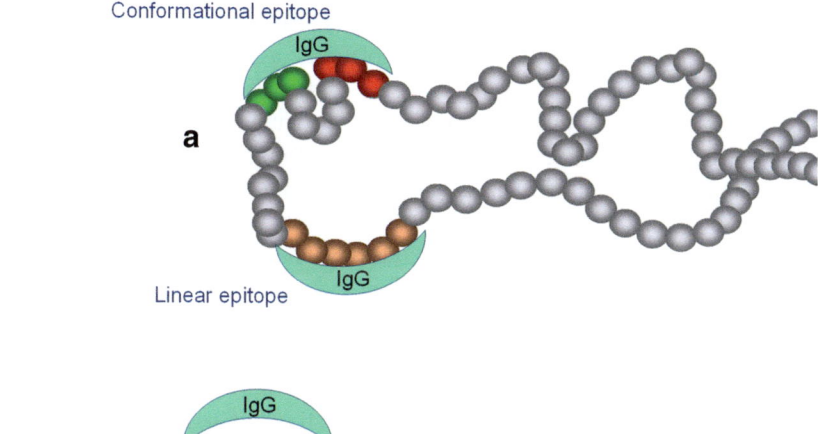
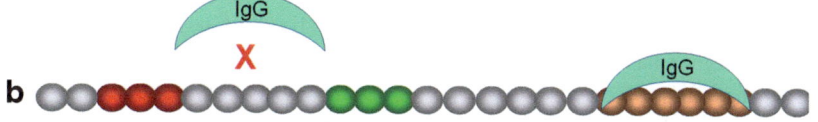

Fig. 6.2 Two classes of epitopes. (**a**) A native protein with a conformational epitope (red, green) is formed by two different parts of the molecule, while a linear epitope is formed by a continuous stretch of amino acids (orange). (**b**) A denatured protein looses its native conformation. Therefore IgG cannot bind anymore to the conformational epitope as it is destroyed while the linear epitope is still available

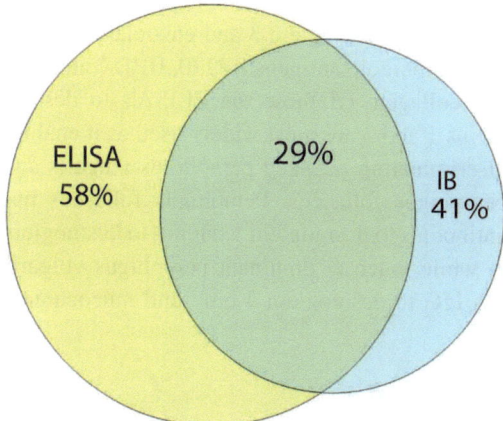

Fig 6.3 Venn diagram showing detection of anti-BP180 IgG antibodies in 357 patients with bullous or mucous membrane pemphigoid. When combined anti-BP180 IgG was found in 70% of the cases

Immunoprecipitation

Immunoprecipitation has played an important role in identification of the autoantigens involved in AIBD, the last one being alpha-2-macroglobulin-like-1 protein in PNP [4]. However as it is a labor intensive technique it is expensive and therefore not much used in routine diagnostics of AIBD.

The advantage of immunoprecipitation over immunoblotting is that the protein extracts for immunoprecipitation are prepared with soft soaps that do not denature proteins and the conformational epitopes therefore remain intact. Classical immunoprecipitation is performed with radioactive labeled proteins. Patient serum is first incubated with protein G-coupled beads. Protein G is a molecule that specifically binds IgG from the serum. After washing the beads are then added to the radioactive extract where the patient IgG will bind to the autoantigen(s) in question. The beads are then removed by centrifugation, washed and the IgG and the radioactive antigen(s) are eluted in SDS-PAGE sample buffer. The sample is then are separated and sorted on molecular size by polyacrylamide gel electrophoresis. Next the radioactive bands are visualized by fluorography and as in immunoblot indentified on basis of

reported to contain the major immunodominant epitopes. In contrast in immunoblotting the full length BP180 molecule is available. When ELISA and immunoblotting are compared immunoblotting detects 12% of the tested cases additional to ELISA (Fig. 6.3). Conversely immunoblotting misses half the cases found by ELISA indicating that also here loss of conformational epitopes plays a role.

molecular mass. Also unknown antigens can be identified by analyzing the radioactive band with advanced mass spectrometry methods. As working with radiochemicals is subject to strict regulations it is an easier option is to perform non-radioactive immunoprecipitation that is a combination of immunoprecipitation and immunoblotting. The procedure is largely the same but with non-radioactive substrates. After immunoprecipitation and gel electrophoresis the gel is blotted and the filter is incubated with a cocktail of antibodies that are specific for the antigens in question. After washing the blot can is stained to visualize which antigens have been precipitated from the extract (Fig. 6.4).

Immunoprecipitation has a higher sensitivity than immunoblot.

ELISA

Enzyme-linked immunosorbent assay (ELISA) is a technique that enables to measure the autoantibody response to a single autoantigen in a quantitative manner. ELISA's are commercially available and easy to perform, so can be introduced in every diagnostic lab. As all serological assays ELISA is based on the binding of patient IgG to the autoantigen. Principle of ELISA is that a small plastic well (200 μl volume) on a plastic plate is coated with a single antigen. The coated molecules are recombinantly produced and consists of the whole or particular part(s) of an antigen. The antigen is not denatured before coating and therefore contains both linear and conformational epitopes. Serum is brought into the coated well and if IgG to the antigen is present it will become bound. Next an anti-human IgG to which a special enzyme is conjugated is brought into the well. This will bind to the IgG and the more IgG is bound to the well the more of the enzyme will be bound. After washing the unbound IgG, a substrate is brought in the well that can be converted by the enzyme into a colored product. The more patient IgG is bound the more color will be produced and the amount of color is thus an indication of the amount of specific autoimmune IgG in the serum of the patient. This enables serological disease monitoring (Fig. 6.5). At January 2015 six different ELISA's were commercially available to respectively the pemphigus antigens desmoglein 1, desmoglein 3 and envoplakin, and to the pemphigoid antigens BP230, BP180 and type VII collagen. Of these the ELISA's to desmogleins 1 and 3 are most widely used as it enables discriminating between pemphigus vulgaris and pemphigus foliaceus. Pemphigus foliaceus has antibodies to desmoglein 1 but not to desmoglein 3, while mucosal dominant pemphigus vulgaris has IgG to desmoglein 3 only and mucocutane-

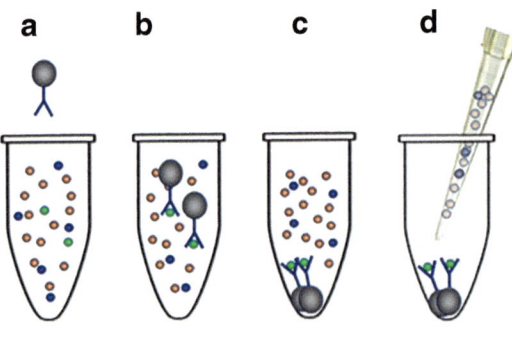
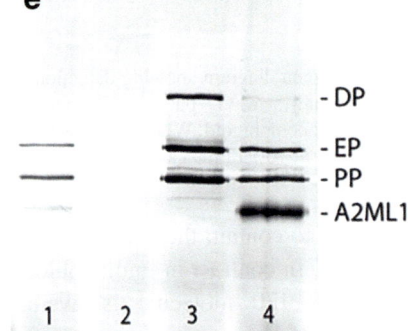
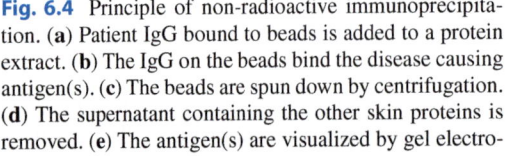

Fig. 6.4 Principle of non-radioactive immunoprecipitation. (**a**) Patient IgG bound to beads is added to a protein extract. (**b**) The IgG on the beads bind the disease causing antigen(s). (**c**) The beads are spun down by centrifugation. (**d**) The supernatant containing the other skin proteins is removed. (**e**) The antigen(s) are visualized by gel electrophoresis followed by immunoblotting. Here sera were analyzed for IgG to PNP antigens. Lane 1 PNP patient, lane 2 PV patient, lane 3 PNP patient, lane 4 PNP patient. *DP* desmoplakin, *EP* envoplakin, *PP* periplakin, *A2ML1* alpha-2-macroglobulin-like-2

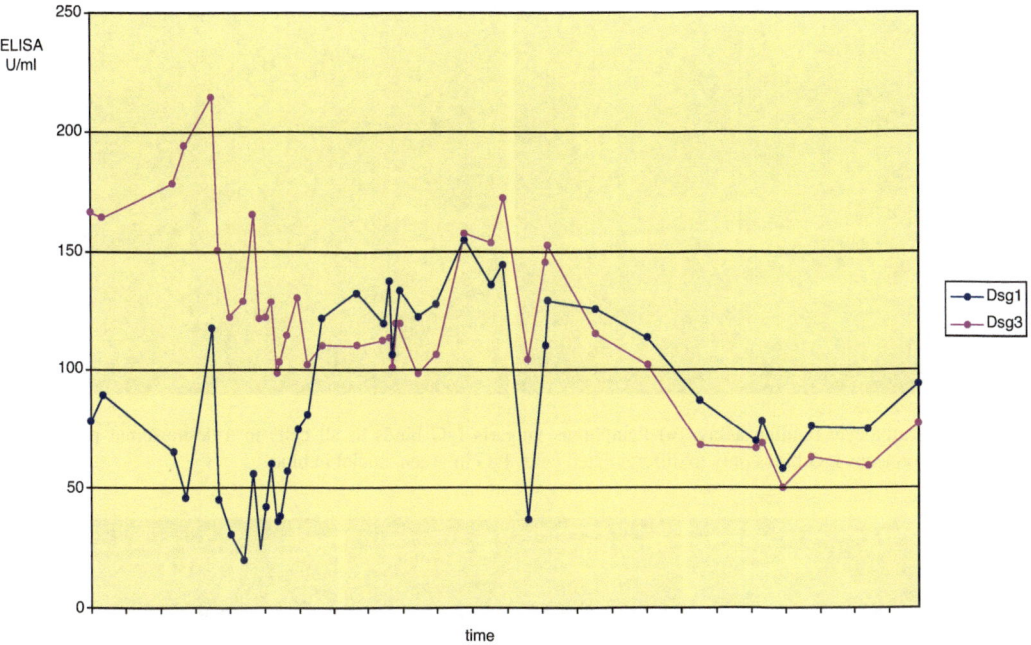

Fig. 6.5 Titer monitoring in pemphigus by ELISA to Dsg1 and 3. The patient was followed for eight years

ous pemphigus vulgaris to both desmogleins 1 and 3 [5]. The sensitivity to detect pemphigus is 89% by ELISA, which is slightly better than 86% by indirect immunofluorescence microscopy on monkey esophagus in our hands. Being quantitative these ELISA's are well suited to follow antibody titers (expressed as relative arbitrary units). The change in titer values from the desmoglein 1 ELISA fairly well corresponds to the activity of skin disease. However the results of the desmoglein 3 ELISA should be interpreted with more caution [6]. For about two-thirds of the patients there is a correlation with mucosal involvement but for the other third ELISA's may stay unchanged despite clinical improvement. Evidence is building that this is due to the presence of non-pathogenic antibodies to desmoglein 3 [7]. ELISA however cannot discriminate between pathogenic and non-pathogenic antibodies. Be aware that ELISA's may be false positive, desmoglein ELISA's up to 13% of tested samples and the NC16A ELISA for 11.3% [8, 9].

ELISA is a quantitative assay for monitoring disease activity.

The envoplakine ELISA has been developed to diagnose paraneoplastic pemphigus. Its sensitivity is estimated to be 63% and lower than immunoblotting [3]. The ELISA to type VII collagen was found to have 54% sensitivity due to approximately half of the patients having a very low undetectable serum titer [10]. For patients that have an ELISA detectable serum titer the type VII collagen ELISA values correspond well with disease activity. Above we already discussed the BP180 ELISA. This ELISA contains a small recombinant fragment NC16A, approximately 6.5% of the entire extracellular domain of BP180, but contains the immunodominant domains. Exact figures of its sensitivity are not know but based on the comparison with immunoblot results it can be estimated to be in the order of 70%. The BP230 ELISA is less sensitive and its diagnostic added value has to be found only 5% [11].

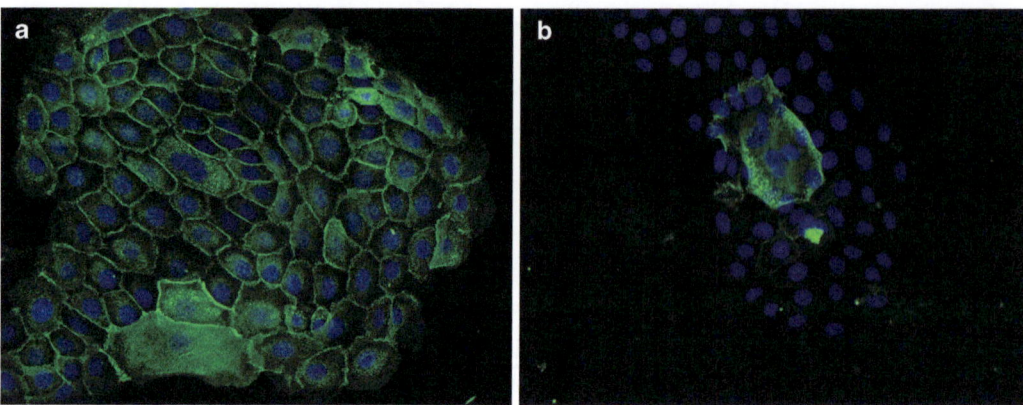

Fig. 6.6 Keratinocyte binding assay. (**a**) Pemphigus vulgaris IgG binds to all cells in a desmosomal pattern. (**b**) Pemphigus foliaceus IgG binds only to differentiated cells. IgG in green, nuclei in blue

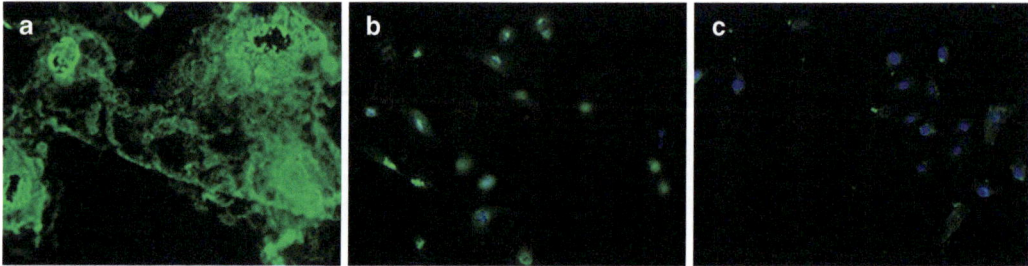

Fig. 6.7 Keratinocyte footprint assay. (**a**) IgG from anti-laminin-332 mucous membrane pemphigoid binds to the migration trails, but IgG from (**b**) epidermolysis bullosa aquisita and (**c**) anti-p200 pemphigoid do not. IgG in green, nuclei in blue

Keratinocyte Binding Assay

The Keratinocyte Binding Assay is the most sensitive and specific assay for pemphigus antibodies [12]. In this assay patient serum is added to keratinocytes cultured on high-calcium medium and incubated for 1 hour. If anti-desmosomal antibodies are present the IgG will bind in a desmosomal pattern. The assay is able to discriminate between pemphigus vulgaris and pemphigus foliaceus as all cells express desmoglein 3 but only differentiated cells express desmoglein 1 (Fig. 6.6). The sensitivity of the assay is 97%. The assay is useful to check for presence of antibodies if the desmoglein ELISA is negative, either because the titer is below the cut-off of the ELISA, or if antibodies to desmocollins are present, or if for some reason the IgG will not bind to the recombinant desmoglein on the ELISA plate, and to rule out false-positive ELISA's. It is not a quantitative assay thus not useful for monitoring antibody titers.

Keratinocyte binding assay is the most sensitive serum assay for pemphigus antibodies.

Keratinocyte Footprint Assay

The Keratinocyte Footprint Assay is a test that is specific for anti-laminin-332 antibodies [12]. Keratinocytes in culture need laminin-332 to attach to the surface of the culture dish. When migrating, the cells polarize and deposit precursor laminin-332 at the rear of the moving cell. This laminin-332 is left behind and forms a unique footprint trail. Keratinocytes are cultured on glass coverslips in low-calcium medium for three days after which coverslips are dried. The coverslips are then incubated with patient serum and bound IgG is visualized by immunofluorescence (Fig. 6.7). The footprint trails do not contain other autoimmune bullous diseases antigens thus the specificity is 100%. Its sensitivity is estimated to be also almost 100%.

Keratinocyte footprint assay is a 100% specific for anti-laminin-332 mucous membrane pemphigoid.

Review Questions

1. Which assay is quantitative?
   a. Immunoblot
   b. ELISA
   c. Immunoprecipitation
   d. All three
2. The size of an epitope is on average
   a. 15 amino acids
   b. 50 amino acids
   c. 150 amino acids
3. ELISA values ……..parallel disease activity
   a. Always
   b. Most times
   c. Seldom
4. You have treated a patient with rituximab. What assay would you request to evaluate your therapy?
   a. Immunoblot
   b. ELISA
   c. Immunoprecipitation
   d. All three

Answers

1. b
2. a
3. b
4. b

References

1. Pas HH. Immunoblot assay in differential diagnosis of autoimmune blistering skin diseases. Clin Dermatol. 2001;19:622–30.
2. Kringelum JV, Nielsen M, Padkjaer SB, Lund O. Structural analysis of B-cell epitopes in antibody:protein complexes. Mol Immunol. 2013;53:24–34.
3. Poot AM, Diercks GF, Kramer D, Schepens I, Klunder G, Hashimoto T, Borradori L, Jonkman MF, Pas HH. Laboratory diagnosis of paraneoplastic pemphigus. Br J Dermatol. 2013;169:1016–24.
4. Schepens I, Jaunin F, Begre N, Laderach U, Marcus K, Hashimoto T, Favre B, Borradori L. The protease inhibitor alpha-2-macroglobulin-like-1 is the p170 antigen recognized by paraneoplastic pemphigus autoantibodies in human. PLoS One. 2010;5:e12250.
5. Mahoney MG, Wang Z, Rothenberger K, Koch PJ, Amagai M, Stanley JR. Explanations for the clinical and microscopic localization of lesions in pemphigus foliaceus and vulgaris. J Clin Invest. 1999;103:461–8.
6. Abasq C, Mouquet H, Gilbert D, Tron F, Grassi V, Musette P, Joly P. ELISA testing of anti-desmoglein 1 and 3 antibodies in the management of pemphigus. Arch Dermatol. 2009;145:529–35.
7. Ishii K, Harada R, Matsuo I, Shirakata Y, Hashimoto K, Amagai M. In vitro keratinocyte dissociation assay for evaluation of the pathogenicity of anti-desmoglein 3 IgG autoantibodies in pemphigus vulgaris. J Invest Dermatol. 2005;124:939–46.
8. Giurdanella F, Nijenhuis AM, Diercks GFH, Jonkman MF, Pas HH. Keratinocyte binding assay identifies anti-desmosomal pemphigus antibodies where other tests are negative. Front Immunol. 2018 Apr 24;9:839.
9. Meijer JM, Diercks GFH, de Lang EWG, Pas HH, Jonkman MF. Assessment of diagnostic strategy for early recognition of bullous and nonbullous variants of pemphigoid. JAMA Dermatol. 2019 Feb 1;155(2):158–65.
10. Terra JB, Jonkman MF, Diercks GF, Pas HH. Low sensitivity of type VII collagen enzyme-linked immunosorbent assay in epidermolysis bullosa acquisita: serration pattern analysis on skin biopsy is required for diagnosis. Br J Dermatol. 2013;169:164–7.
11. Charneux J, Lorin J, Vitry F, Antonicelli F, Reguiai Z, Barbe C, Tabary T, Grange F, Bernard P. Usefulness of BP230 and BP180-NC16a enzyme-linked immunosorbent assays in the initial diagnosis of bullous pemphigoid: a retrospective study of 138 patients. Arch Dermatol. 2011;147:286–91.
12. Giurdanella F, Nijenhuis AM, Diercks GFH, Jonkman MF, Pas HH. Keratinocyte footprint assay discriminates antilaminin-332 pemphigoid from all other forms of pemphigoid diseases. Br J Dermatol. 2020 Feb;182(2):373–81.

Structure of Desmosomes

7

Ena Sokol

Introduction and Aim

Importance of desmosomes for the architecture and mechanical strength of epithelial tissue is demonstrated in several blistering diseases. Perturbation of a desmosomal structure by autoantibodies, toxins or gene mutations can disrupt the architecture and strength of the skin and mucous membranes. Therefore proper function of all the proteins that are part of the complex desmosomal structure is important for tissue integrity. In this chapter we aim in explaining the components of a desmosome and their organization into an adhesive structure.

> **Learning Objectives**
> After studying this chapter, you should be able to:
>
> – Know the structure of a desmosome
> – Know desmosomal proteins and their isoforms
> – Learn the distribution of isoforms of desmosomal proteins

E. Sokol (✉)
Center for Blistering Diseases, University Medical Center Groningen, Groningen, The Netherlands
e-mail: e.sokol@isala.nl

Desmosomes: Cell-Cell Adhesion Structures

Cell junctions are specialized structures that interconnect neighbouring cells to each other (cell-cell junctions) or cells to the matrix (cell-matrix junctions). They can serve as strong sealing points involved in tissue barrier (tight junctions), or as mechanical cell attachment (adherens junctions, desmosomes and hemidesmosomes) or as communication channels (gap junctions).

Desmosomes (desmo-bond, soma-body) are cell-cell junctions that interconnect intermediate filament networks of neighbouring cells and provide strong mechanical strength [1, 2]. They are abundant in stratified epithelium, such as epidermis and epithelium of mucosa, and in heart muscle, but are also present in simple epithelium and in non-epithelial cells like meningeal cells of the arachnoid and the follicular dendritic cells of lymph follicles [3].

Desmosomes can be easily recognized by electron microscopy by their extracellular core domain (ECD) and two opposite dense plaques. Within each plaque two zones can be distinguished: the outer dense plaque (ODP) and the inner dense plaque (IDP) (Fig. 7.1a and b). Proteins that make distinctive zones of desmosomes are transmembrane proteins which belong to cadherin family and cytoplasmic plaque proteins which belong to armadillo and plakin family of proteins. Desmosomal cadherins are desmogleins and desmocollins, armadillo proteins in

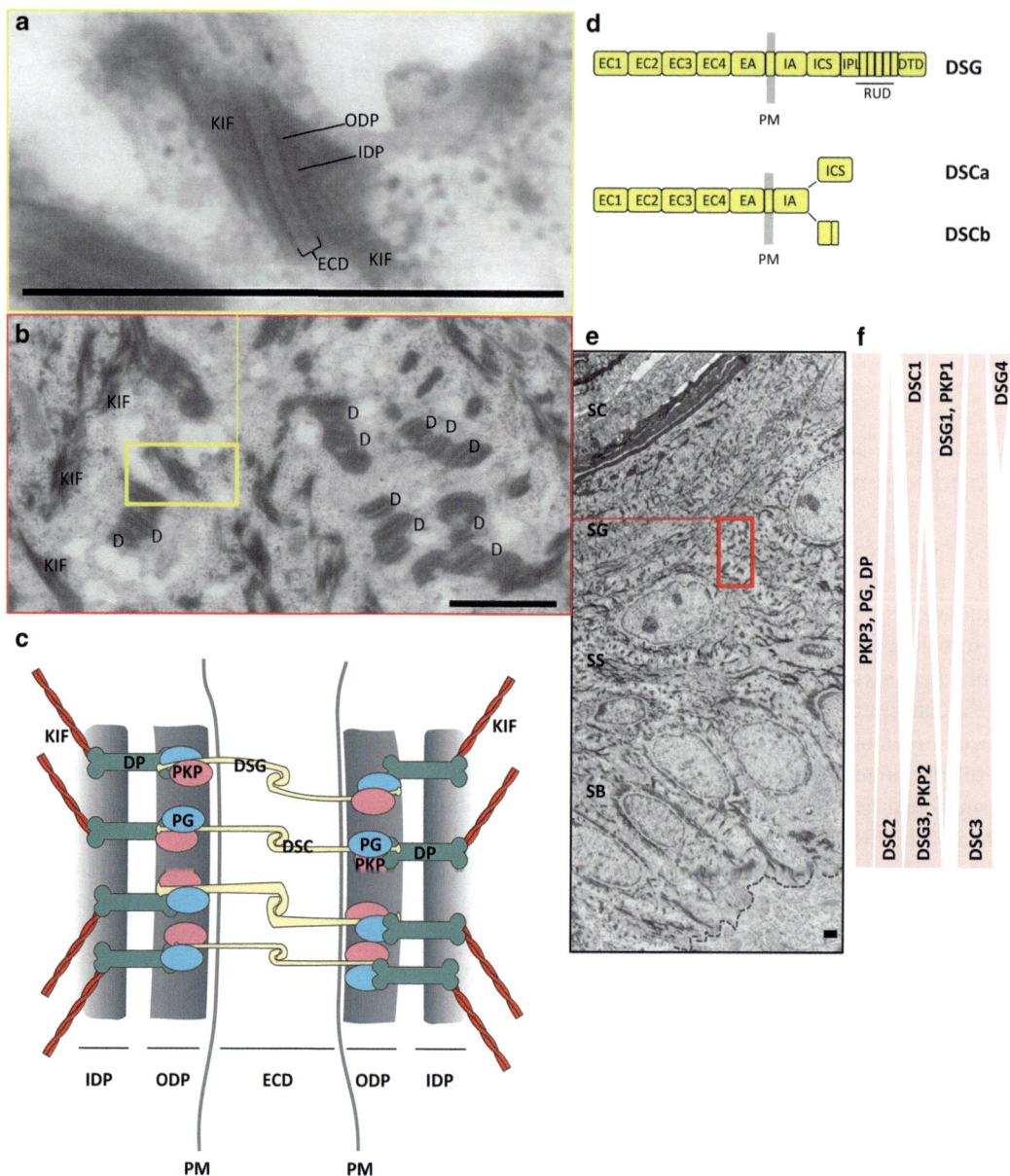

Fig. 7.1 Desmosomal structure, structure of desmosomal cadherins and expression of desmosomal proteins in human epidermis. (**a**) Magnified desmosome and desmosomal distinctive zones. (**b**) Magnified region of epidermis with multiple desmosomes. Yellow box is magnified in panel **a**. (**c**) Schematic presentation of a complete desmosome. Desmosomal proteins are presented in different shapes and colors. Note the organization of desmosomal proteins in ECD, ODP and IDP. (**d**) Structure of desmosomal cadherins: desmoglein and desmocollin 'a' and 'b' form. Desmogleins differ in number of RUD domains. (**e**) Human skin and epidermal layers. Dotted line presents border between dermis and epidermis. Red box is magnified in panel **b**. (**f**) Expression of isoforms of desmosomal proteins through epidermal layers that are shown in panel **e**. *DSG* desmoglein, *DSC* desmocollin, *PG* plakoglobin, *PKP* plakophilin, *DP* desmoplakin, *SB* stratum basale, *SS* stratum spinosum, *SG* stratum granulosum, *SC* stratum corneum, *D* desmosome, *KIF* keratin intermediate filaments, *ECD* extracellular core domain, *ODP* outer dense plaque, *IDP* inner dense plaque, *PM* plasma membrane, *EC* extracellular domain, *EA* extracellular anchor, *IA* intracellular anchor, *IPL* proline-rich linker, *RUD* repeat unit domains, *DTD* desmoglein terminal domain. Panel **a**, **b** and **e** are electron microscopy images that were taken from a nanotomy dataset of normal human skin (Reprinted with permission from reference [4]). Scale bar 1 μm

desmosomes compromise plakoglobin and plakophilins, while main plakin protein in desmosomes is desmoplakin [1–3]. Other members of plakin family such as plectin, periplakin and envoplakin are also found in desmosomes [3]. Extracellular domains of desmosomal cadherins compose ECD where they mediate adhesion, while their intracellular domains together with plakoglobin and plakophilins make ODP. IDP compromises of desmoplakin that couples to the intermediate filament network [Fig. 7.1c]. Pre-structure of a complete desmosome is so called half desmosome which is made of a desmosomal plaque and desmosomal cadherins at one side not connected to its opposite part [5]. Half desmosomes and desmosomes should be distinguished from hemidesmosomes which are cell- matrix junctions and are explained in Chap. 13.

Autoimmune blistering diseases with antibodies against certain desmosomal proteins demonstrate the importance of desmosomes for tissue integrity.

Desmosome are cell-cell junctions that provide strong intercellular adhesion.

Desmosomal Proteins and Their Isoforms

Desmosomal cadherins are calcium dependent glycoproteins and are desmogleins (Dsgs) and desmocollins (Dscs). They require calcium for binding to their opposites. In conditions without calcium half desmosomes will still be formed, but will be soon internalized and complete desmosomal structure will not be achieved [5]. In humans there are 4 types of Dsgs and 3 types of Dscs which are differently distributed. All Dscs isoforms have 2 forms: form 'a' and shorter form 'b', which are results of alternative splicing (Fig. 7.1d). Both Dsgs and Dscs have extracellular part consisting of 4 cadherin repeats (EC1-4) and fifth domain termed extracellular anchor (EA), as well as transmembrane domain (TM) located in the plasma membrane and intercellular part starting with an intracellular anchor (IA) (Fig. 7.1d). Rest of the intercellular part differs were intercellular cadherin-like sequence (ICS) that binds plakoglobin is present in Dsc a form and Dsgs. Dsgs have additional intracytoplasmic regions: intercellular proline rich-linker (IPL), variable number of repeat unit domain (RUD) and glycine rich desmoglein terminal domain (DTD)[1–3].

Plakoglobin also termed as γ- catenin, is an armadillo protein that localizes both to desmosomes and to adherens junctions. Plakoglobin contains 12 armadillo repeats flanked by distinct amino- and carboxy- terminal domain. In desmosomes plakoglobin binds to cytoplasmatic tail of desmosomal cadherins and it is reported that it binds desmoplakin [1–3].

Plakophilins (Pkp) are armadillo proteins that contain 9 armadillo repeats with an insert between repeat 5 and 6 that bend the whole structure. There are 3 isoforms of Pkps. Pkps can bind all other desmosomal components and it is shown that they can bind intermediate filaments or enhance interactions in the desmosomal plaque [1–3].

Desmoplakin belongs to plakin family proteins and it is a key linker between the desmosomal plaque and intermediate filaments. Desmoplakin has 2 isoforms in which globular amino- and carboxy- parts are connected with central α-helical coiled-coil rod domain. Amino- terminal domain contains binding sides for plakoglobin and Pkp, while carboxy- terminal domain contains binding side for intermediate filaments [1–3].

Periplakin, envoplakin and plectin are also found in desmosomes, but it is not clear how important they are for the structure and function [3].

Isoforms of desmosomal proteins are differently distributed in human tissues [6]. All desmosomes bearing tissues express plakoglobin and desmoplakin. Dsg2, Dsc2, Pkp2 are mostly found in simple epithelia. Dsg1 and 3, Dsc1 and 3 are specific for stratified epithelia. Expression of isoforms of desmosomal proteins in the epidermis is cell layer dependent and it is shown in Fig. 7.1e and f. Expression of Dsg1 decreases from upper towards lower epidermal layers, while Dsg3 is present in the basal and suprabasal layers. Dsg4 is found in the upper layers of the epidermis and in the hair follicle [7]. Different expression of isoforms of desmosomal proteins explains localization of lesions in certain autoimmune blistering diseases.

Desmosomal proteins are desmogleins, desmocollins, plakoglobin, plakophilins and desmoplakin.

Review Questions

1. Which cytoskeleton filaments desmosomes interconnect?
    a. Microtubules
    b. Intermediate filaments
    c. Actin filaments
    d. All above
2. Which desmosomal proteins require calcium molecules for their activation and formation of complete desmosome?
    a. Plakophilins
    b. Plakoglobin
    c. Desmogleins and desmocollins
    d. Desmogleins and plakoglobin
3. What is the expression pattern of Dsg1 and Dsg3 in the epidermis?
    a. Dsg1 and Dsg3 are expressed in all layers of the epidermis
    b. Dsg1 and Dsg3 are expressed in the basal and granular layer of the epidermis
    c. Dsg3 is expressed in the basal and suprabasal layers, while Dsg1 expression decreases from the upper to the lower layers of the epidermis.
    d. Dsg1 expression decreases from the basal to the upper layers of the epidermis, while Dsg3 expression decreases from the upper to the lower layers of the epidermis.

Answers

1. b
2. c
3. c

References

1. Garrod D, Chidgey M. Desmosome structure, composition and function. Biochim Biophys Acta. 2008; 1778:572–87.
2. Delva E, Tucker DK, Kowalczyk AP. The desmosome. Cold Spring Harb Perspect Biol. 2009;1:a002543.
3. Waschke J. The desmosome and pemphigus. Histochem Cell Biol. 2008;130:21–54.
4. Sokol E, Kramer D, Diercks GF, Kuipers J, Jonkman MF, Pas HH, Giepmans BN. Large-scale electron microscopy maps of patient skin and mucosa provide insight into pathogenesis of blistering diseases. J Invest Dermatol. 2015;135:1763–70.
5. Demlehner MP, Schafer S, Grund C, Franke WW. Continual assembly of half-desmosomal structures in the absence of cell contacts and their frustrated endocytosis: a coordinated sisyphus cycle. J Cell Biol. 1995;131:745–60.
6. Harmon RM, Green KJ. Structural and functional diversity of desmosomes. Cell Commun Adhes. 2013;6:171–87.
7. Mahoney MG, Hu Y, Brennan D, Bazzi H, Christiano AM, Wahl JK 3rd. Delineation of diversified desmoglein distribution in stratified squamous epithelia: Implications in diseases. Exp Dermatol. 2006;15: 101–9.

Additional Reading

Kowalczyk AP, Green KJ. Structure, function, and regulation of desmosomes. Prog Mol Biol Transl Sci. 2013;116:95–118.

Dusek RL, Godsel LM, Green KJ. Discriminating roles of desmosomal cadherins: beyond desmosomal adhesion. J Dermatol Sci. 2007;45:7–21.

Pemphigus Vulgaris

8

Gerda van der Wier, Marcel F. Jonkman, and Barbara Horváth

Introduction and AIMS

Short Definition in Layman Terms

Pemphigus vulgaris (PV) is a chronic autoimmune blistering disease that affects the mucous membranes only (mucosal dominant PV) or both the mucous membranes and the skin (mucocutaneous PV) (Fig. 8.1; Table 8.1).

> **Learning Objectives**
> After reading this chapter you know how to recognize a patient with pemphigus vulgaris, which specific tests and diagnostics should be done to confirm your diagnosis en how to treat a patient with pemphigus vulgaris.

G. van der Wier (✉)
Center for Blistering Diseases, Department of Dermatology, University Medical Center Groningen, University of Groningen,
Groningen, The Netherlands

Scheper Hospital, Emmen, The Netherlands
e-mail: g.vanderwier@treant.nl

M. F. Jonkman (Deceased) · B. Horváth
Center for Blistering Diseases, Department of Dermatology, University Medical Center Groningen, University of Groningen,
Groningen, The Netherlands
e-mail: b.horvath@umcg.nl

> **Case Study: Part 1**
> A 67-year-old female was referred to our clinic with an 18-month history of crusted erosions on the lip, which was previously treated as lichen planus. Later, she developed multiple itchy erosions located on the scalp, neck, breasts, groin and umbilicus. Dermatological examination revealed painful erosions on the oral and nasal mucosa in addition to the skin lesions. Nikolsky's sign was positive on the skin. The past medical history reported a TIA and she received various cardiovascular medication for several years.

Didactical Questions: Cross Section of Questions to Prime the Readers Interest

Why do some patients with pemphigus vulgaris have only mucous membranes affected, while others have both skin and mucous membranes affected? What is the histopathology of PV? How do autoantibodies cause acantholysis in skin and mucous membranes?

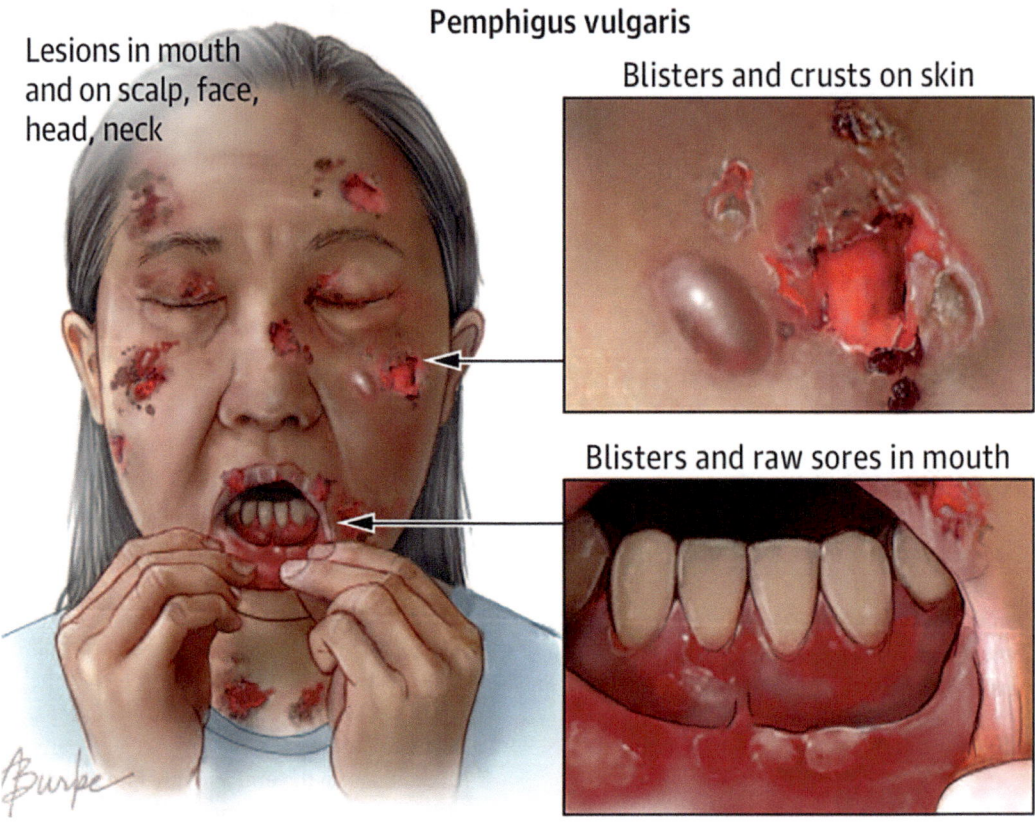

Fig. 8.1 Typical features of patient with pemphigus vulgaris. Drawings by Alison E. Burke adapted from [1]

Table 8.1 IF findings and clinical symptoms of subtypes of pemphigus

	Target antigens	DIF	Clinical symptoms
Pemphigus vulgaris, mucosal-dominant	Dsg3	ECS IgG, IgA ± C3c	Painful erosions of the oral mucosa
Pemphigus vulgaris, mucocutaneous	Dsg1, Dsg3	ECS IgG, IgA ± C3c	Painful blisters and erosions of the oral mucosa and skin
Pemphigus vegetans, Hallopeau type	Dsg3	ECS IgG, IgA ± C3c	Pustules accumulate in body folds and around orifices, easily secondarily infected
Pemphigus vegetans, Neumann type	Dsg3	ECS IgG ± C3c	Papillomas accumulate in body and around orifices, easily secondarily infected
Pemphigus foliaceus Chapter 9	Dsg1	ECS IgG ± C3c	Crusted plaques with multiple layers of scaling, which easily erodes at the scalp, temples, periorbicular area, neck, upper chest and back
Endemic pemphigus Chapter 9	Dsg1	ECS IgG ± C3c	Localized form (form fruste) and generalized form (bullous invasion, keratotic, hyperpigmented, pemphigus herpetiformis and exfoliative erythroderma)

Table 8.1 (continued)

	Target antigens	DIF	Clinical symptoms
Pemphigus erythematosus Chapter 9	Dsg1	ECS/ BMZ IgG ± C3c	Lupus-like butterfly rash and seborrheic distribution. Evoked by UV-light
Pemphigus herpetiformis Chapter 9	Dsg1, Dsg3	ECS IgG, IgA ± C3c	Grouped (herpetiform) distribution of itching erythematous vesicular/bullous/papular lesions, often in an annular-shaped pattern. Nikolsky's sign is negative
IgA pemphigus, subcorneal pustular dermatosis type Chapter 11	Dsc1	ECS IgA ± C3c	Erythematous skin lesions with tiny superficial circinate pustules, desquamation from the edges surfacing the entire body, particularly in the intertriginous areas
IgA pemphigus, intraepidermal neutrophilic IgA dermatosis type Chapter 11	Unknown	ECS IgA ± C3c	Annular erythematous plaques with circinate pustules and crusts that spread outwards and heal inwards in a sunflower-like appearance
Drug-induced pemphigus Chapter 12	Dsg1, Dsg3	ECS IgG, IgA ± C3c	Prodromal stage with pruritis and nonspecific lesions preceding the genuine pemphigus lesions, mimicking all variants of pemphigus
Paraneoplastic pemphigus Chapter 10	Envoplakin, periplakin, desmoplakin, BP230, A2ML1, Dsg1, Dsg3	ECS/ BMZ IgG, IgA ± C3c	Painful severe oral stomatitis, with hemorrhagic crusts. Flaccid to tense blisters at the face, trunk and extremities. Generalised lichenoid erythema. Sporadically shortness of breath. Underlying neoplasm

Dsg1 desmoglein 1, *Dsg3* desmoglein 3, *ECS* epithelial cell surface pattern

Facts and Figures

Definitions and Classification

The term pemphigus is derived from the Greek word *pemphix*, which means blister. Pemphigus is a group of heterogenic chronic mucocutaneous blistering diseases caused by autoantibodies directed against the desmosomal cadherins desmoglein 1 (Dsg1) and/or desmoglein 3 (Dsg3) (Table 8.1) [2]. Pemphigus can be divided into two major forms, based on the level of the blister in the epidermis. The superficial forms of pemphigus are grouped under pemphigus foliaceus, the deep forms under pemphigus vulgaris (mucosal-dominant pemphigus vulgaris and mucocutaneous pemphigus vulgaris) and its variant pemphigus vegetans.

> Blistering in pemphigus is caused by autoantibodies directed against desmoglein 1 and/or 3.

Epidemiology

Pemphigus is rare and its incidence has been estimated to about of 0.2 cases per 100,000 per year in Central Europe. The incidence of the different subtypes of pemphigus varies from 0.076 in Finland to 0.67 in Tunisia. Countries with high incidence of pemphigus are Bulgaria, Greece and the Mediterranean region of Turkey. Pemphigus vulgaris (PV) is the most common subtype comprising 83.1% of all cases in Southern Turkey [3]. The mean age of onset of the disease is approximately 40–50 years of age. There is a slight female predominance.

Pathogenesis

In 1964 Beutner and Jordan observed circulating antibodies directed against the cell surface of keratinocytes in the sera of patients with PV [4]. Later it was demonstrated that autoantibodies in pemphigus are pathogenic and induce blister formation in skin organ culture systems and in neonatal mice. In 1982 Stanley et al characterized the PV antigen at the molecular level by immunoprecipitation using cultured keratinocytes extracts as a substrate. All the PV sera identified a glycosylated 130 kDa glycoprotein [5]. In 1991 Amagai et al isolated a cDNA clone for the PV antigen by immunoscreening a human keratinocytes expression library with autoantibodies prepared from the sera of patients with PV [6]. Analysis of the deduced amino acid sequences of the cDNA clones revealed the nature of pemphigus antigens being desmoglein 1 (Dsg1) and desmoglein 3 (Dsg3). Both antigens are member of the cadherin family of calcium-dependant homodimeric 'adherins' that are located in epithelial cell-cell contacts such as adherens junctions and desmosomes.

Desmoglein Compensation Hypothesis

The desmoglein compensation hypothesis explains why skin or mucous membranes are affected in various forms of pemphigus. This theory states that Dsg1 and Dsg3 can compensate for each other and prevent acantholysis when autoantibodies bind to either molecule (Fig. 8.2) [7]. In skin, Dsg1 is expressed throughout the whole epidermis, but more intense in the superficial layers, whereas Dsg3 is confined to the basal and suprabasal layers. Antibodies to Dsg1 therefore cause blisters in the superficial epidermis since in this area Dsg3 is not present to compensate for the loss of Dsg1. The result is PF, which clinically only affects skin.

In mucosa, Dsg3 is expressed throughout the whole epithelium, whereas Dsg 1 is confined to the superficial layers. Antibodies to Dsg3 therefore cause blisters deep in the mucosa, since in this area Dsg1 is not present to compensate for the loss of Dsg3. The skin remains unaffected, because Dsg1 is present throughout the epidermis and compensates for loss of Dsg3. The result is mucosal dominant PV.

If both Dsg1 and Dsg3 are targeted by antibodies, no compensation is possible. The level of blistering is suprabasal, since 'melting' of desmosomes starts in both skin and mucosa in the lower epithelium at entry point of IgG. The result is mucocutaneous PV.

The desmoglein compensation hypothesis explains the localization and the level of the blister in pemphigus

The exact cellular mechanism by which pemphigus IgG induces acantholysis has been a subject of debate since the discovery of pemphigus autoantibodies by Beutner and Jordan. Since then acantholysis has been explained by several theories: (1) steric hindrance, (2) deranged cell signalling, (3) impairment of desmosome assembly and increased desmosome disassembly

Steric Hindrance

Steric hindrance theory is based on the idea that there is direct interference of pemphigus IgG with the amino-terminal extracellular domain of desmogleins, which form the trans-adhesive interface between keratinocytes. This would lead to a lengthwise splitting of the desmosomes which has indeed been observed by electron microscopy in pemphigus patients and mouse models.

Cell Signalling

Signalling pathways that play a role in the pathogenesis of pemphigus involve complicated interactions between p38-mitogen activated protein kinase (p38MAPK), RhoA, protein kinase C (PKC), epidermal growth factor receptor (EGFR), plakoglobin and c-Myc [8].

Assembly and Disassembly

PV IgG leads to depletion of non-junctional Dsg3 by endocytosis. Eventually, assembly of desmosome fails due to shortage of non-junctional Dsg3 building blocks. Besides binding of PV IgG to non-junctional Dsg3, it might also be possible that PV IgG binds to junctional Dsg3 in the core domain of desmosomes. This leads to disassem-

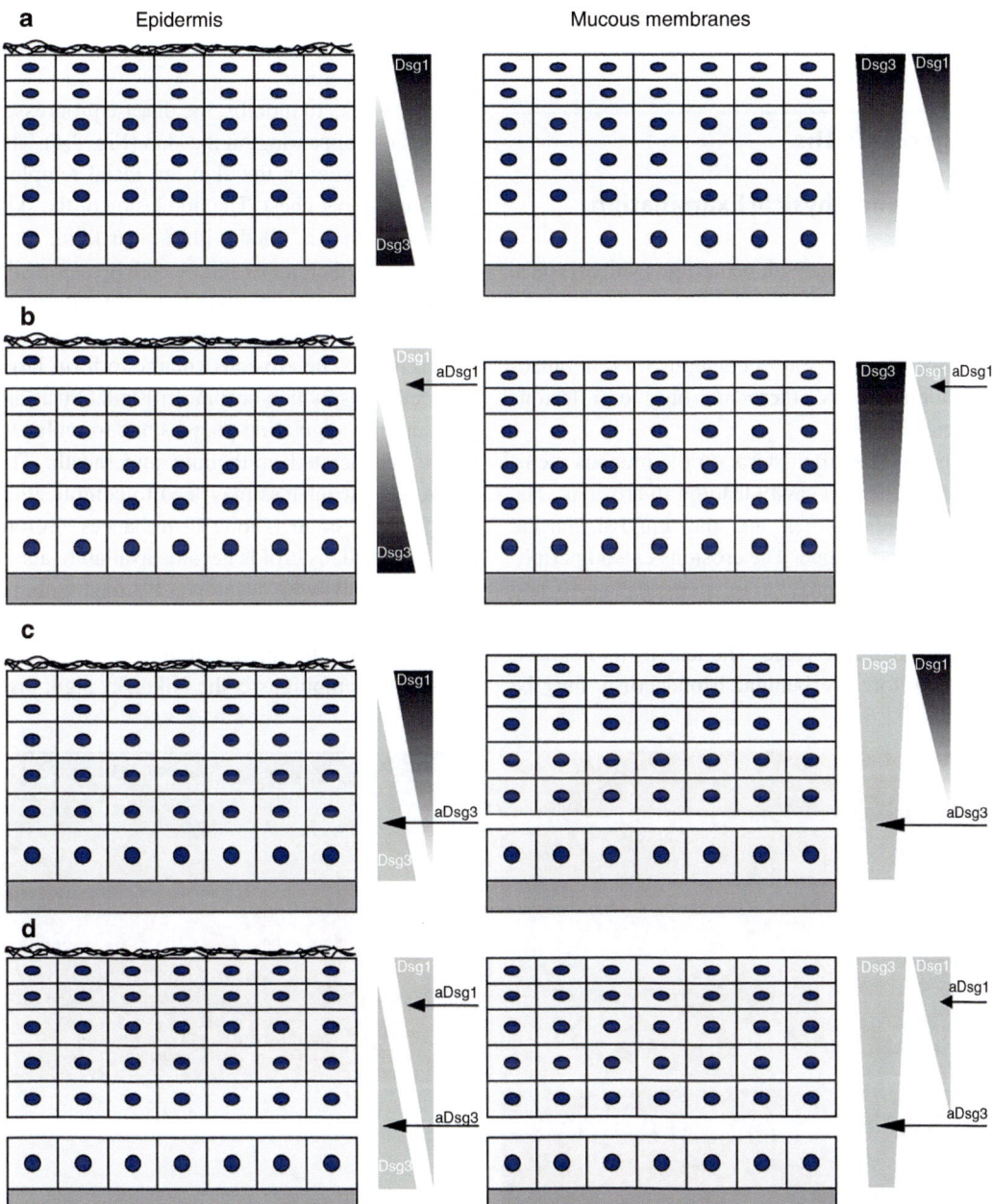

Fig. 8.2 Desmoglein compensation hypothesis. (**a**) Normal distribution of desmoglein (Dsg)1 and Dsg3 in the epidermis and mucous membrane. (**b**) In pemphigus foliaceus, IgG directed against Dsg1 causes subcorneal blistering in skin because in the lower layers Dsg3 compensates for the loss of function of Dsg1. In mucosa however anti-Dsg1 antibodies do not cause blistering, because there is sufficient Dsg3 present throughout all the layers to compensate for Dsg1. (**c**) In mucosal-dominant pemphigus vulgaris (PV), IgG directed against Dsg3 does not cause blistering of the skin because Dsg1 compensates for the loss of function of Dsg3. However there is suprabasal blistering of the mucous membranes because there is not sufficient Dsg1 present to compensate for Dsg3. (**d**) In mucocutaneous PV antibodies directed against both Dsg1 and Dsg3 cause blistering of the skin and the mucous membranes

bly of Dsg3 from the desmosomes, and possible internalization into endosomes.

Diagnosis Paths

History and Physical Examination

Almost all patients with pemphigus vulgaris have painful erosions of the oral mucosa. More than half of the patients also develop blisters and erosions on the skin (mucocutaneous PV). In mucosal dominant PV, there are only oral lesions present (Fig. 8.3).

The disease often starts on the mucous membranes in the oral cavity leading to erosions. The most common sites are the gingiva, buccal mucosa, and tongue. The erosions extend peripherally and may spread to involve the pharynx and larynx with difficulty in eating and drinking and hoarseness of the voice. The lesions do not scar, and therefore are benign. Blood crusts may be present on the nasal septum. Other mucosal surfaces include conjunctiva, oesophagus, vagina, urethra and rectum.

After weeks to months, the disease progresses with lesions appearing on the skin (Fig. 8.4). The predeliction site on the skin are facial temples, scalp, and upper chest. The first lesion of the skin is a blister that is filled with a clear fluid, on a normal or erythematous skin, which breaks easily resulting in painful erosion. The fluid within the blisters may become hemorrhagic, turbid or even seropurulent. The erosions enlarge to form large denuded areas, which become crusted. Crusts are piled up into vegetating plaques due to reblistering of regenerated epithelium underneath. The cutaneous barrier loss may lead to complication as infections or metabolic disturbances. Before systemic corticosteroids became available, about 75% of patients who developed PV died within a year.

A characteristic feature of all forms of active and severe pemphigus is the Nikolsky sign, pro-

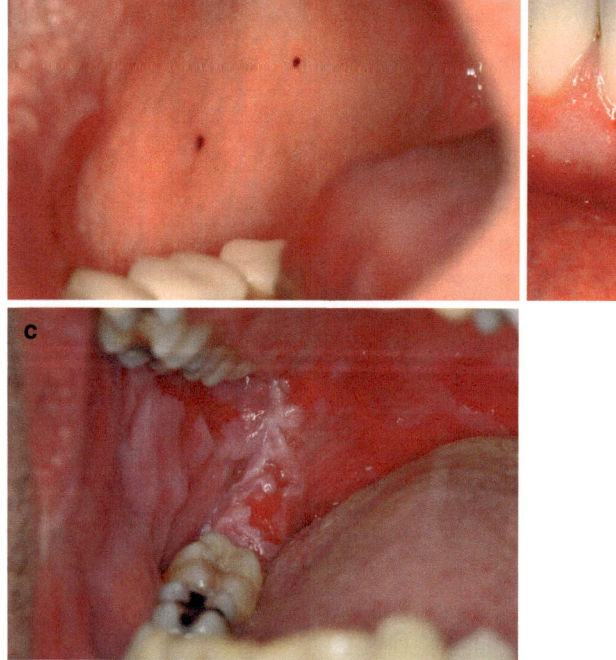

Fig. 8.3 Mucosal-dominant pemphigus vulgaris. Early phase shows (**a**) hemorrhagic vesicles on buccal mucosa, and (**b**) desquamative gingivitis. Late phase shows (**c**) whitish blister roofs (like bacon) and erosions on buccal mucosa and soft palate

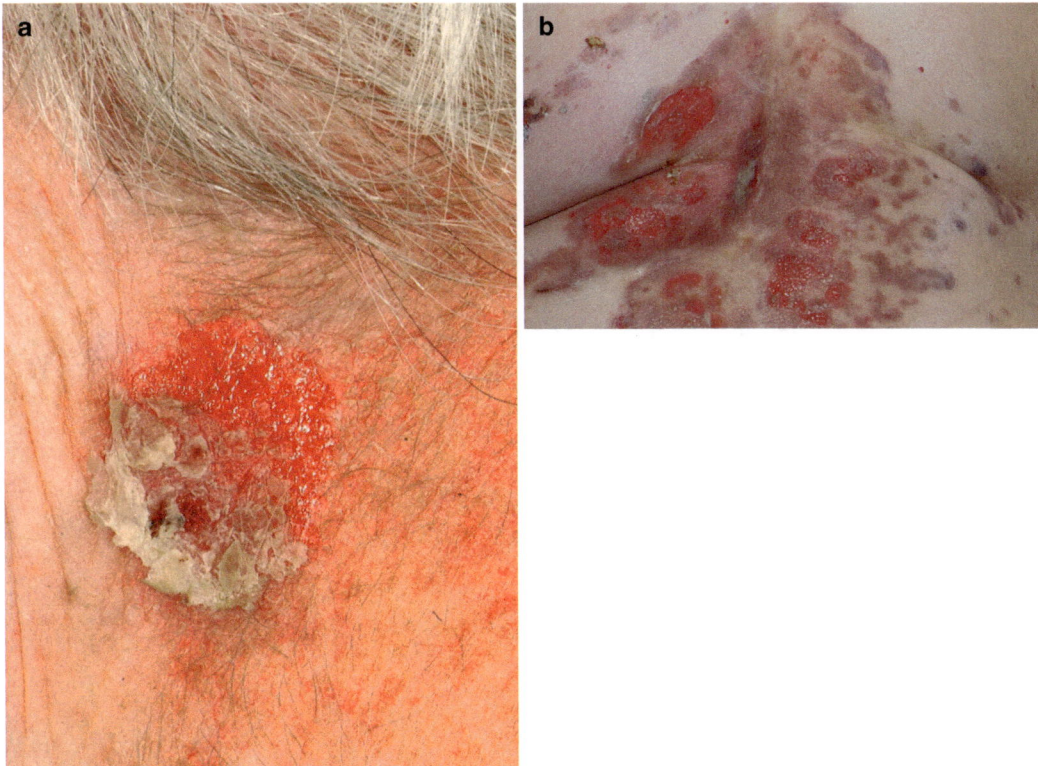

Fig. 8.4 Mucocutaneous pemphigus vulgaris. (**a**) Positive Nikolsky's sign type II on a crust of the temple. (**b**) Symmetrical erosions in dusky erythema on the back

duced when lateral pressure is applied adjacent to a lesion leading to separation of the epidermis.

Lesions of PV generally heal with crusts followed by re-epithelialisation. There is no scarring, although postinflammatory hyperpigmentation may persist for months in patients with Fitzpatrick skin types IV and V. Mild forms of the disease may regress spontaneously. Most patients with pemphigus vulgaris eventually enter a phase of complete remission in which they can be maintained lesion-free with minimum doses of corticosteroids (i.e. prednisolone <10 mg) or without therapy. As medications are tapered, flares in disease activity with development of new lesions and itching are not uncommon.

Pemphigus vegetans is a subtype of PV in which lesions accumulate in body folds (axillae, submammary, and groin) and around orifices (lips, anus). The lesions consist of pustules (Hallopeau type) (Fig. 8.5a) or papillomas (Neumann type) (Fig. 8.5b) or a combination of both (Fig. 8.5c). The affected skin is easily secondarily infected, which explains the foul smelling. As mentioned before, vegetating plaques are common in PV (Fig. 8.6), but the presence of sterile pustules or papillomas in the forementioned regions make it pemphigus vegetans.

General Diagnostics

The initial histopathological finding in pemphigus is intercellular widening between keratinocytes in the epidermis, accompanied by invasion of eosinophilic granulocytes (*eosinophylic spongiosis*). Characteristic for PV is an intraepidermal blister usually just above the basal layer due to loss of cell-cell contact (*suprabasilar acantholysis*) (Fig. 8.7). A few rounded-up acantholytic keratinocytes (*acanthocytes*) as well as clusters of detached epidermal cells float in the blister cavity. The basal cells loose lateral desmosomal

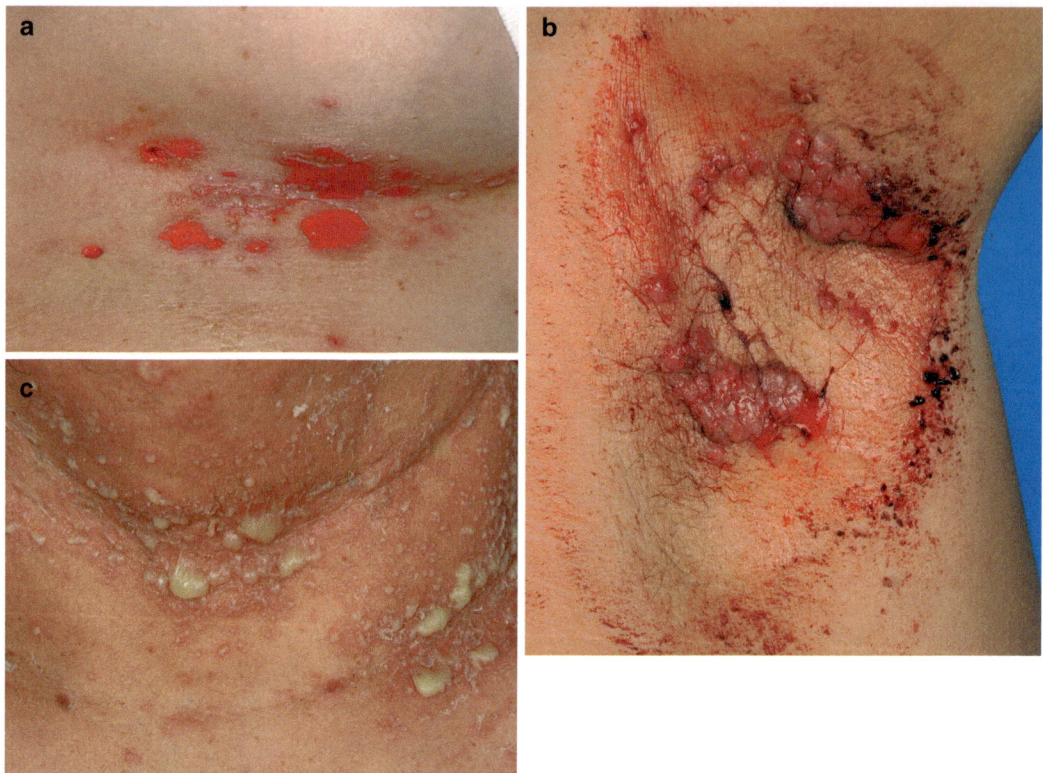

Fig. 8.5 Pemphigus vegetans. (**a**) Hallopeau type with pustules in the body folds. (**b**) Neumann type with papillomas in the axilla (**c**) Hallopeau type with pustules in the body folds

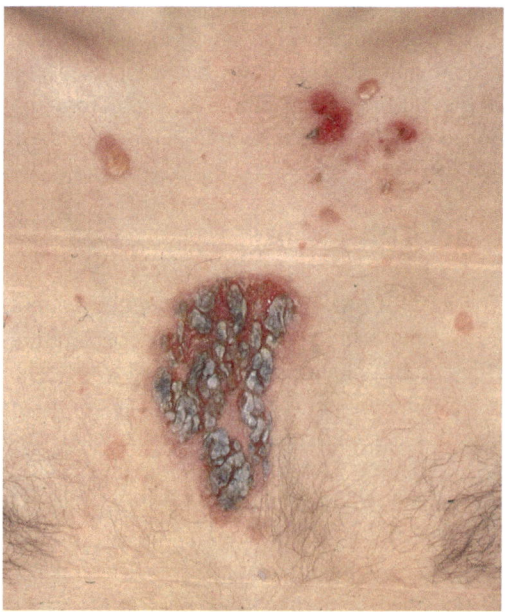

Fig. 8.6 Pemphigus vulgaris: a common vegetating plaque

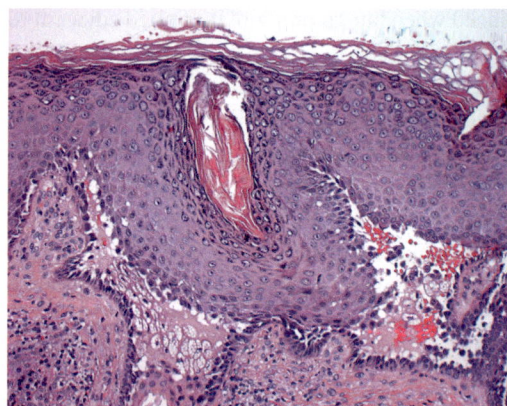

Fig. 8.7 Histopathology of pemphigus vulgaris. Suprabasal acantholysis with basal cells lining the blister floor like 'tombstones' (H&E)

contact with adjacent keratinocytes, but remain attached to the basement membrane via hemidesmosomes, thus giving the appearance of a row of tombstones. The acantholytic process may also involve the hair follicles.

Pemphigus is microscopically characterized by acantholysis

Specific Diagnostics

Immunological Tests
All forms of pemphigus are associated with the presence of skin-bound and circulating antibodies against epithelial cell surface antigens.

Direct Immunofluorescence
Tissue-bound intercellular antibodies are present in lesions and adjacent healthy skin in virtually all patients with pemphigus as detected by direct immunofluorescence microscopy (IF). They are usually IgG, but IgM and IgA with or without complement may also be deposited. See Chap. 4 for more on direct IF in pemphigus.

Indirect Immunofluorescence
Circulating epithelial cell surface (ECS) antibodies in the serum are detectable in up to 89% of patients by ELISA and/or indirect IF.

ELISA
Enzyme-linked immunosorbent assays (ELISA) are available to detect antibodies directed against Dsg1 and Dsg3 (See Chap. 6). The presence of antibodies directed against Dsg3 is associated with mucosal PV, whereas antibodies directed against Dsg1 are associated with PF. Both types of antibodies are present in mucocutaneous PV. ELISA kits are available with the ectodomain of desmoglein produced in insect cells (company) or in human cells (company). The latter has the advantage of containing the mature protein only and not the propeptide as well. It is thought that pathogenic antibodies are directed against conformational epitopes only and these epitopes are present in the mature desmogleins, while non-pathogenic antibodies recognize both mature and propeptide isoforms, correlating with binding of nonconformational epitopes.

There is a correlation between the titre of desmoglein 1 antibodies and skin activity of the disease. Serum monitoring of antibody titres may be useful in guiding therapy, since a rise in their titre usually precedes a recurrence in disease activity, while they usually decrease with successful treatment and disappear in patients in remission.

> **Case Study: Part 2**
> Histopathology of lesional skin sampled from the edge of a blister showed suprabasal acantholysis. Direct immunofluorescence microscopy staining of lesional peribullous skin and healthy skin revealed deposition of IgG and C3c along the ECS. Indirect immunofluorescence microscopy on monkey esophagus was positive for ECS IgG antibodies. ELISA identified positive values of anti-Dsg1 and anti-Dsg3 titers (>150). A diagnose was made of mucocutaneous pemphigus vulgaris.

Treatment Tricks

Initial Treatment and Escalator

Systemic Corticosteroids
The treatment of pemphigus was symptomatic until the introduction of corticosteroids in the 1950s. The majority of patients in the pre-steroid era usually died from overwhelming sepsis within 1 year after disease onset. The use of systemic corticosteroids has transformed an almost invariably fatal disease into a chronic disease whose mortality is less than 6%. However the side effects of systemic steroids; including infection, diabetes, osteoporosis, myopathy, gastrointestinal bleeding, cataracts or central nervous system toxicity result in substantial morbidity and also mortality in pemphigus vulgaris. Therefore later other immunosuppressive agents were introduced to reduce side effects of systemic corticosteroids (see below)

Systemic corticosteroids have an important role at the initial treatment to achieve disease control as their effect is quick and pronounced.

Rituximab

Rituximab has revolutionized the treatment of pemphigus turning the chronic disease to an almost curable disease, where patients can experience a long-term complete remission without any medication. Rituximab is recently registered for pemphigus vulgaris, based on the large randomized controlled trial showing superiority in efficacy and safety above systemic prednisolone alone [9]. According to the S2K European guideline, rituximab is the first line treatment for pemphigus vulgaris, in the initial phase in combination with prednisolone [10].

> Rituximab is a chimeric murine-human monoclonal anti-CD20 antibody, originally developed for the treatment of B-cell malignancies. CD20 is an antigen expressed on the surface of pre-B and mature B cells. Rituximab binds to transmembrane CD20, reduces circulating B cells and prevents their maturation into all antibody-secreting plasma cells, not just those making pathogenic antibodies. It has shown efficacy in patients with refractory antibody-mediated autoimmune disorders. Rituximab is registered for pemphigus vulgaris. The recommended dosage regime by the European guideline is, a cycle of 2 × 1000 mg with a 2-week interval. The cycle is restarted after 6 months in case of absence of complete remission. In patients with complete remission, a maintenance infusion of 500 mg is advised at month 6, 12 and 18. When patients are treated with rituximab and use 2 or more immunosuppressive agents besides this, then treatment to prevent *Pneumocystis jirovice* pneumonia and herpes pneumonia should be started with cotrimoxazole 480–960 mg/day and valaciclovir 500 mg/day during the 3 months following the rituximab infusion.

Rituximab is the first line treatment for pemphigus vulgaris, at the initial phase eventually in combination with systemic corticostreoids

Immunosuppressive Agents

Immunosuppressive agents are commonly used in combination with systemic corticosteroids in order to increase efficacy and may have a steroid-sparing effect, thereby allowing reduced maintenance doses and less side effects of systemic corticosteroids. The most commonly used adjuvants are azathioprine (2–3 mg/kg), mycophenolate mofetil (2000 mg/day), mycophenolic acid (1440 mg/day), cyclophosphamide (≤ 2 mg/kg), methotrexate (10–15 mg/week) and dapsone.

High Dose Human Intravenous Immunoglobulin

Intravenous immunoglobulin (IVIG) neutralizes autoantibodies by several mechanism including anti-idiotypic antibodies, interference with the cytokine network, modulation of B- and T-cell functions, inhibition of complement and cytokine production, and blocking activation and upregulation of inhibitory Fc receptors. A major advantage if IVIG compared with other treatment options is its excellent safety profile. Adverse events are generally mild and reported side effects include headache, fever, chills, myalgia, flushing, hypotension, tachycardia and gastrointestinal symptoms. The standard dose is 2 g/kg/month in 2–4 gifts. The costs of IVIG medication monthly are as high as $10 000 months. Low dose IVIG (0.2 mg/kg/month) may be effective in selected cases [11].

Plasmapheresis and Immunoadsorption

Rapid removal of circulating autoantibodies can be achieved by plasmapheresis (exchanging plasma by fresh-frozen plasma or human albumin) or by immunoadsorption (only removing immunoglobulin). In the past years immonoadsorption replaced plasmapheresis in the treatment of pemphigus. Immunoadsorption allows the processing of the two- to threefold plasma volume per treatment session and is associated with a lower rate of adverse events like infections and allergic reactions [12].

Follow-Up and Tapering

Treatment should be started with rituximab in combination with high dose predniso(lo)ne in a dosage of 1.0–1.5 mg/kg per day. Taper by 25% reduction in biweekly steps (at <20 mg more slowly!). A rule of the thumb quick tapering schedule is 80–60–40–30–25–20–15–12.5–10–7.5–5–2.5–0 mg in steps of 2-weeks. Raise dose by two steps dose when new lesions occur, or continue dose if tapering is not possible.

When patients are treated with rituximab and use 2 or more immunosuppressive agents besides this, then treatment to prevent *Pneumocystis jirovice* pneumonia and herpes pneumonia should be started with cotrimoxazole 480–960 mg/day and valaciclovir 500 mg/day during the 3 months following the rituximab infusion.

> **Case Study: Part 3**
>
> First-line treatment consisted of prednisolone (1 mg/kg) in combination with two intravenous infusions of 1000 mg rituximab separated by 2 weeks, which was preceded by screening according to protocol. The dosage of prednisolone was tapered with 10 mg per 2 weeks until 30 mg per day and after that by 5 mg per 2 weeks. The erosions on the skin healed promptly whereas the oral mucosal erosions persisted and healed more slowly. Oral swabs for bacterial and fungal culture as well as Herpes simplex (HSV) PCR were frequently performed to rule out superinfection causing delayed healing of the mucosa. At month 6, the patient showed complete remission off-therapy and a maintenance infusion of 500 mg of rituximab was administered followed by 500 mg of rituximab at month 12. After 18 months, the patient was discharged from outpatient care and instructed to contact us in case of clinical signs of relapse.

Review Questions

1. What is the most common location of mucocutaneous pemphigus vulgaris is?
   (a) Temples
   (b) Feet
   (c) Genitals
2. The most important risk factor for pemphigus is
   (a) Hair colour
   (b) Country of birth
   (c) Profession
3. Patients with mucosal dominant PV have antibodies directed against
   (a) desmoglein 1
   (b) desmoglein 3
   (c) desmoglein 1 and 3
4. First line treatment of pemphigus is
   (a) superpotent topical corticosteroids
   (b) systemic corticosteroids
   (c) azathioprine
   (d) rituximab

Answers

1. (a)
2. (b)
3. (b)
4. (d)

On the Web

JAMA Dermatology Patient Page, Pemphigus http://archderm.jamanetwork.com/article.aspx?articleid=1879985

International Pemphigus & Pemphigoid Foundation http://www.pemphigus.org/

Van der Wier G. Acantholysis in pemphigus [dissertation]. Groningen: University of Groningen; 2014. http://irs.ub.rug.nl/ppn/38300196X

References

1. Jonkman MF. JAMA dermatology patient page. Pemphigus. JAMA Dermatol. 2014;150(6):680.
2. Schmidt E, Kasperkiewicz M, Joly P. Pemphigus. Lancet. 2019;394(10201):882–94.

3. Uzun S, Durdu M, Akman A, Gunasti S, Uslular C, Memisoglu HR, Alpsoy E. Pemphigus in the Mediterranean region of Turkey: a study of 148 cases. Int J Dermatol. 2006;45:523–8.
4. Beutner EH, Jordon RE. Demonstration of skin antibodies in sera of pemphigus vulgaris patients by indirect immunofluorescent staining. Proc Soc Exp Biol Med. 1964;117:505–10.
5. Stanley JR, Yaar M, Hawley-Nelson P, Katz SI. Pemphigus antibodies identify a cell surface glycoprotein synthesized by human and mouse keratinocytes. J Clin Invest. 1982;70:281–8.
6. Amagai M, Klaus-Kovtun V, Stanley JR. Autoantibodies against a novel epithelial cadherin in pemphigus vulgaris, a disease of cell adhesion. Cell. 1991;67:869–77.
7. Mahoney MG, Wang Z, Rothenberger K, Koch PJ, Amagai M, Stanley JR. Explanations for the clinical and microscopic localization of lesions in pemphigus foliaceus and vulgaris. J Clin Invest. 1999;103:461–8.
8. Li X, Ishii N, Ohata C, Furumura M, Hashimoto T. Signalling pathways in pemphigus vulgaris. Exp Dermatol. 2014;23:155–6.
9. Joly P, Maho-Vaillant M, Prost-Squarcioni C, Hebert V, Houivet E, Calbo S, Caillot F, Golinski ML, Labeille B, Picard-Dahan C, Paul C, Richard MA, Bouaziz JD, Duvert-Lehembre S, Bernard P, Caux F, Alexandre M, Ingen-Housz-Oro S, Vabres P, Delaporte E, Quereux G, Dupuy A, Debarbieux S, Avenel-Audran M, D'Incan M, Bedane C, Bénéton N, Jullien D, Dupin N, Misery L, Machet L, Beylot-Barry M, Dereure O, Sassolas B, Vermeulin T, Benichou J, Musette P. French study group on autoimmune bullous skin diseases. First-line rituximab combined with short-term prednisone versus prednisone alone for the treatment of pemphigus (Ritux 3): a prospective, multicentre, parallel-group, open-label randomised trial. Lancet. 2017;389(10083):2031–40. https://doi.org/10.1016/S0140-6736(17)30070-3.
10. Joly P, Horvath B, Patsatsi A, Uzun S, Bech R, Beissert S, Bergman R, Bernard P, Borradori L, Caproni M, Caux F, Cianchini G, Daneshpazhooh M, De D, Dmochowski M, Drenovska K, Ehrchen J, Feliciani C, Goebeler M, Groves R, Guenther C, Hofmann S, Ioannides D, Kowalewski C, Ludwig R, Lim YL, Marinovic B, Marzano AV, Mascaró JM Jr, Mimouni D, Murrell DF, Pincelli C, Squarcioni CP, Sárdy M, Setterfield J, Sprecher E, Vassileva S, Wozniak K, Yayli S, Zambruno G, Zillikens D, Hertl M, Schmidt E. Updated S2K guidelines on the management of pemphigus vulgaris and foliaceus initiated by the European academy of dermatology and venereology (EADV). J Eur Acad Dermatol Venereol. 2020;34(9):1900–13. https://doi.org/10.1111/jdv.16752.
11. Toth GG, Jonkman MF. Successful treatment of recalcitrant penicillamine-induced pemphigus foliaceus by low-dose intravenous immunoglobulins. Br J Dermatol. 1999;141:583–5.
12. Kasperkiewicz M, Schmidt E, Zillikens D. Current therapy of the pemphigus group. Clin Dermatol. 2012;30:84–94.

Pemphigus Foliaceus

Laura de Sena N. Maehara, Marcel F. Jonkman, and Barbara Horváth

Pemphigus Foliaceus

Introduction and AIMS

Short Definition in Layman Terms

Pemphigus foliaceus is an autoimmune blistering disease that affects the skin in middle-aged patients. Pemphigus foliaceus causes red spots with crusts and scale on the skin (Fig. 9.1). Foliaceus means, "squamous like fallen leafs". The spots commonly start on the scalp and may spread over the entire body (Fig. 9.2). Mucosal lesions or scars do not develop. The disease cannot spread to other people (it is not contagious). The disease is caused by autoantibodies directed against the adhesion molecule desmoglein 1 on the surface of skin cells. Treatment involves finding ways to "calm down" the body's immune system. Prednisone, an oral form of steroid, is usually the first treatment used. The CD20 antibodiy rituximab, may provide months of disease relief and reduce the need for prednisone. Other immunosuppressive drugs can be added in mild cases to allow earlier discontinuation of prednisone treatment.

> **Learning Objectives**
> After reading this chapter you should be able to recognize PF, understand the pathogenesis and the clinics, choose complementary diagnostic procedures, and suggest a plan for therapy.

L. d. S. N. Maehara
Center for Blistering Diseases, Department of Dermatology, University Medical Center Groningen, University of Groningen, Groningen, The Netherlands

Medical School, Centro Universitario de Jaguariuna – Unifaj, Jaguariuna – Sao Paulo, Brazil
e-mail: laura.maehara@prof.unieduk.com.br

M. F. Jonkman (Deceased) · B. Horváth (✉)
Center for Blistering Diseases, Department of Dermatology, University Medical Center Groningen, University of Groningen, Groningen, The Netherlands
e-mail: b.horvath@umcg.nl

> **Case Study: Part 1**
> A 42-year-old man presented with crusted plaques and erosions since 1 month on his face, trunk, arms and legs. The lesions started as 'bubbles' that become wounds. The lesions were painful, and slightly itchy. After further questioning, he recalled having desquamation of the scalp for about 1 year.

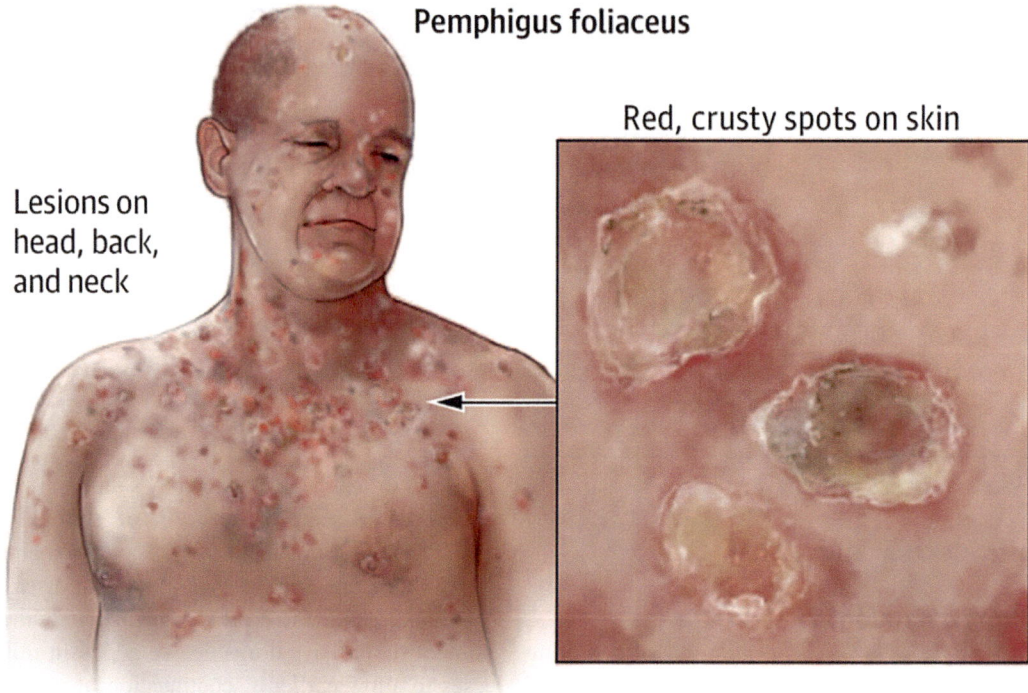

Fig. 9.1 Pemphigus foliaceus with typical distribution of crusted scaly erythematous plaques. Drawings by Alison E. Burke adapted from [1]. Copyright © 2014 American Medical Association. All rights reserved

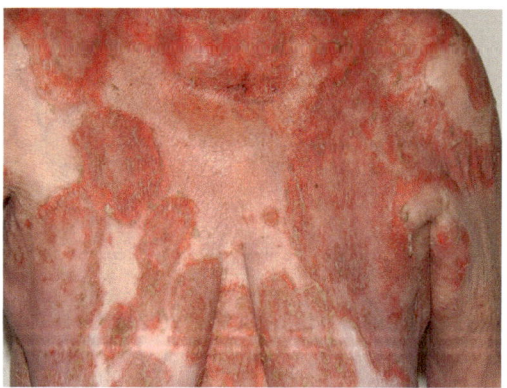

Fig. 9.2 Pemphigus foliaceus: circinate crusted scales and erosions on polycyclic erythema on the trunk

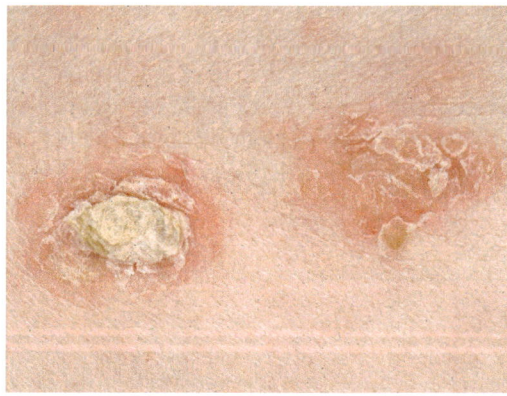

Fig. 9.3 Pemphigus foliaceus: crusted scales resembling pastry puff, or in French 'milles feuilles'

Didactical Questions: Cross Section of Questions to Prime the Reader's Interest

What is the differential diagnosis? Which are the diagnostic tests that should be performed? Would you prescribe any therapy? What other questions should be asked before prescription?

Facts and Figures

Definitions and Classification

Pemphigus foliaceus Cazenave (commonly called PF) is the classical form of PF that is defined by acantholysis in the upper epidermis that leads to crusted, scaling plaques (Fig. 9.3)

and erosions, and contra wise to pemphigus vulgaris has no mucosal involvement. The disease is caused by autoantibodies against desmoglein 1 on the epithelial cell surface [2].

Epidemiology

The age of onset of PF is in the 5th decade. Men and women are equally affected. PF comprises about 17% of all cases with pemphigus. The incidence of PF in non-endemic areas is approximately 0.04 new cases per 100,000 per year.

Pathogenesis

Pathogenic desmoglein 1 (Dsg1) autoantibodies bind the cell membrane and induce loss of cell-cell contact (*acantholysis*) [3]. The compensation theory states that a subcorneal cleft is formed due to the absence of compensatory desmoglein 3 (Dsg3) in the upper part of the epidermis. Likewise, mucosal lesions are not present in PF because of the presence of Dsg3 in the entire mucosal epithelium, which compensates for the loss of Dsg1.

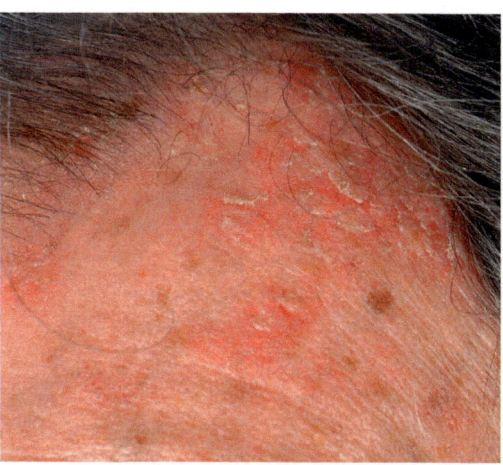

Fig. 9.4 Pemphigus foliaceus: erosions and crusted scales on the forehead mimicking actinic keratosis

Diagnosis Paths

History and Physical Examination

The patient is mostly in good general conditions and may complain of itch or pain that may be localized on the scalp or temples for years. Scaly erythema in the scalp may be misdiagnosed for seborrheic dermatitis or actinic keratosis (Fig. 9.4). A clue to diagnosis is a positive Nikolsky sign (see box Chap. 8). Typical presentation is the crusted plaque with multiple layers of scaling (Fig. 9.3), which easily erodes. The diseases may spread over the trunk and extremities. Predilection sites are the seborrheic area's; scalp, temples, periorbicular area, neck, upper chest and back. The oral cavity is not affected. The extent of the disease may reach erythroderma in severe cases.

General Diagnostics

After the suspicion of an autoimmune disease like pemphigus, careful medical history (hematologic, oncologic, endocrine, cardiovascular and infectious) must be taken to search for risk factors of oral corticosteroid treatment and evolving complications of immunosuppressive therapy. Any medication in use should be listed, in order to detect possible triggers (see Chap. 12, Drug-induced pemphigus) and future interactions of drugs.

Specific Diagnostics

The diagnosis of PF is established by histopathological examination of a skin biopsy demonstrating a subcorneal split. In the lower epidermis epidermal cell-cell widening not commencing to acantholysis is visible. Direct immunofluorescence of peribullous lesional skin demonstrates patient's IgG in an epithelial cell surface (ECS) pattern (Fig. 4.2c). Likewise, patient's serum may contain circulating IgG capable of binding monkey esophagus in an ECS pattern. Autoantibodies specific to Dsg1 are demonstrable by ELISA.

> **Case Study: Part 2**
> The patient was healthy and was not receiving any medication. Two skin biopsies were taken: (1) from the edge of a bulla, not being erosive, for histopathology, and (2) from peribullous erythematous skin for direct immunofluorescence (DIF) micros-

copy. Histology showed a subcorneal blister, and on DIF ECS IgG depositions in a coarse granular pattern were seen. IIF on monkey esophagus showed ECS IgG in a smooth pattern. The ELISA index for antibodies to Dsg1 was >150, and to Dsg3 0. A diagnosis of PF was made (mild to moderate severity based on extensiveness).

Treatment Tricks

Initial Treatment and Therapeutic Ladder

Systemic corticosteroid is the first-line of therapy of PF to achieve disease control within days. The recent published S2K guideline by the European Academy of Dermatology and Venereology (EADV) on pemphigus differentiate clearly between the treatment of mild and moderate to severe PF [4].

In limited disease, topical corticosteroids (class III, IV) can be applied. In mild disease, dapsone in a start dose of 50–100 mg/day, later adjusted to clinical response up to 1.5 mg/kg bodyweight can be initiated in combination with systemic prednisolone 0.5–1.0 mg/kg. In refractory/relapsing cases, also rituximab can be added as 2nd line treatment.

The treatment of moderate to severe PF is similar to PV. First line treatment is prednisolone in 1.0 mg/kg per day (eventually adjusted up to 1.5 mg/kg per day) in combination with rituximab (see box Rituximab Chap. 8) a cycle of 2 × 1000 mg with a 2-week interval, followed by maintaince doses of 500 mg rituximab at month 6, 12 and 18.

Follow-Up and Tapering

Since the skin lesions in PF clear more slowly than in PV, one can expect long-term corticosteroid therapy. Tapering of corticosteroids should be started when no new lesions had developed for a minimum of 2 weeks, and approximately 80% of lesions had healed—that is, at the end of consolidation phase with 25% of the dose, until 20 mg/day, when tapering should be performed more slowly. In responsive cases the tapering schedule is 40–35–30–25–20–15–12.5–10–7.5–5–2.5–0 mg in steps of 2-weeks. Take two steps back if new lesions develop. Start again if disease is not controlled. Tapering on alternating days to avoid repression of the adrenal-hypothalamic axis is not recommended, since the skin will flare up on reduced days.

Other adjuvants therapy used commonly in the treatment of PF are azathioprine 2–3 mg/kg, mycophenolate mofetil 2000 mg, mycophenolic acid 1440 mg. Alternatives are dapsone <150 mg, cyclophosphamide 2 mg/kg, and methotrexate <25 mg/week.

> **Case Study: Part 3**
>
> Therapy was started with prednisolone 0.5 mg/kg. Two weeks later, the patient had improvement of 50% of the lesions, and did not present new lesions. After 2 weeks, tapering was possible. In addition azathioprine was given at a dose of 3 mg/kg. After 16 weeks while reaching a dose of 10 mg prednisolone no improvement was seen. The prednisolone dose was raised to 15 mg (2 steps back). No further tapering was possible. Since the patient was dependent on more than minimal (>10 mg) corticosteroid therapy, it was decided to start rituximab treatment with two intravenous infusions of 1000 mg rituximab separated by 2 weeks, which was preceded by screening according to protocol.

Endemic Pemphigus

Introduction and AIMS

Endemic pemphigus foliaceus, also referred as *fogo selvagem* ('wildfire') is a subtype of PF first mentioned as *pemphigus brasiliensis* in the medical lexicon in 1763 by François Boissier de Sauvages. In endemic PF the same pathogenic antibodies to Dsg1 were demonstrated as in PF Cazenave. *Fogo selvagem* patients are young rural workers, children or relatives living in endemic areas in Brazil. In Colombia, two groups of endemic patients have been described: (1) Indian tribes in the southern areas of the

Amazonian and Orinoquian forest regions, and (2) endemic PF in gold-mining regions of El Bagre [5]. Patients with the new variant present not only antibodies to Dsg1, but also to other adhesion molecules. In Tunisia, endemic areas are also rural, and patients are mostly women. Use of traditional cosmetics was suggested as a risk factor [6]. Recently, a small focus of endemic PF was noticed in Tanzania [7].

Facts and Figures

Endemic PF in Brazil was reported in deforested rural areas, close to rivers, affecting workers and their relatives, including young children. Black fly bites were shown to increase the risk [8], as many studies have been confirmed the link between the fly and other hematophagous insects and the disease. The theory is that insect's saliva, through molecular mimicry, triggers the synthesis of IgM and IgG1 to Dsg1, and later a class switch results in pathogenic IgG4. Moreover epitope spreading is needed, anon-pathogenic IgG1 bind extracellular domain 5 (EC5) of Dsg1, whereas pathogenic IgG4 bind EC1 and EC2 of Dsg1.The risk factor for the disease would be some specific HLA alleles (DRB1*0404, 1402 and 1406). Although endemic PF is common in Brazil, a recent report showed that pemphigus vulgaris, and not endemic PF, is more frequent in one endemic area in São Paulo [9].

Diagnosis Paths

Endemic pemphigus patients present with crusted plaques similar to PF (Fig. 9.5). Clinical presentations include localized form (form fruste) and generalized forms (bullous invasion, keratotic, hyperpigmented, pemphigus herpetiformis and exfoliative erythroderma). For histological and immunological exams refer to PF.

Treatment Tricks

Patients diagnosed with endemic pemphigus are treated similarly those with PF.

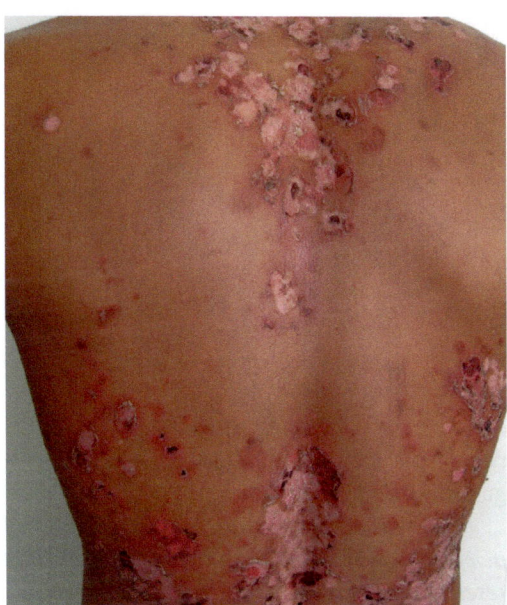

Fig. 9.5 Fogo selvagem: erosions and circinate crusted scales symmetrical on the back in young male

Pemphigus Herpetiformis

Introduction

The diagnostic criteria of pemphigus herpetiformis (PH) were first reported by Jablońska et al. in 1975 [10]. Before the use of immunofluorescence the clinical presentation was named dermatitis herpetiformis with acantholysis. The skin disease is remarkable itchy, which is uncommon for pemphigus. Moreover, Nikolsky's sign is negative.

Facts and Figures

Pemphigus herpetiformis (PH) is a variant of pemphigus with arciform (Fig. 9.6) and annular lesions and severe itch that resembles clinically dermatitis herpetiformis, however all immunological findings fit with pemphigus. The main autoantigen is desmoglein 1, and for that reason PH is called a variant of pemphigus foliaceus. In a minority of the cases one may find autoantibodies against desmoglein 3and also suprabasilar acantholysis resembling a variant of pemphigus vulgaris. PH can be the initial presentation of a disease what later evolves to classic nonendemic

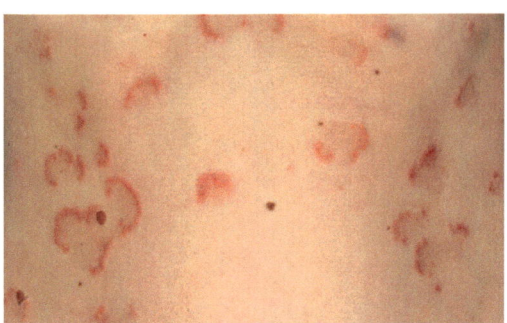

Fig. 9.6 Pemphigus herpetiformis: arciform erythematous papules and beginning vesiculation on the trunk

pemphigus foliaceus, fogo selvagem or pemphigus vulgaris [11, 12].

Pemphigus herpetiformis (PH) is variant of pemphigus with annular lesions and itch that resembles clinically dermatitis herpetiformis

Case Study: Part 1
A 70-year-old female was hospitalized because of a very itchy dermatosis. Dermatological examination showed erythematous macules that became confluent to large symmetrical areas. Many crusts and some vesicles were present. Nikolsky sign was negative.

Diagnosis Paths

The diagnosis is based on the criteria listed in Table 9.1.

The differential diagnosis of PH includes dermatitis herpetiformis, pemphigus foliaceus, pemphigus vulgaris, bullous pemphigoid, IgA pemphigus, and linear IgA bullous dermatosis.

Case Study: Part 2
Histopathology showed intra-epidermal pustules with neutrophilic granulocytes and some acanthocytes (Fig. 9.7). Direct immunofluorescence detected tissue-bound epithelial cell surface IgG and IgA in rough desmo-pattern in the lower 2/3 of the epidermis. Indirect immunofluorescence on monkey esophagus was positive for circulating epithelial cell surface IgG and IgA. ELISA revealed IgG and IgA antibodies against desmoglein1. A diagnosis was made of pemphigus herpetiformis.

Additional workup revealed the presence of heart failure and normal-iron anemia.

Table 9.1 Suggested diagnostic criteria for pemphigus herpetiformis [10]

Characteristic appearances	Mandatory
Grouped (herpetiform) distribution of itching erythematous vesicular/bullous/papular lesions, often in an annular-shaped pattern	**Yes**
Eosinophilic/neutrophilic spongiosis/intraepidermal pustules with or without acantholysis	No
Skin-bound epithelial cell surface IgG and/or C3	**Yes**
Circulating epithelial cell surface IgG[a]	No
Detection of circulating IgG autoantibodies against desmoglein 1 and/or 3, desmocollin 1 and/or 3[a]	No

[a]At least 1 of the 2 criteria (positive indirect immunofluorescence microscopy or detection of specific autoantibodies) should be fulfilled if direct immunofluorescence microscopy is not available

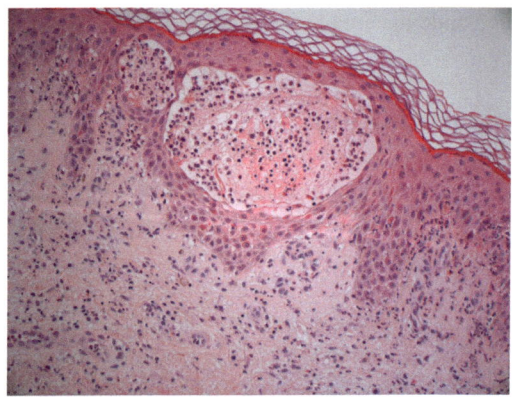

Fig. 9.7 Histopathology of pemphigus herpetiformis. Two intra-epidermal pustules filled with neutrophilic granulocytes

Treatment Tricks

PH is considered to be less life threatening than other types of pemphigus. It usually responds well to monotherapy with dapsone, which is considered the drug of first choice.

> **Case Study: Part 3**
> Because of anemia and heart failure dapsone was relatively contraindicated. Treatment consisted of minocycline 200 mg and topical whole body ultrapotent corticosteroid. Itch was treated by hydroxyzine 10 mg bd. Captopril was changed to losartan, since it might induce pemphigus. The skin lesions resolved and the patient was discharged from hospitalization after 4 weeks. Complete remission was maintained while on minocycline 100 mg bd and topical lesional corticosteroids. Prednisolone could be avoided.

Pemphigus Erythematosus

Introduction

Pemphigus erythematosus (PE) was first described in 1926 by Senear and Usher [13] as a condition with a lupus-like butterfly rash or severe seborrheic dermatitis, which they suggested was a combination of pemphigus vulgaris and lupus erythematosus (LE). Investigatingthe differences between pemphigus vulgaris and PF, it became clear that PE is rather an early form of PF. After introducing the routine immunofluorescence as a diagnostic tool, the association with LE revived. Chorzelski et al. [14] described a "lupus-band" deposition in sun-exposed skin areas of patients with PE, together with antinuclear antibodies (ANAs) as in LE. Later it was clarified that the gross findings in patients with PE do not meet the criteria for systemic LE as published by the American College of Rheumatology.

Pemphigus erythematosus is not related to lupus erythematosus

Facts and Figures

The nature of the "lupus-band phenomenon" in PE was disclosed by Oktarina et al. [13]. The granular BMZ depositions located below the lamina densa consist of IgG, complement, and the shed desmoglein 1 ectodomain. It was hypothized that shedding of the Dsg1 ectodomain was the result of UV-induced apoptosis. Patients with PE are often erroneously treated by UV phototherapy for a presumed psoriasis [15].

Pemphigus erythematosus is a localized form of pemphigus foliaceus often elicited by UV exposure

> **Case Study: Part 1 [15]**
> An 80-year-old woman was admitted to our hospital with a 3-year history of generalized progressive erythemato-squamous skin lesions with pustules and flaccid blisters. She had been diagnosed elsewhere as psoriasis pustulosa complicated by secondary infection with *Staphylococcus aureus*. The patient had received several therapies including methotrexate, systemic erythromycin, acitretin and cyclosporine. Due to methotrexate related hepatotoxicity and inefficacy of the other therapies, the patient switched over to a twice-weekly regimen of psoralen-UVA (PUVA) therapy with 40 mg methoxsalen. During PUVA therapy, the skin lesions worsened and therapy was stopped after 3 weeks.
>
> Physical examination revealed suberythroderma, consisting of confluent and scattered red macules with scales and purulent crusts. In the face a malar distribution was present (Fig. 9.8). Multiple erosions and flaccid blisters were seen and Nikolsky sign was positive. The mucous membranes were not involved.

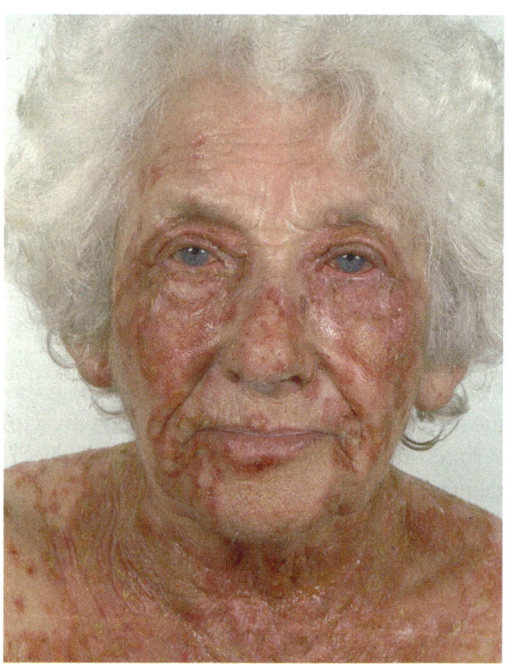

Fig. 9.8 Pemphigus erythematosus: typical facial butterfly eruption. Copyright © 2021 American Medical Association. All rights reserved

Diagnosis Paths

The diagnosis is based on the criteria listed in Table 9.2. The differential diagnosis of PE includes pemphigus foliaceus, acute cutaneous lupus erythematosus, and psoriasis.

Immunofluorescence of pemphigus erythematosus shows a pseudolupus-band that consists of IgG, complement, and desmoglein 1 ectodomain

Table 9.2 Suggested diagnostic criteria for pemphigus erythematosus

Characteristic appearances	Mandatory
Malar erythemato-squamous plaques and vesicles in a 'butterfly' pattern	Yes
Recent UV exposure	No
Subcorneal blister	No
DIF: IgG and/or C3 depositions at epithelial cell surface	Yes
DIF: granular IgG and C3 depositions at epithelial basement membrane zone	Yes
IIF: Circulating epithelial cell surface IgG	No
ELISA: detection of circulating IgG autoantibodies against desmoglein 1	No
Absence of raised ANA titer	Yes

Case Study: Part 2

Histopathology revealed subcorneal blisters. Direct immunofluorescence microscopy showed intra-epidermal epithelial cell surface depositions of IgG and C3c and in addition coarse granular depositions of IgG and C3c that colocated to the shed desmoglein 1 ectodomain in the lower epidermal basement membrane zone (Fig. 9.9). Indirect immunofluoresence on monkey esophagus showed ECS IgG antibodies with a titer of >1:320 and retrospective ELISA analysis demonstrated anti-Dsg1 antibodies. Blood tests were negative for antinuclear, anti-ENA, anti-dsDNA, anti-SSA, anti-smooth muscle and anti-striated muscle antibodies. A diagnosis of pemphigus erythematosus was made.

Treatment Tricks

The treatment of PE is similar to that of PF. Protection to UV light should be advised.

Case Study: Part 3

The patient received multidisciplinary care. Geriatric doctor was consulted for drug therapy advice because of previous hepatotoxicity. Specialized nurses provided dressings for painful erosions. The patient was kept in a dark room. Therapy was started with prednisolone 0.5 mg/kg (20 mg). Three weeks later, the patient had improvement of 80% of the lesions, and did not present new lesions since 2 weeks, so tapering was possible. Adjuvant therapy was not necessary and after 12 weeks the patient was in complete remission on minimal therapy (5 mg prednisolone). Six months later, the patient was in complete remission off therapy. In 2 years of follow up, the lady was in partial remission off therapy and died 5 years later for other medical reason.

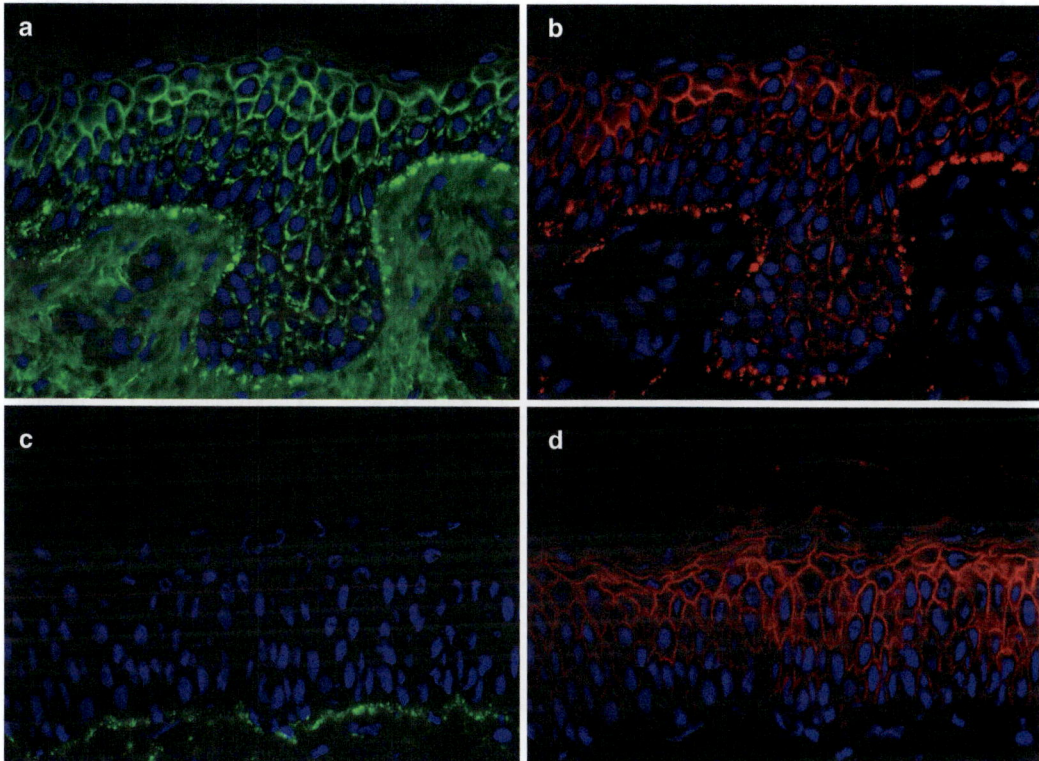

Fig. 9.9 Direct immunofluorescence of pemphigus erythematosus (PE) reveals granular depositions of IgG (green in **a**) along the epidermal basement membrane zone (EBMZ), that co-localize with the Dsg1 ectodomain (red in **b**). In the skin from a patient with systemic lupus erythematosus (SLE), a lupus band is detected of granular IgG alon the EBMZ (green in **c**), without Dsg1 ectodomain precipitations (red in **d**). Note that the epithelial cell surface shows clusters of IgG and Dsg1 in PE (**a, b**), whereas negative IgG and smooth Dsg1 in SLE

Review Questions

1. Which localization of lesions is more likely to be present in a pemphigus foliaceus patient?
   (a) Abdomen
   (b) Feet
   (c) Upper trunk
2. The most prevalent area for endemic pemphigus is
   (a) Rural
   (b) Urban
   (c) none
3. First line treatment of pemphigus foliaceus is
   (a) dapsone
   (b) cyclophosphamide
   (c) systemic corticosteroids

Answers

1. (c)
2. (a)
3. (c)

On the Web

JAMA Dermatology Patient Page, Pemphigus http://archderm.jamanetwork.com/article.aspx?articleid=1879985

International Pemphigus & Pemphigoid Foundation http://www.pemphigus.org/

References

1. Jonkman MF. JAMA dermatology patient page. Pemphigus. JAMA Dermatol. 2014;150:680.
2. Schmidt E, Kasperkiewicz M, Joly P. Pemphigus. Lancet. 2019;394(10201):882–94.
3. Amagai M. Desmoglein as a target in autoimmunity and infection. J Am Acad Dermatol. 2003;48:244–52.
4. Joly P, Horváth B, Patsatsi A, Uzun S, Bech R, Beissert S, Bergman R, Bernard P, Borradori L, Caproni M, Caux F, Cianchini G, Daneshpazhooh M, De D, Dmochowski M, Drenovska K, Ehrchen J, Feliciani C, Goebeler M, Groves R, Guenther C, Hofmann S, Ioannides D, Kowalewski C, Ludwig R, Lim YL, Marinovic B, Marzano AV, Mascaró JM Jr, Mimouni D, Murrell DF, Pincelli C, Squarcioni CP, Sárdy M, Setterfield J, Sprecher E, Vassileva S, Wozniak K, Yayli S, Zambruno G, Zillikens D, Hertl M, Schmidt E. Updated S2K guidelines on the management of pemphigus vulgaris and foliaceus initiated by the european academy of dermatology and venereology (EADV). J Eur Acad Dermatol Venereol. 2020;34(9):1900–13.
5. Abreu-Velez AM, Reason IJ, Howard MS, Roselino AM. Endemic pemphigus foliaceus over a century: part I. N Am J Med Sci. 2010;2:51–9.
6. Bastuji-Garin S, Turki H, Mokhtar I, Nouira R, Fazaa B, Jomaa B, Zahaf A, Osman AB, Souissi R, Hémon D, Roujeau JC, Kamoun MR. Possible relation of Tunisian pemphigus with traditional cosmetics: a multicenter case-control study. Am J Epidemiol. 2002;155:249–56.
7. de Waard M, Jonkman MF. Chapter 14. Bullous diseases. In: Hamerlinck F, Lambert J, Neumann H, editors. Textbook of ethnic dermatology Haarlem. DCHG Medical Communication: The Netherlands; 2012. p. 157.
8. Lombardi C, Borges PC, Chaul A, Sampaio SA, Rivitti EA, Friedman H, Martins CR, Sanches Júnior JA, Cunha PR, Hoffmann RG, Diaz LA. Environmental risk factors in endemic pemphigus foliaceus (Fogo selvagem). "The Cooperative Group on Fogo Selvagem Research". J Invest Dermatol. 1992;98:847–50.
9. Goncalves GA, Brito MM, Salathiel AM, Ferraz TS, Alves D, Roselino AM. Incidence of pemphigus vulgaris exceeds that of pemphigus foliaceus in a region where pemphigus foliaceus is endemic: analysis of a 21-year historical series. An Bras Dermatol. 2011;86:1109–12.
10. Jablonska S, Chorzelski TP, Beutner EH, Chorzelska J. Herpetiform pemphigus, a variable pattern of pemphigus. Int J Dermatol. 1975;14:353–9.
11. Santi CG, Maruta CW, Aoki V, Sotto MN, Rivitti EA, Diaz LA. Pemphigus herpetiformis is a rare clinical expression of nonendemic pemphigus foliaceus, fogo selvagem, and pemphigus vulgaris. Cooperative Group on Fogo Selvagem Research. J Am Acad Dermatol. 1996;34:40–6.
12. Kasperkiewicz M, Kowalewski C, Jabłońska S. Pemphigus herpetiformis: from first description until now. J Am Acad Dermatol. 2014;70:780–7.
13. Senear FE, Usher B. An unusual type of pemphigus combining features of lupus erythematosus. Arch Dermatol Syphilol. 1926;13:761–81.
14. Chorzelski T, Jabłońska S, Blaszczyk M. Immunopathological investigations in the Senear-Usher syndrome (coexistence of pemphigus and lupus erythematosus). Br J Dermatol. 1968;80:211–7.
15. Oktarina DAM, Poot AM, Kramer D, Diercks GFH, Jonkman MF, Pas HH. The IgG "lupus-band" deposition pattern of pemphigus erythematosus: association with the desmoglein 1 ectodomain as revealed by 3 cases. Arch Dermatol. 2012;148:1173–8.

Further Reading

Hertl M, Jedlickova H, Karpati S, Marinovic B, Uzun S, Yayli S, Mimouni D, Borradori L, Feliciani C, Ioannides D, Joly P, Kowalewski C, Zambruno G, Zillikens D, Jonkman MF. Pemphigus. S2 guideline for diagnosis and treatment—guided by the European Dermatology Forum (EDF) in cooperation with the European Academy of Dermatology and Venereology (EADV). J Eur Acad Dermatol Venereol. 2014;29:405–14.

Paraneoplastic Pemphigus

Angelique M. Poot, Gilles F. H. Diercks, Hendri H. Pas, Marcel F. Jonkman, and Barbara Horváth

Introduction and AIMS

Short Definition in Layman Terms

Paraneoplastic pemphigus (PNP) is an autoimmune disease, with severe blistering of the lips and oral mucosa, and occurs in the presence of an underlying neoplasm.

A. M. Poot
Center for Blistering Diseases, Department of Dermatology, University Medical Center Groningen, University of Groningen, Groningen, The Netherlands

Department of Dermatology, Medisch Centrum Twente (MST), Enschede, The Netherlands

G. F. H. Diercks
Center for Blistering Diseases, Department of Dermatology, University Medical Center Groningen, University of Groningen, Groningen, The Netherlands

Center for Blistering Diseases, Department of Pathology, University Medical Center Groningen, University of Groningen,
Groningen, The Netherlands
e-mail: g.f.h.diercks@umcg.nl

H. H. Pas · M. F. Jonkman (Deceased)
B. Horváth (✉)
Center for Blistering Diseases, Department of Dermatology, University Medical Center Groningen, University of Groningen, Groningen, The Netherlands
e-mail: h.h.pas@umcg.nl; b.horvath@umcg.nl

Learning Objectives
After reading this chapter you will:
1. Be able to recognize the spectrum of clinical manifestations of paraneoplastic pemphigus.
2. Know which neoplasms are most often associated with paraneoplastic pemphigus.
3. Know the tools and pitfalls in the diagnostic approach of paraneoplastic pemphigus.

Case Study: Part 1
A 69-year old female with painful erosions and hemorrhagic crusts covering her lips and buccal mucosa was seen at the emergency department. Erythematous macules and erosions were seen on her trunk and extremities. In addition, bullae were present on palms and soles. The patient mentioned having lost 10 kg in the last 6 months.

Didactical Questions

The manifestations of paraneoplastic pemphigus may be clinically indistinguishable from those of other blistering diseases.

How can we differentiate between paraneoplastic pemphigus and other clinically similar diseases? And why is this differentiation important?

Facts and Figures

Definitions and Classification

PNP is characterized by a painful oral stomatitis, a variety of skin manifestations, and a complex autoimmune response. It occurs in the presence of an underlying neoplasm, of which it may be the first sign in 10–30% of cases. PNP is sometimes be referred to as paraneoplastic autoimmune multiorgan syndrome (PAMS), because next to the mucous membranes and the skin, other organs such as the lungs may be affected, and because the histological hallmark for pemphigus, i.e. intraepidermal acantholysis, is not always present in PNP [1, 2].

The clinical hallmark of PNP is a painful stomatitis

Epidemiology

Up to-date around 500 PNP cases have been described worldwide, since 1990. It comprises 3–5% of all pemphigus cases. The underlying neoplasm is most often lymphoproliferative in nature, such as non-Hodgkins lymphoma, thymomas and leukemia. Sarcomas and other solid malignancies may also be found. In addition benign lymphoproliferative diseases may be underlying, such as Castlemans disease, which is most prevalent in young-adults and children with PNP [1–3].

The underlying neoplasm in PNP is most often lymphoproliferative in nature

Pathogenesis

The autoantibody response in PNP is directed against multiple antigens found in skin and mucosa, including the proteins of the plakin family (such as envoplakin, periplakin, desmoplakin and BP230), the protease inhibitor alpha-2-macroglobulin-like 1 protein (A2ML1) and the desmosomal cadherins desmoglein 3 and less often desmoglein 1. These antigens are involved in cell-cell or cell-matrix adhesion. The source of these autoantibodies and their exact role in the pathogenesis of PNP is not yet fully understood. Neoplastic cells may produce these autoantibodies themselves, or may stimulate B-cells to do so. The autoantibodies are thought to induce blisters of mucosa and skin, via acantholysis or other means. Cellular auto-immunity also plays a role in PNP. The variety of clinical manifestations of PNP is attributed to the balance between the cellular and humoral response. A cellular autoimmune reaction produces more lichenoid clinical features, whereas the humoral autoimmune reaction leads to more pemphigus and pemphigoid-like clinical manifestations [3, 4].

The balance between the humoral and cellular autoimmune response determines the type of cutaneous manifestations in PNP

Diagnosis Paths

History and Physical Examination

PNP usually affects adults, with an average age of onset being 60 years. Rarely children may also be affected.

The most characteristic clinical feature of PNP, is a painful severe oral stomatitis, with hemorrhagic crusts and erosions of the intra-oral mucosa, extending to include the vermilion border of the lips. Conjunctival and genital mucosa may also be involved. Cutaneous manifestations range from flaccid to tense blisters as seen in pemphigus vulgaris and bullous pemphigoid, painful erythema and skin detachment as seen in toxic epidermal necrolysis, targetoid lesions as seen in erythema multiforme, and lichenoid papules and plaques as seen in lichen planus, or the variable manifestations of graft versus host disease, but may also be absent in a subset of patients. The distribution typically involves the face, trunk and extremities, but may also include palms and soles, which distinguishes it from the classical pemphigus variants. A subset of patients, ranging from 8 to 93%, may develop shortness of breath or even respiratory failure, due to bronchiolitis obliterans [5, 6]. Not frequently, also other auto-immune disease can develop, as myasthenia gravis, glomerulosclerosis or paraneoplastic neurological syndrome [2].

A subset of PNP patients develop bronchiolitis obliterans

Diagnostics

Diagnosis of PNP is based on three main features (Table 10.1). The demonstration of envoplakin and periplakin antibodies is most sensitive and specific. Immunoblotting, immunoprecipitation, and indirect immunofluorescence on rat bladder urothelium (Fig. 10.1) are suitable tools to detect these antibodies [7]. Direct immunofluorescence of patient skin may also be used but is not very sensitive and specific for PNP (Fig. 10.2).

The diagnosis of PNP is confirmed by the demonstration of envoplakin and periplakin, and/or A2ML1 antibodies in patient serum

In a small subset of PNP patients, often with lichenoid skin lesions, no circulating antibodies are detected, probably because the cellular autoimmune response, and not the humoral, dominates in these patients with 'lichenoid PNP'.

Histological features of PNP vary, including intra-epidermal acantholysis, subepidermal blistering, interface dermatitis and keratinocyte apoptosis and necrosis. Therefore histology alone is not sufficient to confirm the diagnosis of PNP [1, 4].

Table 10.1 Diagnostic criteria for paraneoplastic pemphigus [3]

#	Criterium
1	Presence of severe stomatitis (cheilitis)
2	Histology of acantholysis and/or interface dermatitis
3	Presence of an underlying neoplasm
4	The demonstration of envoplakin and periplakin and/or A2ML1 antibodies in the serum of patients

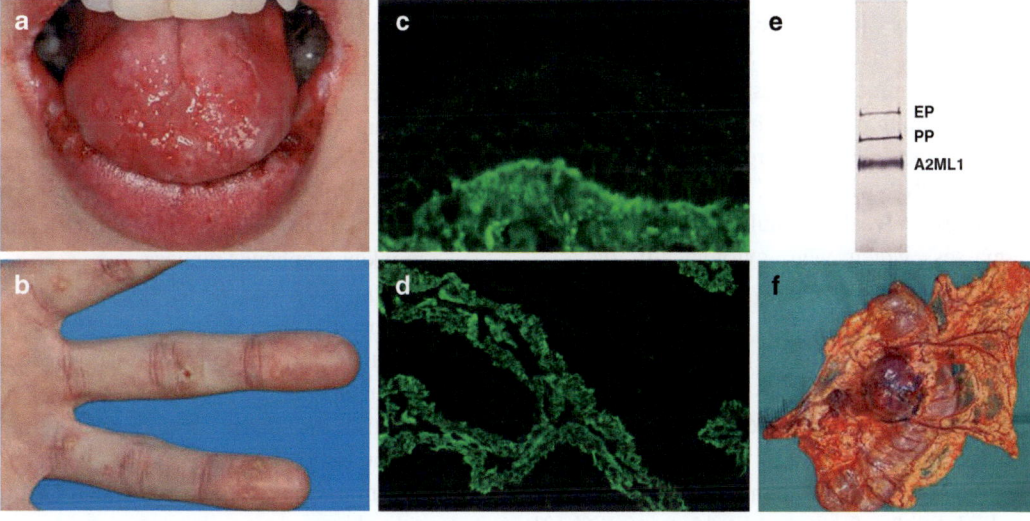

Fig. 10.1 Paraneoplastic pemphigus (**a**) hemorrhagic cheilitis and stomatitis (**b**) punctate keratoses on the palms (**c**) immunodepositions both, on the epithelial cell surface and along the basement membrane zone (**d**) serum immunoassay positivity on rat bladder (**e**) autoantibodies to envoplakin (EP), periplakin (PP) and alpha-2-macroglobulin-like 1 (A2ML1) (**f**) intra-abdominal tumor: follicular dendritic cell sarcoma. Copyright © 2021 John Wiley and Sons. All right reserved

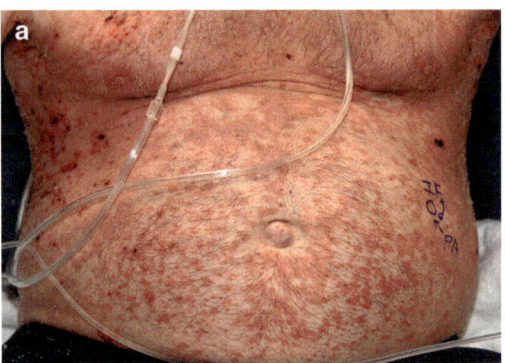
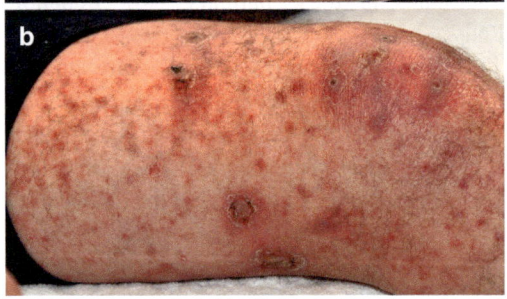

Fig. 10.2 Paraneoplastic pemphigus in a male with lichenoid phenotype showing (**a**) macular erythema with fine scales on the trunk and erosions in the flanks. (**b**) On the upper leg lichenoid plaques are discernable

A small subset of PNP patients are seronegative

Case study: Part 2
Drug history was negative, ruling out toxic epidermal necrolysis. Serology showed negative immunoblot results, but a positive IgG staining of the rat bladder urothelium by indirect immunofluorescence. The diagnosis PNP was made. Further imaging studies revealed multiple abdominal masses, which were cytologically diagnosed as non Hogdkin lymphoma.

Treatment and Prognosis

Despite aggressive treatment, mortality rates are high, with a 5-year survival rate of 38% [3] Rituximab and traditional immunosuppressiva as corticosteroids, cyclosporine, cyclophosphamide, azathioprine and mycophenolate mofetil are used [3]. More recently, several cases are published over PNP treatedwith ibrutinib, a Bruton's kinase inhibitor, alemtuzumab an anti-CD52 monoclonal antibody and tocilizumab, an anti-IL-6 monoclonal antibody with various outcomes [3].

Noteworthy, in addition to the medical treatment, the underlying neoplasm must be treated. The presence of bronchiolitis obliterans or toxic epidermal necrolysis-like clinics seems to be independent negative prognostic factors for death in PNP [3] Deaths occur mainly due to infections and progression of the underlying malignancy [6]. Patients with Castleman disease seem to have a better prognosis for survive.

Case Study: Part 3
The patient was started on R-CHOP chemotherapy (rituximab, cyclophosphamide, hydroxydaunorubicin, oncovin, and prednisolone), but after 1 week developed a *S. aureus* sepsis and respiratory failure. Three weeks later, she died of multi-organ failure.

Review Questions

1. PNP patients are characterized clinically by:
   (a) A severe stomatitis.
   (b) The combination of flaccid and tense blisters.
   (c) lichenoid plaques.
2. Which of the following results confirm the diagnosis PNP?
   (a) Cell surface staining of serum IgG in monkey esophagus mucosa.
   (b) A dual ECS and BMZ IgG deposition pattern in patient skin.
   (c) Serum IgG binding to rat bladder urothelium.
   (d) Positive anti-desmoglein 3 IgG serum antibodies by ELISA.
   (e) Serum IgG binding to the roof of salt-split skin.
3. Theoretically, which subset of PNP patients is more likely to have negative serology?
   (a) Patients with flaccid intraepidermal blisters.

(b) Patients with tense, subepidermal blisters.
(c) Patients with lichenoid plaques, showing interface dermatitis in histology.
4. Which autoantibodies are most sensitive and specific for PNP?
   (a) envoplakin and periplakin antibodies.
   (b) BP230 antibodies.
   (c) desmoglein 3 antibodies.
   (d) A2ML1 antibodies.

Answers

1. a
2. c
3. c
4. a

References

1. Anhalt GJ. Paraneoplastic pemphigus. J Investig Dermatol Symp Proc. 2004;9:29–33.
2. Amber KT, Valdebran M, Grando SA. Paraneoplastic autoimmune multiorgan syndrome (PAMS): beyond the single phenotype of paraneoplastic pemphigus. Autoimmun Rev. 2018;17(10):1002–10.
3. Kim JH, Kim SC. Paraneoplastic pemphigus: paraneoplastic autoimmune disease of the skin and mucosa. Front Immunol. 2019;10:1259.
4. Czernik A, Camilleri M, Pittelkow MR, Grando SA. Paraneoplastic autoimmune multiorgan syndrome: 20 years after. Int J Dermatol. 2011;50:905–14.
5. Leger S, Picard D, Ingen-Housz-Oro S, Arnault JP, Aubin F, Carsuzaa F, Chaumentin G, Chevrant-Breton J, Chosidow O, Crickx B, D'incan M, Dandurand M, Debarbieux S, Delaporte E, Dereure O, Doutre MS, Guillet G, Jullien D, Kupfer I, Lacour JP, Leonard F, Lok C, Machet L, Martin L, Paul C, Pignon JM, Robert C, Thomas L, Weiller PJ, Ferranti V, Gilbert D, Courville P, Houivet E, Benichou J, Joly P. Prognostic factors of paraneoplastic pemphigus. Arch Dermatol. 2012;148:1165–72.
6. Zimmermann J, Bahmer F, Rose C, Zillikens D, Schmidt E. Clinical and immunopathological spectrum of paraneoplastic pemphigus. J Dtsch Dermatol Ges. 2010;8:598–606.
7. Poot AM, Diercks GF, Kramer D, Schepens I, Klunder G, Hashimoto T, Borradori L, Jonkman MF, Pas HH. Laboratory diagnosis of paraneoplastic pemphigus. Br J Dermatol. 2013;169:1016–24.

IgA Pemphigus

11

Barbara Horváth and Marcel F. Jonkman

Introduction and AIMS

Short Definition in Layman Terms

IgA pemphigus is a distinct form of pemphigus characterized by tissue-bound and circulating IgA autoantibodies against desmosomal and non-desmosomal surface antigens.

IgA pemphigus is a rare disease mediated by IgA autoantibodies against desmosomal and non-desmosomal epithelial cell surface antigens

Learning Objectives
After reading this chapter you will be able to diagnose and differentiate pustular dermatoses and to recognize the classic clinics of IgA pemphigus. You will be able to perform and interpret the immunological tests and to make a treatment algorithm.

Case Study: Part 1
77-year old male patient presented with widespread annular erythematous plaques with tiny pustules at the periphery on the trunk and extremities (Fig. 11.1). There was erythema, edema and desquamation on the palms and footpads. The body folds like armpits, groin were not affected. Patients had malaise, but no fever was detected.

Previously there were no changes in medication. Medical history was negative for atopic disease and psoriasis. No drug allergy was previously documented.

Didactical Questions: Cross Section of Questions to Prime the Readers Interest

How can you diagnose a sterile pustular dermatosis? What would you see in the histopathological section? How can you make the difference between autoimmune and autoinflammatory diseases? In this section the focus is on the clinical differential diagnostics and work up of patients with extensive pustular dermatosis.

B. Horváth (✉) · M. F. Jonkman (Deceased)
Center for Blistering Diseases, Department of Dermatology, University Medical Center Groningen, University of Groningen,
Groningen, The Netherlands
e-mail: b.horvath@umcg.nl

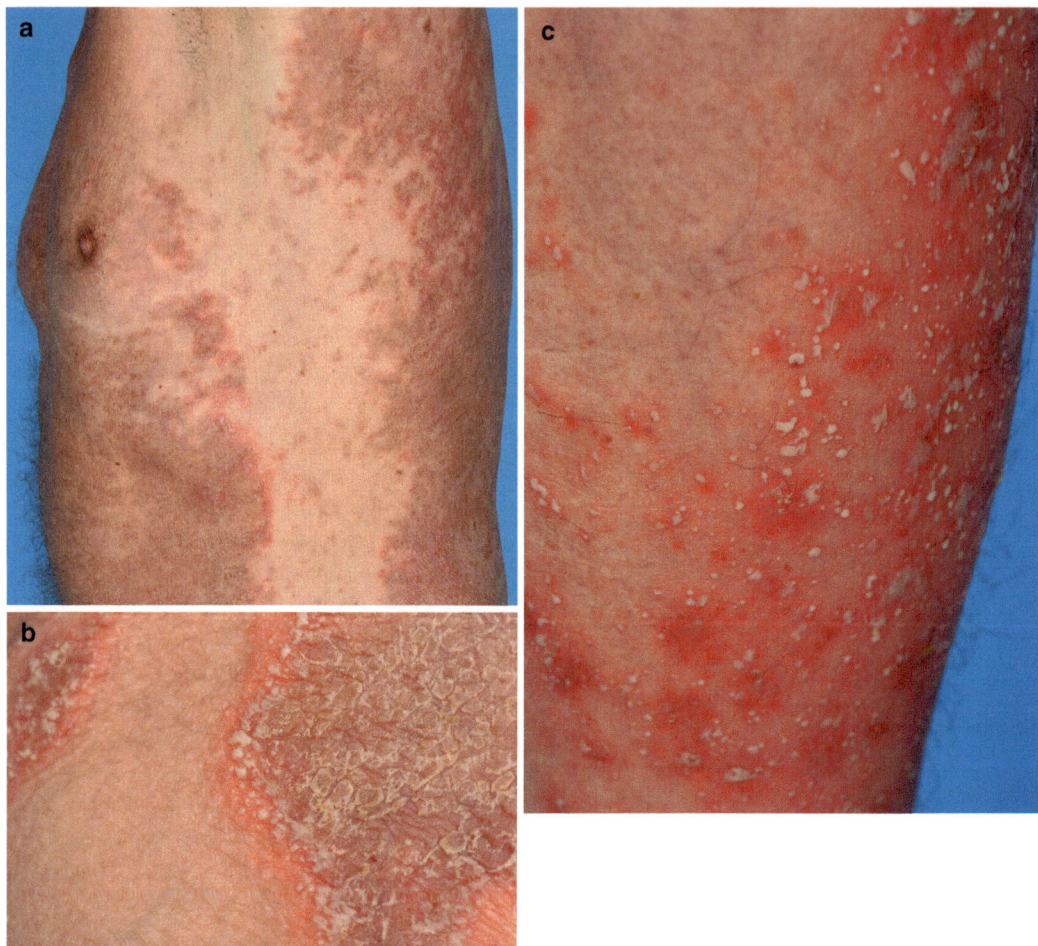

Fig. 11.1 IgA pemphigus in a patient with erythematous plaques with miliary to lenticular pustules over (**a**) the trunk, and (**c**) extremities. (**b**) In detail, the pustules are distributed on the advancing edge (circinate) of the erythematous plaques

Facts and Figures

Definitions and Classification

IgA pemphigus (IGAP) is an autoimmune blistering disease characterized by tissue-bound and circulating autoantibodies exclusively from de IgA class against desmosomal and non-desmosomal surface proteins of the epidermis [1, 2]. Based on the clinics, histology and the autoantibody pattern it is divided into two major forms; the *subcorneal pustulosis dermatosis* type (SPD-type) and the *intraepidermal neutrophilic IgA dermatosis* type (IEN-type). However, there are still cases of atypical overlapping phenotype of IGAP which can't be classified into these two forms [3]. Moreover, in classic subcorneal pustular dermatosis or Sneddon-Wilkinson's disease no autoantibodies are detected in skin or serum.

Sneddon-Wilkinson's disease is similar to IgA pemphigus SPD type but without the IgA depositions in the skin

Epidemiology

IGAP has several synonyms such as intraepidermal neutrophilic IgA dermatosis, intercellular IgA dermatosis, IgA pemphigus foliaceus, intraepidermal IgA pustulosis, and IgA herpetiform pemphigus. A recent systemic review identified around 100 cases of IGAP [3]. IGAP has a slight female predominance with an age distribution of 1-month to 92-years, with an average of 51.5 years [3, 4]. It seems widely distributed all over the word as several cases are reported from all over the world.

Pathogenesis

In the SDP-type the IgA autoantibodies target the desmosomal cadherins. In most cases the major autoantigen is desmocollin 1 (Dsc1) which is expressed in the upper part of the epidermis [4, 5], but also other desmocollins can be targeted like desmocollin 2 (Dsc2) and desmocollin 3 (Dsc3). The autoantigen profile of the IEN-type more heterogeneous, no major autoantigen is identified yet. Some studies report reactivity against desmogleins 1 and 3, desmocollins 1–3, as well as other, still unknown, non-desmosomal proteins on the epithelial cell surface [6].

Using immunoelectron microscopy gold particles are mostly seen in the extracellular spaces between keratinocytes at desmosomes in SDP-type IGAP. In contrast, in IEN type, the gold particles are mainly in the intercellular spaces in non-desmosomal areas [6].

Once IgA is bound to the keratinocyte surface neutrophils accumulate in the epidermis leading to intraepidermal blister, later pustule formation. However the exact pathomechanism is still unknown.

In the SDP-type IGAP the IgA autoantibodies target mostly desmocollin 1, whereas the autoantigen profile of the IEN-type are heterogeneous; the major autoantigen is still not revealed.

Diagnosis Paths

History and Physical Examination

Onset of IgA pemphigus is subacute [1], first small fragile vesicles appear but soon they transform to pustules. The lesions spread centrifugal and form annular plaques with collarette-like scaling. The **SPD-type** is undistinguishable from the classic SPD; there are erythematous skin lesions with **tiny superficial** circinate pustules, and later desquamation from the edges surfacing the entire body, particularly in the intertriginous areas. In contrast the **IEN-type** is characterized by annular erythematous plaques with circinate pustules and crusts that spread outwards and heal inwards, giving the lesions a so-called **sunflower-like appearance**. Mucous membranes are almost always spared [1].

General Diagnostics

Routine histopathology in the SPD-type IGAP shows infiltration of neutrophils in the epidermis and upper dermis with subcorneal pustules, acantholysis can be seen, but not always. The IEN-type is characterized by blisters filled with neutrophils in the middle layers of the epidermis, acantholysis is sparse or absent. Sometimes eosinophils are seen in the intraepidermal pustules [7].

A recent systematic review revealed that 18% of the IGAP patient has a coexistent malignancy (mostly IgA gammopathy), but also concomitant appearance of solid tumors, autoimmune diseases, like ulcerative colitis, Crohn's disease, Sjogren syndrome and also HIV infections were reported. As none of the patient had a known IgA gammopathy before the diagnosis of IGAP, despite the low evidence, screening for IgA gammopathy is advisable [3].

In IGAP screening for IgA gammopathy is advisable.

Specific Diagnostics

By direct immunofluorescence, the SPD-type IGAP shows IgA depositions on cell surfaces in the uppermost layers of the epidermis. Conversely, in the IEN-type the IgA depositions are distributed over the whole thickness of the epidermis [8]. As mentioned before in 10% of the cases a combined IgA/IgG and C3 deposition is detectable.

The circulating IgA antibodies are detectable only about 66.7% of the cases on indirect immunofluorescence [3]. Using normal human skin sections, autoantibodies react with the upper part of the epidermis in the SPD-type, whereas with the whole epidermis in the IEN-type [2].

Standard immunoblotting technique can be disappointing, as no consequent reactivity can be seen, maybe due to the conformation sensitive epitopes in IGAP. Only some cases with anti-Dsg3 showed reactivity in immunoblot [2]. ELISA testing for IgA to desmoglein 1 and 3 is not standard [2]. The most useful assay to detect IgA antibodies targeting conformation dependent epitopes on desmocollin 1 is using cDNA transfected COS-7 [4]. However this technique is available only in specific laboratories.

Case Study: Part 2

Routine laboratory examination showed leukocytosis (WBC: 16.9 10^9/ml) with neutrophilia (15.46 10^9/ml), elevated ESR (71 mm per hour) and CRP (177 IU/ml).

Common bacterial swab of the pustule and blood showed no microorganism. On histopathological examination were intra-en subcorneal neutrophil accumulations (pustules) seen in the epidermis without the presence of eosinophil granulocytes.

Direct immunofluorescence microscopy showed fine granular ECS depositions of IgA (2+) in the upper epidermal layers (Fig. 11.2). On indirect immunofluorescence no circulating autoantibodies either of IgA or IgG class were detected on monkey esophagus. Further serological examinations on salt-split skin, Western blot, and desmogleins 1 and 3 ELISA were all negative for both IgA and IgG.

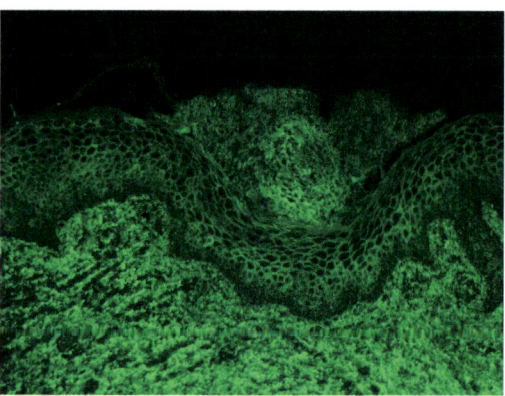

Fig. 11.2 Direct immunofluorescence of skin biopsy reveals epithelial cell surface (ECM) depositions of IgA in the epidermis. Note the pustule in the center due to subcorneal accumulation of neutrophils

Treatment Tricks

Initial Treatment and Therapeutic Ladder

Due to its rarity treatment protocols are missing. Treatment algorithm is adapted and from pemphigus and from the neutrophil dermatoses.

The first line therapy is dapsone (25–125 mg/day) because it suppresses several functions of neutrophils (see box Dapsone Chap. 20) [9]. If dapsone is contraindicated or not effective retinoids are the drugs of choice. Previously etretinate was given with success, nowadays several success is reported by acitretin [10] or isotretinoin.

Topical or systemic corticosteroid are also used. There are single case reports describe positive effect of adalimumab and mycophenolate mofetil, colchicine, tetracycline, sulfamethoxazole/trimethoprim, methotrexate, cyclosporine. Surprisingly positive effect of UVA photochemotherapy (PUVA) is observed [11].

The first line therapy is dapsone because it suppresses several functions of neutrophils

Case Study: Part 3

After excluding glucose-6-phosphat dehydrogenase (G6PD) deficiency patient received dapsone orally. The initial dose was 50 mg per day, which was increased up to 75 mg daily after 1 week under blood controls. Unfortunately soon after patient developed dyspnoe and acral cyanosis. Blood examination showed a slightly elevated methemoglobin within the normal range and elevated sulfahemoglobin, patient still had good hemoglobins levels, but the reticulocytes were low (not compensating hemolysis). After tapering and stopping dapsone the cyanosis improved, but patient was not able to restart dapsone because of the return of acrocyanosis and dyspnoe. In the next step patients received topical clobetasol ointment daily with acceptable result.

Follow-Up and Tapering

IGAP seems to be recalcitrant disease, so frequently combined therapy is needed [11].

Review Questions

1. What is not a subtype of IGAP?
    (a) Subcorneale pustulosus dermatosis type
    (b) Intraepidermal neutrophilic IgA dermatosis type
    (c) Sneddon-Wilkinson disease
2. Which form of IGAP is characterized by erythematous skin lesions with tiny superficial pustules, particularly in the intertriginous areas?
    (a) SPD-type
    (b) IEN-type
    (c) Both types
3. Which form of IGAP is characterized by the so called sunflower-like appearance?
    (a) SPD-type
    (b) IEN-type
    (c) Both types
4. First line treatment of IGAP is
    (a) dapsone
    (b) systemic corticosteroids
    (c) azathioprine
5. Which medication is the 2nd choice?
    (a) Super potent topical corticosteroids
    (b) retinoids
    (c) azathioprine

Answers

1. c.
2. a.
3. b.
4. b.
5. a.

On the Web

http://www.emedicine.medscape.com/article/1063776-overview.

References

1. Tsuruta D, Ishii N, Hamada T, Ohyama B, Fukuda S, Koga H, Imamura K, Kobayashi H, Karashima T, Nakama T, Dainichi T, Hashimoto T. IgA pemphigus. Clin Dermatol. 2011;29:437–42.
2. Hashimoto T. Immunopathology of IgA pemphigus. Clin Dermatol. 2001;19:683–9.
3. Kridin K, Patel PM, Jones VA, Cordova A, Amber KT. IgA pemphigus: a systematic review. J Am Acad Dermatol. 2020;82(6):1386–92.
4. Suzuki M, Karube S, Kobori Y, Usui K, Murata S, Kato H, Nakagawa H. IgA pemphigus occur-

ring in a 1-month-old infant. J Am Acad Dermatol. 2003;48:S22–4.
5. Hashimoto T, Kiyokawa C, Mori O, Miyasato M, Chidgey MA, Garrod DR, Kobayashi Y, Komori K, Ishii K, Amagai M, Nishikawa T. Human desmocollin 1 (Dsc1) is an autoantigen for the subcorneal pustular dermatosis type of IgA pemphigus. J Invest Dermatol. 1997;109:127–31.
6. Ishii N, Ishida-Yamamoto A, Hashimoto T. Immunolocalization of target autoantigens in IgA pemphigus. Clin Exp Dermatol. 2004;29:62–6.
7. Nishikawa T, Hashimoto T. Dermatoses with intraepidermal IgA deposits. Clin Dermatol. 2000;18:315–8.
8. Hashimoto T, Ebihara T, Nishikawa T. Studies of autoantigens recognized by IgA anti-keratinocyte cell surface antibodies. J Dermatol Sci. 1996;12:10–7.
9. Hirata Y, Abe R, Kikuchi K, Hamasaka A, Shinkuma S, Ujiie H, Nomura T, Nishie W, Arita K, Shimizu H. Intraepidermal neutrophilic IgA pemphigus successfully treated with dapsone. Eur J Dermatol. 2012;22:282–3.
10. Ruiz-Genao DP, Hernandez-Nunez A, Hashimoto T, Amagai M, Fernandez-Herrera J, Garcia-Diez A. A case of IgA pemphigus successfully treated with acitretin. Br J Dermatol. 2002;147:1040–2.
11. Yasuda H, Kobayashi H, Hashimoto T, Itoh K, Yamane M, Nakamura J. Subcorneal pustular dermatosis type of IgA pemphigus: demonstration of autoantibodies to desmocollin-1 and clinical review. Br J Dermatol. 2000;143:144–8.

Further Reading

Hashimoto T, Komai A, Futei Y, Nishikawa T, Amagai M. Detection of IgA autoantibodies to desmogleins by an enzyme-linked immunosorbent assay: the presence of new minor subtypes of IgA pemphigus. Arch Dermatol. 2001;137:735–8.

Ishii N, Ishida-Yamamoto A, Hashimoto T. Immunolocalization of target autoantigens in IgA pemphigus. Clin Exp Dermatol. 2004;29:62–6.

Geller S, Gat AA, Zeeli T, Hafner A, Eming R, Hertl M, Sprecher E. The expanding spectrum of IgA pemphigus: a case report and a review of the literature. Br J Dermatol. 2014;171:650–6.

Moreno AC, Santi CG, Gabbi TV, Aoki V, Hashimoto T, Maruta CW. IgA pemphigus: case series with emphasis on therapeutic response. J Am Acad Dermatol. 2014;70:200–1.

Drug-Induced Pemphigus

12

Sylvia H. Kardaun
and Laura de Sena Nogueira Maehara

Short Introduction in Layman Terms

Pemphigus can be induced or triggered by drugs. In drug-induced pemphigus (DIP) the disease was not present before exposure to the putative drug, whereas in drug-triggered pemphigus (DTP) the autoimmune process was already programmed by a predisposed genetic background, and only facilitated by the drug. Contrary to the latency time in most other cutaneous adverse drug reactions, latency between start of new medication and onset of the reaction can sometimes be long, up to several months. This can easily lead to a missed diagnosis. Timely withdrawal of the culprit drug regularly results in full resolution in DIP, whereas in DTP this is generally not the case. Because both DIP/DTP and idiopathic pemphigus mainly occur in the elderly, often using polypharmacy, establishing the culprit can be challenging.

S. H. Kardaun (✉)
Department of Dermatology, Center for Blistering Diseases, University Medical Center Groningen, University of Groningen,
Groningen, The Netherlands

L. de Sena Nogueira Maehara
Department of Dermatology, Center for Blistering Diseases, University Medical Center Groningen, University of Groningen,
Groningen, The Netherlands

Department of Dermatology, Paulista School of Medicine, Federal University of São Paulo,
São Paulo, Brazil

Learning Objectives
After reading this chapter you should be aware that:

- Some drugs can induce or trigger pemphigus; in every patient with pemphigus, and in particular in new cases, a meticulous drug history should be taken to identify and withdraw potential culprits to achieve a potential remission.
- Although clinical and immunopathological features in DIP are rather similar to those in idiopathic pemphigus, itching or absence of mucosal involvement can be clues for the differentiation.
- Different subtypes of pemphigus can preferentially be provoked by different drugs or groups of drugs, sometimes with a different prognosis.

Case Study: Part 1
A 57-year-old woman presented with pruritic, painful erosions and crusts on the upper trunk since 2 weeks. She denied fever and the use of new medication. Careful history learned that captopril had been prescribed for hypertension since 6 months. Moreover, penicillin i.v. had been used for 10 days for erysipelas, 2 weeks before the onset of trunk lesions.

Facts and Figures

To date, more than 100 drugs have been associated with pemphigus, classified in three different functional groups (Table 12.1): (1) thiol-associated drugs (drugs containing a thiol (-SH) group or a disulphide bond that releases SH groups or "masked thiols": non-thiol drugs containing sulphur that metabolizes to an active thiol group), (2) phenol drugs, and (3) non-thiol/non-phenol drugs [1–6]. Next to systemic drugs, some cases of "contact pemphigus" have been ascribed to topical application of e.g. ophthalmic drops or cutaneous ointments such as imiquimod or cantharidin [4].

Although cases of DIP have been regularly published, it is a rare condition occurring in probably 10% of pemphigus, with a slight male predominance, except for penicillamine in which females outnumber males. However, because e.g. penicillins are regularly prescribed and probably often overlooked as a culprit, pemphigus might be more often drug related than previously substantiated.

Clinical presentations of DIP comprise pemphigus vulgaris (PV, most cases), closely followed by pemphigus foliaceus (PF), and few cases of pemphigus erythematosus (PE), pemphigus herpetiformis (PH), IgA pemphigus, polymorphic pemphigus, combined features of pemphigus and pemphigoid, paraneoplastic pemphigus, and unclassified cases [1].

Contrary to idiopathic pemphigus, DIP is often associated with pruritus and has a prodromal stage with nonspecific lesions resembling common drug eruptions, preceding the genuine pemphigus lesions, or e.g. pharyngitis. Full-blown DIP often shows scaling and crusting (PF, Fig. 12.1), seborrheic lesions with a butterfly distribution predominantly on the face (PE), or small vesicles with crusted erosions grouped to annular or gyrate lesions (PH) [2].

It is estimated that up to 7% of patients treated with penicillamine for at least 6 months might acquire pemphigus [2]. Thiol-drugs probably account for the majority of cases of DIP [6]. In a systematic review of 170 reported patients with the reported outcomes, thiol-associated drugs,

Table 12.1 Drugs involved in inducing or triggering pemphigus, grouped according to their chemical structure

Thiol-associated drugs
Penicillamine
Captopril
Bucillamine
Penicillins and its derivatives (aminopenicillins)
Cephalosporins[a]
Piroxicam
Gold sodium thiomalate
Imatinib
Thiamazole
Thiopronin
Pyritinol[a]
5-thiopyridoxine[a]
Phenols (drugs containing a phenol ring)
Cephalosporins[a]
Aspirin
Rifampicin
Levodopa
Heroin
Pentachlorophenol
Phenobarbital
Pyritinol[a]
5-thiopyridoxine[a]
Non-thiol, non-phenol drugs
ACE inhibitors other than captopril
Ca channel blockers
Most NSAIDs
Nifedipine
Biological modifiers of the immune response[b]
Glibenclamide
Psoralens
Imiquimod
Others

ACE: angiotensin-converting enzyme, *NSAID:* nonsteroidal anti-inflammatory drug
[a]Both thiol and phenol drugs
[b]Including rituximab, interferon-α, interleukin-2, vaccins

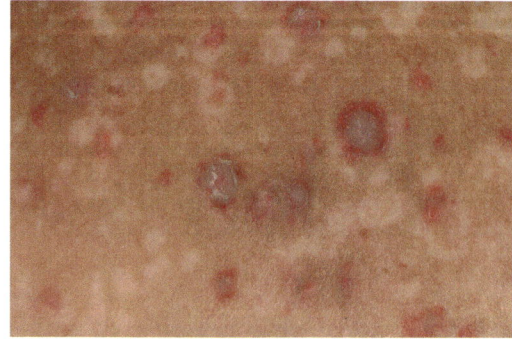

Fig. 12.1 Drug-induced pemphigus foliaceus in a female who received penicillamine for seronegative rheumatoid arthritis

especially penicillamine (33.1%), captopril (7.7%) and bucillamine (6.5%) were the three most reported drugs related to DIP, in which PF was the most common clinical presentation. The mean age was about 57 years, and most cases were less severe and had a better prognosis. Cutaneous, mucocutaneous and mucosal involvement were reported in 68.6, 30.1 resp. 1.3% with a mean latency of 154 days [1].

Where lesions can appear from days to several months after drug initiation with a median latency of 60 days, thiol drugs have a longer latency time compared to non-thiol drugs.

DIP caused by thiol drugs will often subside after drug withdrawal, in contrast to pemphigus due to non-thiol drugs [2]. In a systematic review of 170 reported patients, about 30% of thiol-associated pemphigus did resolve spontaneously after only drug withdrawal, others needed additional or maintenance therapy, while only about 12% did not heal [1]. The median time to remission was significantly longer for penicillamine-induced pemphigus (90 days) compared to captopril (60 days) or bucillamine or other drugs (30 days) [1].

Features of PV are most often seen in DIP and DTP in users of non-thiol drugs. Mucosal involvement is mainly restricted to the PV subtype and is otherwise rare. In the majority of DIP cases, tissue bound antibodies (93%) and less often circulating antibodies (Dsg 3: 34.9% and Dsg 1: 72.7%), although often with low titres are in accordance with idiopathic pemphigus, complicating differentiation [1, 3].

Notably, exacerbations or flares, mainly of PV, most likely caused by drugs. have also been reported, though never ascribed to thiol drugs.

Pathogenesis is not completely known, but probably comprises endogenous (e.g. predisposing genetic background or underlying comorbidities, especially of autoimmune origin, such as rheumatoid arthritis) and exogenous factors (e.g. drugs), acting as a trigger to unmask the disease. Immunologic acantholysis may start with biochemical events resulting in neoantigen formation and autoantibody production. Thiol-associated drugs and immune modulators could also directly interfere with the immune system resulting in release of forbidden B-cell clones. Moreover, autoantibodies could be mediated by enzymes promoting plasminogen activators. Phenol drugs may cause cytokine release, promoting acantholysis and effecting regulation and synthesis of complement and proteases. The non-thiol/non-phenol drugs may promote immune acantholysis in several ways: by overexpression of target antigens, overactivation of the immune system, amplification of the local immune response and release of plasminogen activators [3, 5].

Diagnosis Paths

Apart from idiopathic pemphigus, DIP and DTP should be differentiated from other bullous eruptions, such as bullous pemphigoid, erythema multiforme, Stevens-Johnson syndrome, impetigo, and varicella zoster. Every new case or flare up of pemphigus should be thoroughly investigated for a potential drug-relation. Cases of DIP may present with nonspecific cutaneous manifestations or e.g. pharyngytis before genuine lesions of pemphigus occur [3]. Pruritus or absence of mucosal involvement are important hints for DIP. History including in particular last year's drug use, nonspecific prodromal skin lesions and pruritus, is followed by a thorough dermatological examination of skin and mucosae. Histopathology may reveal eosinophilic spongiosis, epithelial necrosis, irregular acantholysis, variability of the epidermal splitting level, even in a single biopsy, and rather dense dermal infiltrates [3]. Intercellular antibodies are generally found in the skin, similar to in idiopathic pemphigus, but antibodies in the serum are more rare and, if present, of a low titre.

Drug causality in some cases has been strengthened e.g. by a positive patch test and/or lymphocyte transformation test with the suspected drug. Because the gold standard of dechallenge, followed by rechallenge with the suspected culprit is complicated due to the inherent risk, a stepwise dechallenge can be a useful alternative.

> **Case Study: Part 2**
> The patient had pruritus, scaling and small erosions on the face and upper body, while mucosal involvement was absent. Histology revealed cleavage of the epidermis at several levels and dermal mixed infiltrates containing many eosinophils. DIF identified intercellular epidermal staining, mainly confined to the upper layers. The ELISA test detected antibodies to desmoglein 1.

Treatment Tricks

Withdrawal of the suspected culprit drug is mandatory and, sometimes temporarily sustained by additional therapy, will lead to remission in approximately 50% of cases of DIP caused by thiol-associated drugs, opposed to only 15% in those due to non-thiol drugs [3]. However, sometimes maintenance therapy is needed. In DTP, despite elimination of the drug, the disease often continues with all the characteristics of idiopathic pemphigus, in particular when presenting as PV.

> **Case Study: Part 3**
> Captopril was withdrawn, while penicillin had already been stopped a few days earlier. Prednisolone 0.5 mg/kg resulted in remission within a few weeks. The preferred diagnosis was DIP, caused by captopril and/or penicillin. The patient was informed about the diagnosis, possible causes, the need for a careful follow up, and the advice to avoid certain drugs, especially those with "thiol groups" (see Table 12.1).

Review Questions

1. Choose the correct statement about drug-induced pemphigus:
   (a) In drug-induced pemphigus (DIP) the autoimmune disease was not programmed before the drug exposure.
   (b) In drug-triggered pemphigus (DTP) the autoimmune disease was not present before the drug exposure.
   (c) In drug-triggered pemphigus (DTP) the autoimmune process will be stopped after suspension of the culprit drug.
2. In DIP, lesions may appear from days to several months after drug initiation. Which drug is more likely to induce pemphigus with a longer time-latency?
   (a) enalapril
   (b) penicillamine
   (c) none
3. Drug withdrawal, sometimes temporarily sustained by additionally therapy will lead to remission of pemphigus in approximately:
   (a) 50% of cases due to non-thiol drugs
   (b) 50% of cases of DIP caused by thiol drugs
   (c) none of above

Answers

1. (a)
2. (b)
3. (b)

On the Web

Litt's Drug Eruption & Reaction Database. http://www.drugeruptiondata.com

References

1. Ghaedi F, Etesami I, Aryanian Z, Kalantari Y, Goodarzi A, Teymourpour S, Mahmoudi H, Daneshpazhooh M. Drug-induced pemphigus: a systematic review of 170 patients. Int Immunopharmacol. 2021;92:107299.
2. Brenner S, Wolf R, Ruocco V. Drug-induced pemphigus. Clin Dermatol. 1993;11:501–5.
3. Brenner S, Bialy-Golan A, Ruocco V. Drug-induced pemphigus. Clin Dermatol. 1998;16:393–7.
4. Brenner S, Goldberg I. Drug-induced pemphigus. Clin Dermatol. 2011;29:455–7.
5. Ruocco V, Ruocco E, Lo Schiavo A, Brunetti G, Guerrera LP, Wolf R. Pemphigus: etiology, pathogenesis, and inducing or triggering factors: facts and controversies. Clin Dermatol. 2013;31:374–81.
6. Goldberg I, Kashman Y, Brenner S. The induction of pemphigus by phenol drugs. Int J Dermatol. 1999;38:888–92.

Structure of Hemidesmosomes and the Epidermal Basement Membrane Zone

Iana Turcan, Maria C. Bolling, and Marcel F. Jonkman

Introduction and Aims

Learning Objectives
The role of hemidesmosomes and basement membrane in maintaining tissue organization and integrity is demonstrated in several sAIBDs. In this chapter, our aim is to explain the structural complexity and function of hemidesmosomal and basement membrane zone proteins and their relationship to each other and list the sAIBDs that involve them (see Table 13.1).

Facts and Figures

Hemidesmosomes

Hemidesmosomes (HDs) are specialized complexes that provide attachment of the intermediate filament network in epithelial cells to the underlying basement membrane in the skin,

Table 13.1 Targeted molecules and their corresponding autoimmune disease at the site of hemidesmosomes and basement membrane zone

Location	Molecule	Autoimmune blistering disease
Hemidesmosome	Plectin	Anti-plectin pemphigoid Paraneoplastic pemphigus
	BP180 BP230	Bullous pemphigoid Nonbullous cutaneous pemphigoid Brunsting-Perry pemphigoid Lichen planus pemphigoides Pemphigoid gestationis Linear IgA bullous dermatosis Mucous membrane pemphigoid
	LAD-1, LABD-97	Linear IgA bullous dermatosis
	α6β4 integrin	Mucous membrane pemphigoid
Basement membrane	Laminin 332 Laminin 311 (α3 chain)	Mucous membrane pemphigoid
	Type VII collagen	Epidermolysis bullosa acquisita
	p200	Anti-p200 pemphigoid

I. Turcan
Zürich, Switzerland

M. C. Bolling (✉) · M. F. Jonkman (Deceased)
Center for Blistering Diseases, Department of Dermatology, University Medical Center Groningen, University of Groningen,
Groningen, The Netherlands
e-mail: m.c.bolling@umcg.nl

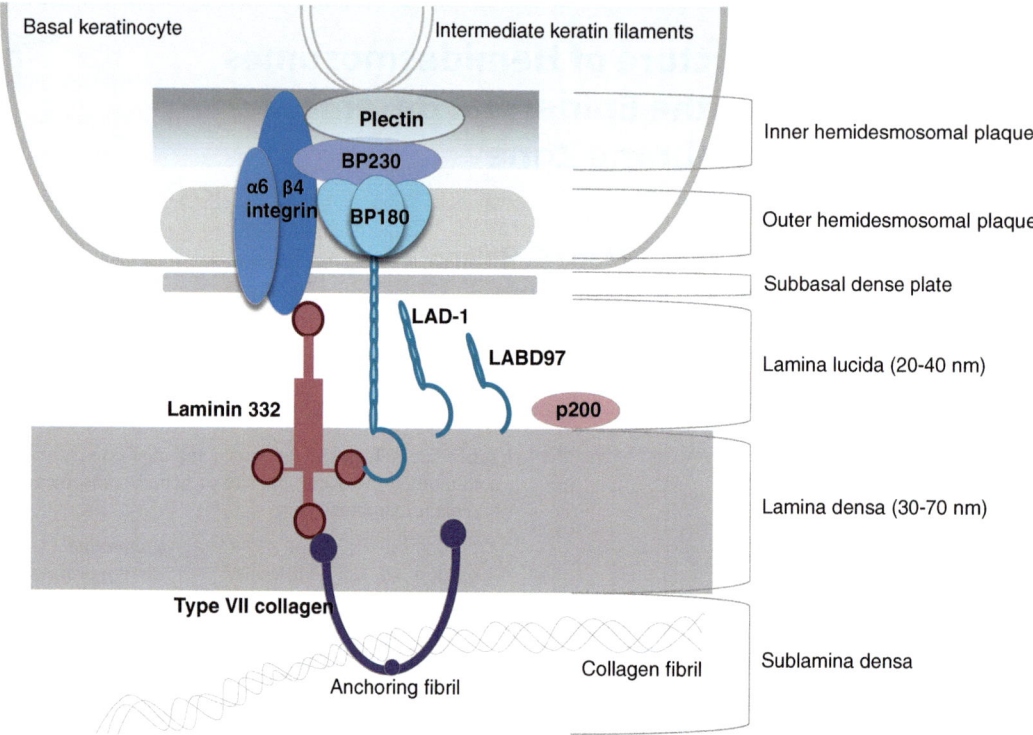

Fig. 13.1 Schematic representation of the hemidesmosome and dermal-epidermal junction including all molecules known to be targeted in autoimmune bullous diseases

mucous membranes of the cornea, pharynx, larynx, esophagus, genitals, and in the amnion. The name originates from its appearance as half of a desmosome, a cell-cell anchoring complex (see Chap. 7). HDs have a tripartite electron-dense plaque structure including the inner hemidesmosomal plaque, the outer hemidesmosomal plaque and the sub-basal dense plaque (Fig. 13.1).

Hemidesmosomes connect intermediate filaments to the basement membrane matrix

Subsequent is a succinct description of the most relevant constituents of HDs.

Plectin is a protein of the plakin family with a molecular mass over 500 kDa. This polypeptide consists of a central coiled-coil rod domain flanked by the globular N-terminal head domain and a C-terminal tail domain at each end, respectively. The N-terminus provides binding sites for integrin β4, BP180 and actin filaments, while the C-terminus connects to intermediate keratin filaments. Furthermore, plectin plays a role in attaching intermediate keratin filaments through association with BP230 [1]. Plectin has many isoforms with a long common rod domain, which are distributed in specific tissues such as stratified squamous epithelia, heart, skeletal muscle, and nerve tissue. Plectin 1a is the dominant isoform in hemidesmosomes in skin. This protein may become target for autoimmunity. Although a rare event, anti-plectin antibodies have been identified in sera from bullous pemphigoid (BP) patients [2]. Plectin has also been implicated as an autoantigen in paraneoplastic pemphigus (PNP).

BP230 is a member of the plakin protein family, like plectin. Also known as BPAG1, this molecule was the first discovered antigen to be targeted in bullous pemphigoid (BP). Structurally, BP230 is composed of a central coiled-coil rod domain flanked by N- and C-termini at each end, respectively. The N-terminus plays an important function in integrating BP230 into the HD and has BP180 and integrinβ4 as ligands; the C-terminus connects to intermediate keratin filaments [3]. Through alternative splicing, the DST gene encoding BP230 generates tissue-specific isoforms expressed in the skin, central nervous system, and muscles, respectively [4]. BP230 has been involved as an autoantigen in several sAIBDs including BP, mucous membrane pemphigoid (MMP), Brunsting-Perry pemphigoid, pemphigoid gestationis (PG), lichen planus pemphigoides (LPP), and linear IgA dermatosis (LAD).

180 kDa bullous pemphigoid antigen or BP180, also known as BPAG1 or type XVII collagen, is a transmembrane hemidesmosomal glycoprotein. The N-terminal is non-collagenous and located intracellular, while the extracellular domain has a triple-helical shape containing collagenous repeats, hence the term type XVII collagen. Intracellularly, BP180 interacts with integrin $\alpha6\beta4$ and plectin and aids the integration of BP230 into the HD. The extracellular domain crosses lamina lucida into the lamina densa where it binds laminin 332 [5]. BP180 is expressed in the skin, mucosa, central nerve tissue, teeth, placenta, and umbilical cord. Specific autoimmunity targeting this antigen leads to a spectrum of subepidermal autoimmune disorders such as BP, MMP, Brunsting-Perry pemphigoid, PG, LPP, and LAD. Notably, the ectodomain of BP 180, by means of stepwise proteolytic cleavage, generates the 120-kDa (LAD-1) and 97-kDa (LABD-97) antigens. These shed ectodomains are deposited in the lamina lucida and may become target of IgA autoantibodies in LAD.

Integrin $\alpha6\beta4$ is a transmembrane molecule at the heart of the HDs. The integrin $\beta4$ subunit has a large intracellular domain which interacts with the intracellular domain of BP180 and links intermediate keratin filaments through plectin and BP230. The extracellular domains of the integrin $\alpha6$ and integrin $\beta4$ subunits bind to laminin 332 in the extracellular matrix [6]. Integrin $\alpha6\beta4$ is expressed in stratified squamous and transitional epithelia such as the skin, mucous membranes, gastro-intestinal, and urinary tract. Both $\alpha6$ and $\beta4$ integrin subunits have been suggested as autoantigens in MMP in some studies; the evidence may benefit from more validation.

Epidermal Basement Membrane Zone

The epidermal basement membrane provides architectural linkage and a functional continuity between epidermis and the underlying dermis. Another important task is the maintenance of a barrier for unrestricted passage of chemical or pathological agents into the body or water and electrolytes out of the body. Basement membrane is too small to be visualized with light microscopy and can be identified only by electron microscopy. It contains an electron-lucent 20–40 nm thick layer named lamina lucida and a 30–70 nm thick electron-dense layer named lamina densa. This division is, nevertheless, a tissue preparation and dehydration artifact resulting from the retraction of plasma membrane and thus exposure of lamina lucida [5]. The structural composition of the basement membrane involves supramolecular aggregates that include laminin isoforms, type IV collagen, type VII collagen, perlecan, and nidogen [7].

Basement membrane zone interfaces epithelial and dermal compartment

Following is a succinct description of the most relevant constituents of the basement membrane.

Laminins represent a family of heterotrimeric molecules consisting of three different chains (α, β, and γ), which assemble into cross-shaped polypeptide. It is found in stratified squamous, transition, and simple epithelia [8]. Laminin 332 is a major component of the epidermal basement membrane and by binding integrin establishes a firm linkage to the underlying matrix. An additional function is mediation of keratinocyte migration [9]. Laminin 332 may become a target antigen in MMP. Also, laminin $\gamma1$ chain has been involved in some cases of anti-laminin $\gamma1$/anti p-200 pemphigoid.

p200 is a 200 kDa polypeptide in the lower lamina lucida, whose exact identity has not yet been fully clarified. The associated sAIBD is anti-p200 pemphigoid.

Type VII collagen is the main, if not the sole, component of anchoring fibrils in the sublamina densa zone. Anchoring fibrils have a semicircular shape and link the lamina densa to the papillary dermis underneath. Structurally, it consists of three identical α-chains which organize into a triple-helical collagenous structure flanked by globular N-terminus (NC1) and C-terminus (NC2). This molecule is expressed in the basement membrane zone of the skin, cornea, pharynx, larynx, genital mucosa, esophagus, and chorioamnion [10]. Autoantibodies targeting type VII collagen are associated with epidermolysis bullosa acquisita (EBA).

Type IV collagen provides an architectural scaffold for other macromolecules by forming a network of interactions. Autoantibodies against the α3 chain of type IV collagen in the basement membrane of the lungs and kidneys are involved in the pathogenesis of antiglomerular basement membrane disease.

Review Questions

1. Which protein is a structural component of the hemidesmosome?
   (a) Integrin α6β4
   (b) Type IV collagen
   (c) Laminin 332
   (d) Type VII collagen
2. Which protein is a structural component of the basement membrane zone?
   (a) BP230
   (b) Type VII collagen
   (c) Integrin α6β4
   (d) BP180
3. BP180 and BP230 proteins associated with the following sAIBDs:
   (a) BP, MMP, Brunsting-Perry pemphigoid, PG, LPP, EBA
   (b) BP, MMP, Brunsting-Perry pemphigoid, PG, LPP, LAD
   (c) BP, MMP, LPP, PG, p-200 pemphigoid, LAD

Answers

1. (a)
2. (b)
3. (b)

On the Web

https://en.wikipedia.org/wiki/Hemidesmosome
https://en.wikipedia.org/wiki/Collagen,_type_XVII,_alpha_1
https://en.wikipedia.org/wiki/Basement_membrane

References

1. Koster J, van Wilpe S, Kuikman I, Litjens SH, Sonnenberg A. Role of binding of plectin to the integrin beta4 subunit in the assembly of hemidesmosomes. Mol Biol Cell. 2004;15:1211–23.
2. Buijsrogge JJ, de Jong MC, Kloosterhuis GJ, Vermeer MH, Koster J, Sonnenberg A, Jonkman MF, Pas HH. Antiplectin autoantibodies in subepidermal blistering diseases. Br J Dermatol. 2009;161:762–71.
3. Koster J, Geerts D, Favre B, Borradori L, Sonnenberg A. Analysis of the interactions between BP180, BP230, plectin and the integrin alpha6beta4 important for hemidesmosome assembly. J Cell Sci. 2003;116:387–99.
4. Leung CL, Zheng M, Prater SM, Liem RK. The BPAG1 locus: alternative splicing produces multiple isoforms with distinct cytoskeletal linker domains, including predominant isoforms in neurons and muscles. J Cell Biol. 2001;154:691–7.
5. Hashmi S, Marinkovich MP. Molecular organization of the basement membrane zone. Clin Dermatol. 2011;29:398–411.
6. Borradori L, Sonnenberg A. Structure and function of hemidesmosomes: more than simple adhesion complexes. J Invest Dermatol. 1999;112:411–8.
7. Turcan I, Jonkman MF. Blistering disease: insight from the hemidesmosome and other components of the dermal-epidermal junction. Cell Tissue Res. 2015;360(3):545–69.
8. Pierce RA, Griffin GL, Mudd MS, Moxley MA, Longmore WJ, Sanes JR, Miner JH, Senior RM. Expression of laminin alpha3, alpha4, and alpha5 chains by alveolar epithelial cells and fibroblasts. Am J Respir Cell Mol Biol. 1998;19:237–44.
9. Rousselle P, Beck K. Laminin 332 processing impacts cellular behavior. Cell Adh Migr. 2013;7:122–34.
10. Uitto J, Pulkkinen L, Christiano AM. Molecular basis of the dystrophic and junctional forms of epidermolysis bullosa: mutations in the type VII collagen and kalinin (laminin 5) genes. J Invest Dermatol. 1994;103:39S–46S.

Additional Reading

Walko G, Castanon MJ, Wiche G. Molecular architecture and function of the hemidesmosome. Cell Tissue Res. 2014;360(2):363–78.

Pemphigoid Diseases Affecting the Skin

14

Joost M. Meijer, Aniek Lamberts, and Jorrit B. Terra

Bullous Pemphigoid

Introduction and Aims

Short Definition in Layman Terms

Bullous pemphigoid (BP) is the most common blistering disease of the skin and mucous membranes (Fig. 14.1). BP mainly affects elderly and is clinically characterized by severe itch with tense blisters, erythema or urticarial plaques. Not all patients have skin blistering, approximately 1 in 5 patients has nonbullous pemphigoid (NBP) with severe itch and eczematous skin lesions. BP and NBP are mediated by an immune response against two structural proteins in the hemidesmosomes that are important for maintaining the integrity of the skin. Dysfunction may lead to subepidermal blistering in BP. Treatment of BP and other subtypes of pemphigoid is based on suppression of the immune system, with corticosteroid creams applied to the skin or oral drugs.

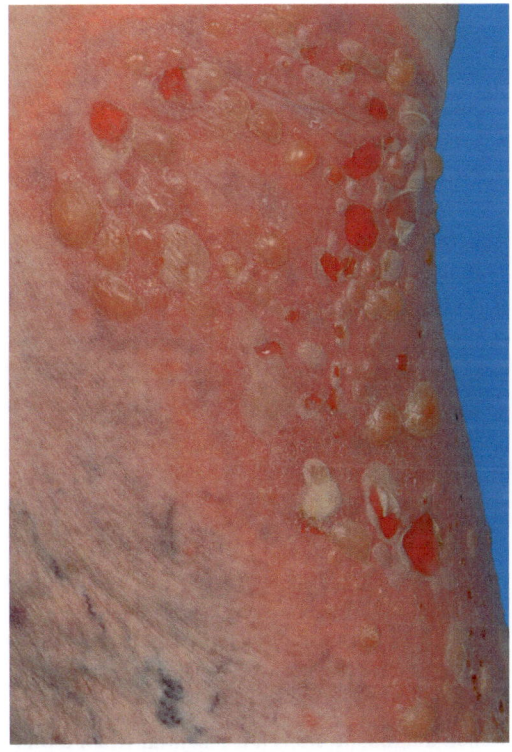

Fig. 14.1 Infiltrated urticarial plaques with tense blisters on predilection sites of BP: the flexural surfaces of the legs and the thighs. Multiple ruptured blisters leave eroded areas

BP is the most common autoimmune blistering disease mainly affecting elderly

> **Learning Objectives**
> After reading this chapter, you should be able to recognize the typical clinical presentation of BP, but also be aware of non-bullous pemphigoid. Moreover, you are familiar with the target antigens, the hallmarks in histopathology and immunofluorescence microscopy and diagnostic criteria. You should also be aware of treatment options in BP.

> **Case Study: Part 1**
> A 83-year-old woman with severe itch for several months is treated by her general practitioner with several ointments. Later on, she also develops erythematous papules and urticarial plaques on her back and extremities, with also some vesicles. Diagnosed as urticaria, she was treated with topical corticosteroids and oral antihistamines, without improvement. The dermatologist noted multiple tense blisters on erythematous skin, and erosions on the flexor aspects of the extremities at physical examination. Nikolsky sign was negative, and mucous membranes were unaffected.

Didactical Questions: Cross Section of Questions to Prime the Reader's Interest

Which diagnostic steps are essential when a blistering disease is suspected? What are the similarities and differences between pemphigus and pemphigoid, can you make the differentiation on clinical symptoms alone? How do you make the diagnosis of BP and NBP and what is the first choice treatment?

Facts and Figures

Definitions and Classification

Pemphigoid: the etymology of the word pemphigoid is 'form of a blister' (*pemphix*, blister and *eidos*, form in Greek). Therefore, the adjective 'bullous' is not strictly necessary. In 1953, Walter F. Lever differentiated pemphigoid diseases from pemphigus, based on histopathology and clinical presentation. He described intraepidermal separation and loss of cell adherence between keratinocytes (acantholysis) in pemphigus, and introduced the term bullous pemphigoid (BP) for diseases with subepidermal splitting [1]. BP is defined by autoantibodies against two hemidesmosomal proteins: BP180 and BP230. The classification of pemphigoid diseases includes several subtypes, based on different clinical symptoms, target antigens and autoantibody isotypes (Table 14.1). BP is the most common pemphigoid disease. BP predominantly affects the skin, involvement of the mucous membranes is seen in up to 20% of cases.

Epidemiology

BP most frequently affects elderly, with onset of disease usually after the age of 70 years. Incidences have been described from 1.21 to 2.17 per 100,000 persons per year. Moreover, the incidence rises substantially with age, up to 15–33 per 100,000 per year in people older than 80 years. The incidence of BP in Europe has more than doubled in the last decade, which might be related to both the increasing age of the general population, multi-drug use and the availability and quality of diagnostics. BP rarely occurs in infancy and childhood (see Chap. 24). BP has been associated with a high morbidity and a considerable 1-year mortality rate ranging from 20 to 40%. Most important risk factors for poor outcome are high age, widespread disease, a low Karnofsky score and high doses of oral corticosteroids [1].

Pathogenesis

BP is characterized by the presence of IgG autoantibodies against components of hemidesmosomes in the EBMZ, BP180 and BP230. Binding of autoantibodies to the antigens initiates a complex process, leading to separation of the epidermis and the dermis with subepidermal blister formation. Additionally, deposits of IgA, IgE and complement may also be found along the EBMZ. Most

Table 14.1 Target antigens, IF findings and clinical symptoms of subtypes of subepidermal autoimmune blistering diseases

Disease type	Target antigens	IF Findings DIF	IIF SSS	Clinical symptoms
Bullous pemphigoid	BP180 BP230	n-serrated EBMZ IgG ± IgA, IgE, C3c	Epidermal	Pruritus, urticaria, tense blisters without predominant mucosal involvement
Nonbullous pemphigoid	BP180 BP230	n-serrated EBMZ IgG ± IgE, C3c	Epidermal	Erythematous papules or nodules, pruritus on primary nondiseased skin, eczematous lesions, urticarial plaques
Brunsting-Perry pemphigoid	BP180	n-serrated EBMZ IgG ± C3c	Epidermal	Erosions and blisters confined to the head, face, neck and upper trunk leaving atrophic scars
Lichen planus pemphigoides	BP180 BP230	n-serrated EBMZ IgG ± C3c	Epidermal	Tense blisters independent of the lichenoid plaques and papules of lichen planus
Pemphigoid gestationis	BP180 BP230	n-serrated EBMZ C3c ± IgG	Epidermal	Intense pruritic urticarial rash, papules and tense blisters starting around umbilicus and then spread over the body
Linear IgA bullous dermatosis	BP180 LAD-1, LABD-97	n-serrated EBMZ IgA ± IgG	Epidermal	Tense blisters and erosions in 'string of pearls', without predominant mucosal involvement
Anti-p200 pemphigoid	p200	n-serrated EBMZ IgG ± C3c	Dermal	Pruritus, tense bullae, vesicles, urticarial plaques, predominantly on the extremities and trunk
Epidermolysis bullosa acquisita	Type VII collagen	u-serrated EBMZ IgG ± IgA	Dermal	Mechanobullous variant: acral blistering that heal with scarring and milia. Inflammatory variant: widespread vesicles and blisters, without scarring or milia

EBMZ epidermal basement membrane zone, *IF* immunofluorescence microscopy, *DIF* direct IF, *IIF SSS* indirect IF salt-split-skin, *IgG/IgA/IgE* immunoglobuline G/A/E, *C3c* complement C3, *BP* is characterized by subepidermal blister formation

BP patients have autoantibodies against the extracellular part of the 16th non-collagenous domain (NC16A) of BP180 (immunodominant region). BP230 is a 230-kDa intracellular component of the hemidesmosomal plaque. However, the pathogenic relevance of autoantibodies against BP230 is not fully elucidated. Isoforms of both BP180 and BP230 are also expressed in the central nervous system, which might explain the association between BP and neurological diseases, such as cognitive impairment, Parkinson's disease and stroke in up to half of patients with BP [1].

Main target antigens in BP are hemidesmosomal proteins BP180 and BP230

Diagnosis Paths

History and Physical Examination

BP typically presents with severe pruritus, localized or generalized tense blisters and erythema or urticarial plaques (Fig. 14.2). Nikolsky sign is negative. Predilection sites are the trunk, abdomen and flexural aspects of the extremities. Blisters may arise on both healthy and erythematous skin, often have a transparent or serous exudate and can persist for several days. Ruptured blisters leave erosions and crusts, but do not heal with scarring. Mucosal involvement is seen in 10–20% of BP patients, mostly the oral mucosa. Clinical and diagnostic clues are summarized in Table 14.2. A pitfall can be the prodromal phase that exists in a number of patients that only have pruritus and excoriated, eczematous or urticarial lesions that precede the development of blisters, or have persistent nonbullous pemphigoid [2]. A detailed medical history should be obtained, including a medication history with recent drug intake. Furthermore, the extent of BP should be assessed, for example with the BP Disease Area Index (BPDAI, see Chap. 2).

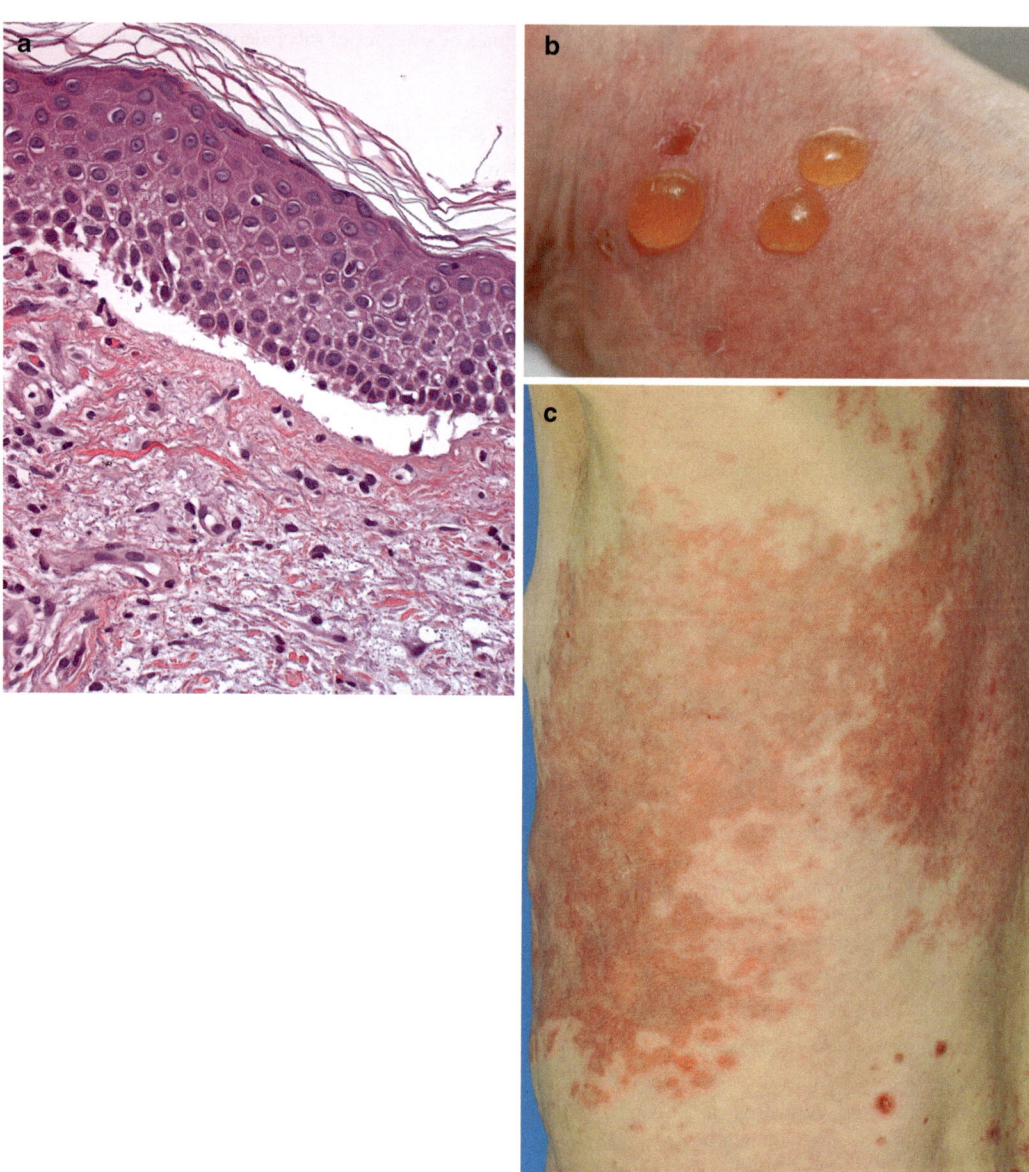

Fig. 14.2 Hallmarks of BP: (**a**) Histopathology of H&E section of lesional skin biopsy with subepidermal blister formation with eosinophils and a dermal inflammatory eosinophilic infiltrate (magnification 400×), (**b**) tense bullae on inflamed, erythematous skin, (**c**) confluent infiltrated urticarial plaques on the trunk

General Diagnostics

Which diagnostic steps are essential when bullous or nonbullous pemphigoid is suspected? The diagnosis of BP and NBP is based on a combination of criteria comprising clinical features and specific findings in direct IF and serology. Both DIF and IIF SSS should be performed for optimal diagnosis of BP and NBP. Based on a large diagnostic accuracy study, diagnostic criteria consist of at least two positive results out of three criteria: (1) pruritus and/or predominant cutaneous blisters, (2) linear IgG and/or C3c deposits (in an n-serrated pattern) by DIF on a skin biopsy specimen, and (3) positive epidermal side staining by IIF SSS on a serum sample [3]. A complete blood count often shows peripheral eosinophilia.

Table 14.2 Clues to diagnosis of BP

Clinical clues for diagnosis of BP	Diagnostic clues for diagnosis of BP
Elderly with severe pruritus	Peripheral eosinophilia
Eczematous lesions, papules or nodules	Subepidermal splitting
Urticarial plaques	Dermal inflammatory infiltrate of eosinophils
Localized or generalized tense blisters	DIF IgG/C3c along EBMZ n-serrated pattern
Mucosal lesions	IIF on monkey esophagus IgG positive
Polypharmacy	IIF SSS IgG positive epidermal binding
Nikolsky sign negative	BP180 NC16A ELISA positive
Good response to oral corticosteroids	Immunoblot BP180 positive

Main clinical symptoms of BP are tense blisters, urticarial plaques and pruritus

Histopathology of a bullous lesion shows subepidermal splitting and an inflammatory infiltrate composed of mainly eosinophils and neutrophils. However, in absence of blistering, the histopathology may be non-specific, and be limited to eosinophilic spongiosis or an eosinophilic infiltrate in the upper dermis. Direct immunofluorescence microscopy reveals a linear n-serrated immunodeposition of IgG and/or complement C3 along the EBMZ. Other Ig subclasses can be found, such as IgA, IgM and occasionally IgE.

Diagnosis of bullous and nonbullous pemphigoid is based on clinical features, DIF and immunoserology

Specific Diagnostics

Diagnosis of BP and NBP can be confirmed with very high specificity by serology using IIF on 1.0 M NaCl-split skin (SSS) substrate showing binding of antibodies to the epidermal side (roof) of the artificial split [3]. IIF on monkey esophagus is less sensitive. Combining the IIF SSS technique (epidermal or dermal binding) with serration pattern analysis (n-serrated versus u-serrated) allows to differentiate between different subtypes of pemphigoid and EBA (see Chap. 4). BP180 NC16A and BP230 ELISA's are not recommended for initial diagnosis, due to frequent borderline findings [3]. After confirmed diagnosis of BP, the BP180 NC16A ELISA can be used to monitor disease activity. Immunoblot can be used to test the patient's serum reactivity to BP180, BP230 and/or other rare targeted antigens.

> **Case Study: Part 2**
> Histopathology of a lesional biopsy of an intact blister showed a subepidermal blister with a dense inflammatory infiltrate of eosinophils. A perilesional skin biopsy for DIF showed linear depositions of IgG 3+, IgA 1+ and C3c 3+ in an n-serrated pattern along the EMBZ. Serologic testing by IIF SSS was positive for IgG on the epidermal side of the salt-split-skin. BP180 NC16A and BP230 ELISA IgG indexes were 51 (positive), and 7 (negative), respectively. Immunoblot was positive on BP180 and BP230 IgG. The diagnosis was made of BP, which initially presented only with pruritus.

Treatment Tricks

Initial Treatment and Therapeutic Ladder

BP can have a clinical course that may last from several months to years. The high age of BP patients and the possible presence of co-morbidities can make the treatment management more difficult. Recommended first-line therapy for mild, moderate and severe disease is superpotent topical steroids (clobetasol propionate) 30–40 g/day applied daily over the whole body, including blisters, erosions and healthy skin, but sparing the face [4]. Whole body application of superpotent topical corticosteroids is considered to be effective and save and has a lower cumulative dose of corticosteroids and less side-effects compared to oral corticosteroids. Patients with localized BP can be treated with superpotent topical corticosteroids applied to lesional skin only. Oral corticosteroids (prednisone 0.5 up to 0.75 mg/kg/day) are often used in treatment of moderate to severe BP and may be accompanied by adjunctive superpotent topical corticosteroids and/or immunosuppressive or -modulating agents [4]. Low-dose methotrexate (2.5–12.5 mg/week) was reported to be an effective and relatively safe therapeutic option in elderly BP patients [5]. Systemic anti-inflammatory antibiotics (doxycycline) may be used as alternative treatment when oral corticosteroids are contraindicated. Other therapeutic options include dapsone, azathioprine, mycophenolate mofetil, or mycophenolic acid. Rituximab treatment may be considered when these agents are contraindicated or in refractory cases of BP (see box XX pemphigus) [6]. Subsequently, the combination of intravenous immunoglobulin (IVIG) and Rituximab may be considered if Rituximab monotherapy is ineffective.

Whole body application of superpotent topical steroids is first-choice therapy in BP

> **Case Study: Part 3**
> First-line therapy with whole body application of superpotent topical corticosteroids (40 g/day) improved her complaints, but appeared to be insufficient. Therefore, the patient received adjunctive treatment with Methotrexate 7.5 mg/day, later increased to 10 mg/day. Pruritus and the frequency of blistering reduced, after 3 month the patient reached complete remission and methotrexate was lowered to 7.5 mg/day again. When mild symptoms of itch returned, adjunctive treatment with lesional superpotent topical corticosteroids was sufficient to maintain complete remission.

Follow-Up and Tapering

BP can last for several years and has the tendency to relapse. Determination of anti-BP180 NC16A IgG antibodies by ELISA follows disease activity and severity and can also be used to identify patients with a high risk of relapse. Current evidence suggests to continue initial topical treatment until 15 days after disease control, when no new lesions arise and lesions begin to heal. Then treatment of superpotent topical corticosteroids should be reduced by a tapering schedule, with daily treatment in the 1st month, every 2 days in the 2nd month, 2 times a week in the 3rd month and once a week starting in the 4th month. Tapering of oral corticosteroids after disease control is based on clinical course, and when available on serum levels of anti-BP180 NC16A IgG [3].

Nonbullous Pemphigoid

Short Definition in Layman Terms

Nonbullous pemphigoid (NBP) is the subset of patients with immunopathological findings of BP and pruritus, but no blister development. Similar to BP, the onset of disease is often at high age. Patients may present with chronic itch or with various nonbullous inflammatory skin lesions. NBP patients are frequently misdiagnosed as drug reaction or dermatitis, and therefore the diagnostic delay is long. Clinicians should be aware of this pemphigoid subtype when encountering elderly patient with pruritus.

Definitions and Classification

In 1953 Walter F. Lever added the pleonasm "bullous" to the name pemphigoid in an attempt to separate it from mucous membrane pemphigoid. We now know that BP is not always bullous. In the literature there is no unanimity on how to name the subset of patients with pemphigoid without blistering. The coined terms include, pruritic nonbullous pemphigoid, pemphigoid nodularis, papular pemphigoid, prurigo-nodularis like pemphigoid, non-bullous BP, prodromal BP and BP incipiens. Because these patients have pemphigoid of the skin without blistering, we classify this subtype as NBP [2].

Epidemiology

Of all patients presenting with BP, approximately 20–25% does not have blistering. The majority of the patients with NBP is above 70 years of age. Probably NBP is underdiagnosed in elderly with chronic itch, because of unfamiliarity of clinicians with the diagnosis of NBP.

Approximately 20% of patients with bullous pemphigoid do not show skin blistering, a variant termed nonbullous pemphigoid

Pathogenesis

The pathogenesis of NBP shows great resemblance to that of BP, and also relies on the production of IgG autoantibodies that target hemidesmosomal proteins BP180 and BP230. It is unknown why patients with NBP do not develop blisters, while the diagnostic immunological findings can be similar to BP. In contrast to BP with mainly BP180 autoreactivity, predominant reactivity to BP230 is seen in NBP that might lead to a less extensive inflammatory response. Moreover, less frequent complement activation is observed in NBP versus BP skin.

Clinical Symptoms

The clinical presentation of NBP is heterogeneous and may mimic other inflammatory diseases. Patients most commonly present with severe pruritus, accompanied by erythematous papules and nodules [2]. Moreover, eczematous lesions, urticarial plaques, and pruritus on primary nondiseased skin could be observed (Fig. 14.3).

Think of NBP in elderly with chronic itch

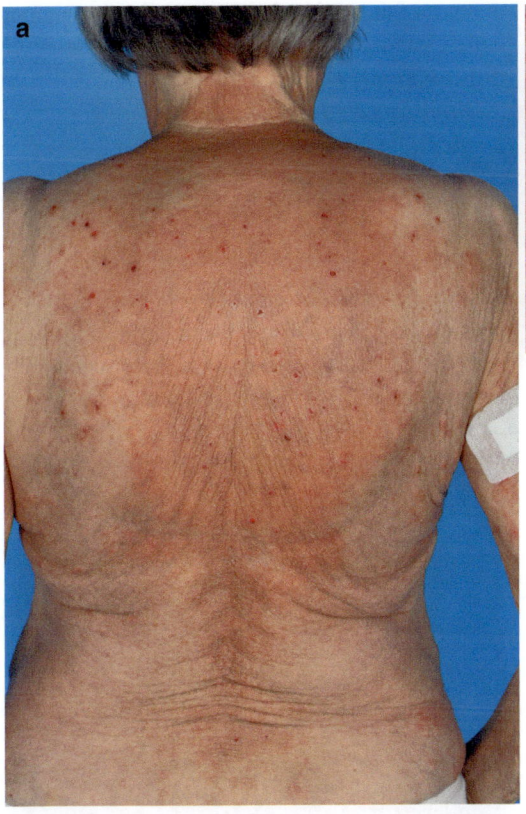
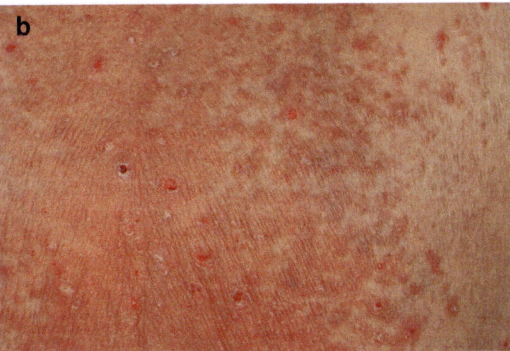

Fig. 14.3 An elderly NBP patient with pruritic, excoriated eczematous lesions on the back (**a**), and in detail (**b**); DIF showed lineair IgG along the BMZ in the n-serrated pattern

Diagnosis Paths

Similar to diagnosis of BP (above), diagnosis of NBP is based on a combination of criteria comprising clinical features and specific findings in direct IF and serology [3]. In the absence of blisters we recommend a biopsy for DIF in NBP from lesional skin. Diagnosis of NBP can be made by positive IIF on SSS (epidermal binding) in combination with a compatible clinical phenotype [3]. Other serological tests like immunoblot or NC16A ELISA can support the diagnosis. However, single positive results by BP180 NC16A or BP230 ELISA should not be considered as having BP or a BP variant, because of frequent borderline results.

Treatment Tricks

Treatment of this intense pruritic condition is essential. Treatment recommendations for NBP are similar as in BP, with first-line treatment of whole body application of superpotent topical corticosteroids. If not responsive, systemic treatment with low-dose methrotrexate is the next recommended step [2]. In other cases maintenance treatment with low dose oral corticosteroids is necessary, or Rituximab might be considered in refractory cases.

Brunsting-Perry Cicatricial Pemphigoid

Short Definition in Layman Terms

Brunsting-Perry cicatricial pemphigoid is a form of localized pemphigoid affecting the skin and limited to the head and neck area, leading to scarring. Brunsting-Perry cicatricial pemphigoid is rare, but difficult to recognize for clinicians. A skin biopsy for DIF must be performed for a correct diagnosis.

Facts and Figures

In 1957, Brunsting and Perry described a rare localized form of cicatricial pemphigoid patients who presented with itchy erosions with blisters that heal with scarring at the site of the scalp, face and neck [7]. Circulating IgG autoantibodies target BP180, and occasionally LAD-1. Subepidermal split formation occurs in most cases at the level of the lamina lucida. The target, the C-terminal domain of BP180 that is located in the lamina densa, might be responsible for the scarring phenotype. The average age at onset of symptoms is 58 years and the male/female ratio is 2:1.

Clinical Symptoms

Brunsting-Perry cicatricial pemphigoid clinically presents with erosions and blisters of the head, neck and shoulder area that heal with scarring and milia (Fig. 14.4). The scarring of the scalp will develop in permanent alopecia. Mucosal involvement is rarely seen. Because of its rarity and resemblance with other diseases like epidermolysis bullosa acquisita, erosive pustular dermatosis of the scalp, chronic infection, squamous cell carcinoma, folliculitis decalvans it may be difficult to recognize.

Brunsting-Perry cicatricial pemphigoid is localized on head, neck and shoulders

Diagnosis Paths

Histopathological biopsy of the border of an erosion of the scalp shows subepidermal blistering with lymphocytes, neutrophils and eosinophils, and the presence of extensive scarring in the der-

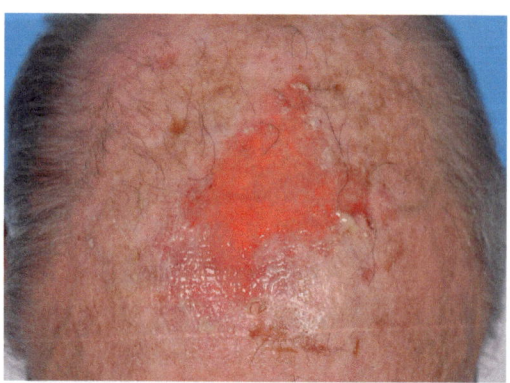

Fig. 14.4 Sharply bordered erosions on the scalp with scarring alopecia in a patient with Brunsting-Perry pemphigoid

mis, with loss of hair follicles. DIF on perilesional skin shows linear deposits of IgG and C3 in the n-serrated pattern along the epidermal BMZ. DIF of normal healthy skin of the upper arm may also show deposits of IgG and C3c. The indirect immunofluorescence examination is often negative.

Treatment Tricks

The disease is responding well to oral corticosteroids (prednisolone 0.5–0.75 mg/kg/day) in combination with immunosuppressive agents like azathioprine (2–3 mg/kg/day). For painful erosions using a wound dressing with a silicon layer is useful.

Lichen Planus Pemphigoides

Introduction and AIMS

Lichen planus pemphigoides (LPP) is a rare variant of pemphigoid diseases characterized by a combination of clinical, histological and immunological features of both lichen planus (LP) and BP. In the bullous form of LP blistering is restricted to LP lesions, however, in LPP blisters appear also on normal appearing skin.

Facts and Figures

The term lichen planus pemphigoides or 'lichen ruber pemphigoides' was first used by Kaposi in 1892, describing a dermatosis with lichen planus lesions with additional blistering. The pathogenesis of LPP is not completely understood yet, LPP is associated with an autoimmune response directed mostly against the NC16A domain of BP180. A suggested theory is that LP lesions damage the basal keratinocytes and expose the BP180 antigens, leading to a secondary autoimmune reponse with autoantibodies to the EBMZ [1]. The mean age of onset is usually younger (50–60 years) than in BP.

Diagnosis Paths

LPP clinically presents with a lichenoid eruption of papules and plaques preceding bullous lesions on both LP lesions and previously normal skin. LPP predominantly affects the extremities and tends to be less severe than BP. Histopathology shows typical findings of LP in papular lesions and subepidermal blistering in biopsies of bullous lesions. The diagnosis of LPP is confirmed by detection of IgG autoantibodies or C3c directed against the EBMZ by DIF of a perilesional biopsy, and detection of circulating IgG autoantibodies against BP180 NC16A, and enables to distinguish LPP from bullous LP.

In LPP blisters may arise on LP lesions and previously normal skin

Treatment Tricks

Simultaneous treatment of LP lesions and bullous lesions is needed to avoid an ongoing stimulation of the autoimmune process at the EBMZ. Treatment follows algorithms as for LP and BP [1]. The prognosis is good, with a reported low rate of recurrence of blistering.

Pemphigoid Gestationis

Short Definition in Layman Terms

Pemphigoid gestationis (PG) is a pregnancy-associated subtype of pemphigoid which manifests in the 2nd or 3rd trimester of pregnancy. Sporadically this disease presents within 4 weeks after birth.

PG usually manifests in the 2nd and 3rd trimester of pregnancy

Facts and Figures

Holmes and Black suggested in 1982 to name the disease pemphigoid gestationis instead of herpes gestationis, because of the correlation of the clinical spectrum and immunlogical findings with pemphigoid diseases. PG is characterized by autoreactivity to the NC16A domain of BP180.

Epidemiology

The annual incidence of PG is 1:50,000 pregnancies. No difference in phenotype is seen in both Caucasians and Afro-Americans. PG can arise at any moment in childbearing age.

Pathogenesis

The pathogenesis of PG is not fully known. It is believed that PG is caused by loss of protection of the feto-placental unit against allogeneic recognition by the mother. In normal pregnancy, there is no expression of MHC II antigens on the trophoblast. This is a mechanism that protects the fetus against recognition by the maternal immune system. Within PG patients, however, there is an aberrant expression of MHC class II molecules in the placenta. Consequently, BP180 present in the placenta is presented to the maternal immune system, leading to an immune response with the formation of autoantibodies against BP180 and affection of the skin [8].

Clinical Symptoms

PG presents with pruritic urticarial plaques, vesicles and tense blisters starting around the umbilicus, followed by expansion over the trunk and the distal extremities (Fig. 14.5). Remission is usually seen within 6 months. In the minority of the patients (<5%) PG persists and converts into BP. Recurrence of PG occurs in more than 90% of the additional pregnancies. Exacerbation may occur prior to menses or after starting oral anticonception. Because of placental insufficiency, there is a risk of growth retardation and premature delivery of the fetus. There is no increased risk of stillbirth or spontaneous abortion. In 10% of the neonates a transient form of BP is seen. Neonatal disease has a mild course with remission within days to weeks [8].

Inform the patient about the possibility of recurrence of PG in following pregnancies

Diagnosis Paths

Histopathology shows subepidermal blistering with eosinophilic infiltrate. Final diagnosis can be made by DIF showing C3c and IgG depositions in the n-serrated pattern along the EBMZ. IgG1 and IgG3 having strong complement binding properties cause the presence of C3c. IIF performed on 1 M NaCl-split skin substrate showing binding of antibodies to the epidermal site (roof) of the split and by immunoblot analysis revealing immunoglobulin binding to the 180-kDa antigen.

Treatment Tricks

The first-line therapy for PG is (super) potent topical corticosteroids in combination with H1-receptor antagonist. Oral corticosteroids can be introduced at an initial dose of 0.25–0.5 mg/kg/day when (super) potent topical corticosteroids are not sufficient enough. A multidisciplinary approach with the gynecologist is recommended.

Anti-p200 Pemphigoid

Introduction

Anti-p200 pemphigoid is a recently defined, rare subtype of pemphigoid diseases characterized by autoantibodies against a 200-kDa protein (p200) of the EBMZ. The molecular identity of the pathogenic autoantigen has yet to be defined. Anti-p200 pemphigoid is probably misdiagnosed and classified as BP or inflammatory EBA, because of low availability of diagnostics test.

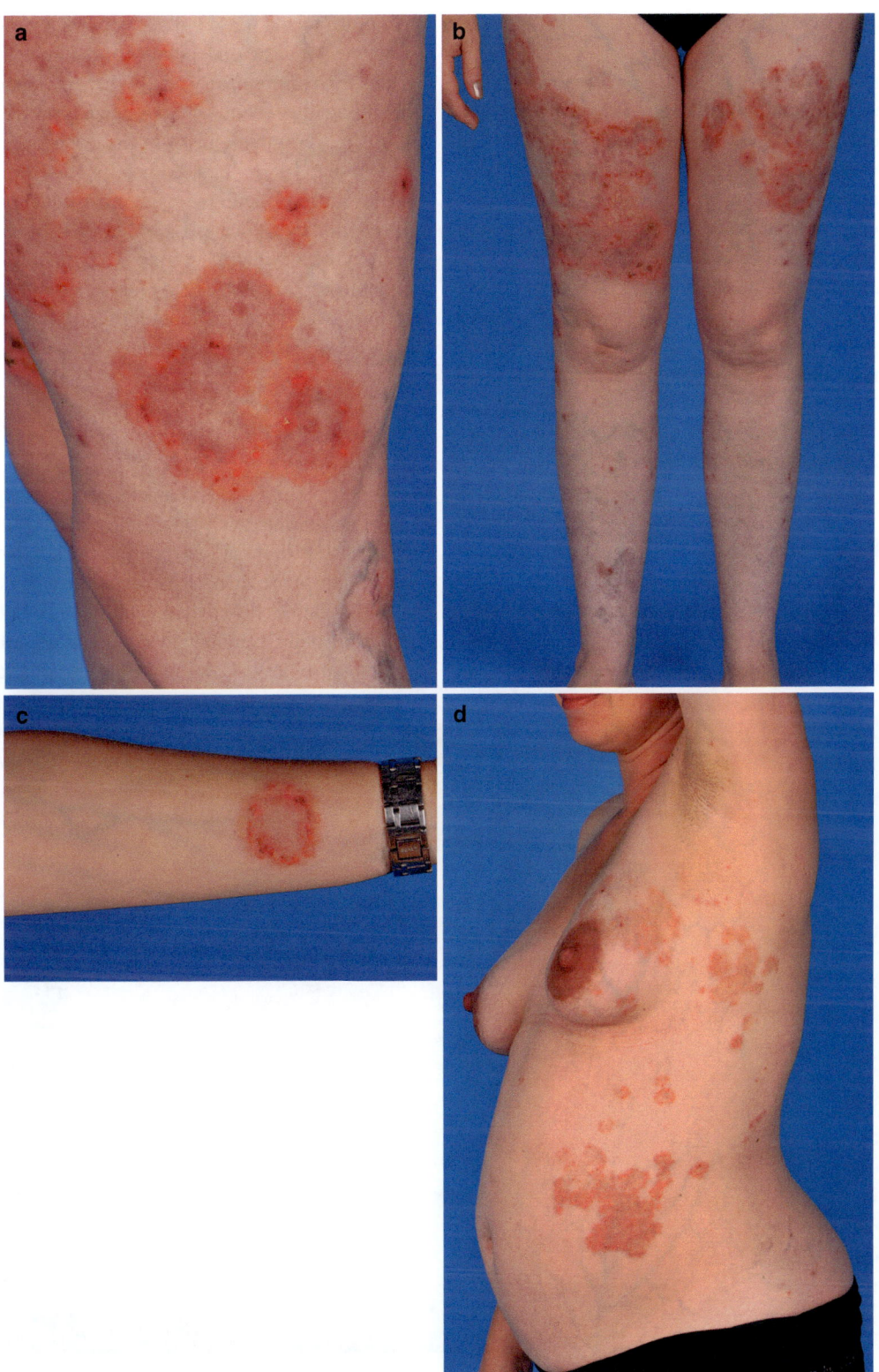

Fig. 14.5 Pemphigoid gestationis in a woman in the 24th week of gestation with pruritic eruption of circinate vesicles on urticarial plaques (**a–d**) [Reprinted with permission from *Ned Tijdschr Geneeskd*. 2009;153: B36. Diagnostic image. A pregnant female with blisters]

Facts and Figures

Originally described in 1996 as a novel subepidermal autoimmune blistering disease with autoantibodies against an unknown 200-kDa component of the EBMZ, the disease was consequently termed anti-p200 pemphigoid [9]. Since then, it was renamed to laminin γ1 pemphigoid as a new entity, because serum samples of 90% of anti-p200 patients appeared to recognize the glycoprotein laminin γ1, mainly the C-terminus region. However, *ex vivo* and *in vivo* studies were unable to show pathogenic activity of laminin γ1 [10].

The autoantigen in anti-p200 pemphigoid is a 200-kDa protein in the lower EBMZ

Clinical Symptoms

The clinical presentation of anti-p200 pemphigoid is heterogeneous and may mimic BP, LAD and inflammatory EBA. Most patients present with pruritus and tense bullae, vesicles and erythematous or urticarial plaques, predominantly on the extremities and trunk. When monomorphic blistering occurs solitary on hands and feet, it may resemble dishydrotic pemphigoid (Fig. 14.6a, b). In approximately 10–20% of patients mucous membranes are involved, but not as predominant as in anti-LN-332 MMP. Lesions normally heal without scarring. Patients tend to be younger than in BP. An association with psoriasis was seen in about 30% of reported cases, mostly in Japanese patients [10].

Diagnosis Paths

Anti-p200 pemphigoid is characterized by subepidermal blistering with a mainly neutrophilic inflammatory infiltrate, in contrast to a typical eosinophilic infiltrate in BP. However, histopathology alone cannot differentiate anti-p200 pemphigoid from other pemphigoid diseases. DIF of a perilesional biopsy shows linear deposits of IgG

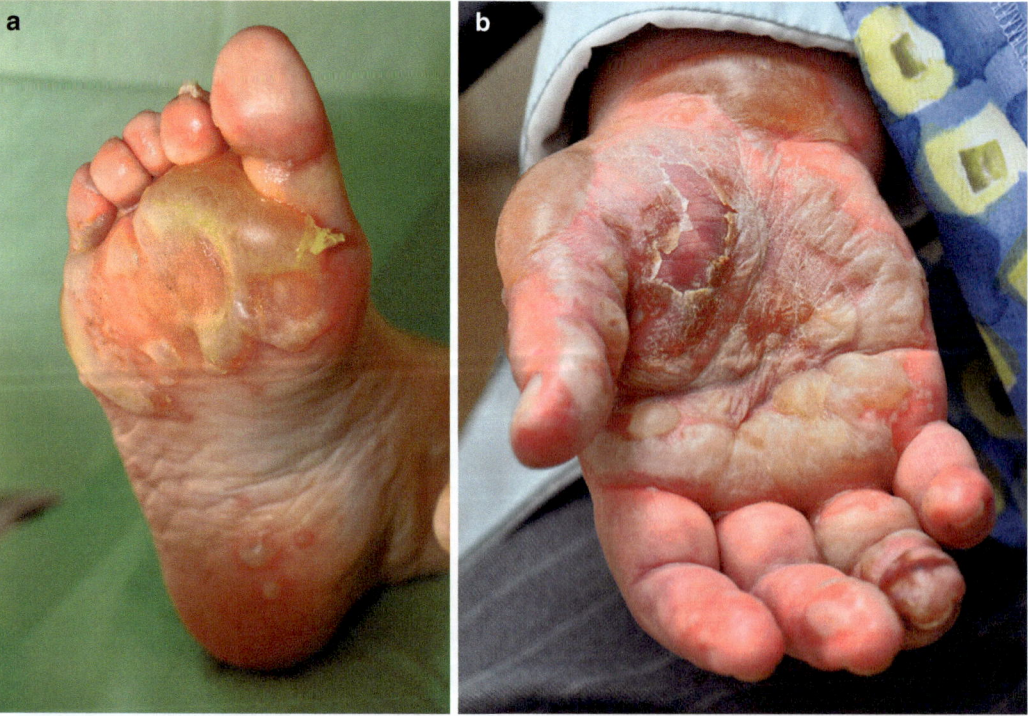

Fig. 14.6 Anti-p200 pemphigoid. Resembling dyshidrotic pemphigoid with multiple tense blisters on (**a**) the right foot and the palm of (**b**) the right hand

and/or IgA and complement C3 along the EBMZ in an n-serrated pattern. Using serration pattern analysis, anti-p200 pemphigoid can be differentiated from EBA with a u-serrated pattern along the EBMZ. Autoantibodies in anti-p200 pemphigoid bind to the lower lamina lucida, therefore IIF on salt-split-skin reveals binding of circulating autoantibodies along the dermal side of the artificial split. This method allows differentiating anti-p200 pemphigoid from BP, but not from anti-LN-332 MMP and/or EBA. Specific serological diagnostic tests are needed to distinguish these subtypes of pemphigoid diseases, such as IIF analysis on knockout skin (see Chap. 5) or immunoblotting of dermal extract with a 200-kDA protein band.

Anti-p200 pemphigoid is characterized by a mainly neutrophilic infiltrate in histology, IgG n-serrated pattern along EBMZ in DIF, and dermal binding in IIF SSS

Treatment Tricks

Treatment of anti-p200 pemphigoid follows the same guidelines as for BP, but anti-p200 pemphigoid is not a milder form of BP. First choice treatment in mild to moderate disease is superpotent topical steroids (clobetasol propionate 0.05%). In severe disease, oral corticosteroids (prednisolone 0.5 mg/kg/day) and adjunctive immunosuppressive therapy can be used (see BP section).

Review Questions

1. What are the three main clinical symptoms of BP?
   (a) Eczema, urticaria and tense blisters
   (b) Pruritus, urticarial plaques and tense blisters
   (c) Pruritus, nodules and tense blisters
   (d) Papules, nodules and tense blisters
2. Nonbullous pemphigoid may mimic:
   (a) Dry skin (xerosis cutis)
   (b) Scabies
   (c) Atopic dermatitis
   (d) All of mentioned above
3. First-line treatment of mild and severe BP is
   (a) Superpotent topical corticosteroids whole body application
   (b) Oral corticosteroids
   (c) Azathioprine
   (d) Dapsone
4. Patients with Brunsting-Perry cicatricial pemphigoid present with:
   (a) Predominant mucosal involvement
   (b) Tense blisters predominantly on the extremities and trunk
   (c) Erosions and blisters at the head, neck and shoulder area
   (d) Itch, urticaria and flat blisters
5. Lichen planus pemphigoides is characterized by:
   (a) Autoantibodies targeting collagen VII
   (b) Blisters on both lichen planus lesions and normal skin
   (c) Blisters solitary on lichen planus lesions
   (d) Vesicles and tense blisters starting around the umbilicus
6. Which statement about pemphigoid gestationis is correct
   (a) Pemphigoid gestationis manifests in the 1st trimester of pregnancy
   (b) The BP180 C-terminal domain is the target antigen.
   (c) Exacerbation may occur before menstruation or after starting oral anticonception
   (d) There is an increased risk of stillbirth
7. Clinical features of anti-p200 pemphigoid include:
   (a) Psoriasis
   (b) Blisters on acral sites
   (c) Predominant mucosal lesions
   (d) Scarring of lesions

Answers

1. (b)
2. (d)
3. (a)
4. (c)
5. (b)
6. (c)
7. (b)

References

1. Schmidt E, Zillikens D. Pemphigoid diseases. Lancet. 2013;381:320–32.
2. Lamberts A, Meijer JM, Pas HH, Diercks GFH, Horváth B, Jonkman MF. Nonbullous pemphigoid: insights in clinical and diagnostic findings, treatment responses and prognosis. J Am Acad Dermatol. 2019;81(2):355–63.
3. Meijer JM, Diercks GFH, de Lang EWG, Pas HH, Jonkman MF. Assessment of diagnostic strategy for early recognition of bullous and nonbullous variants of pemphigoid. JAMA Dermatol. 2019;155(2):158–65.
4. Feliciani C, Joly P, Jonkman MF, Zambruno G, Zillikens D, Ioannidis D, Kowalewski C, Jedlickova H, Karpati S, Marinovic B, Mimouni D, Uzun S, Yayli S, Hertl M, Borradori L. Management of bullous pemphigoid: the European Dermatology Forum consensus in collaboration with the European Academy of Dermatology and Venereology. Br J Dermatol. 2015;172(4):867–77.
5. Fisch A, Morin L, Talme T, Johnell K, Gallais Sérézal I. Low-dose methotrexate use and safety for older patients with bullous pemphigoid and impaired renal function: a cohort study. J Am Acad Dermatol. 2020;82(6):1532–4.
6. Lamberts A, Euverman HI, Terra JB, Jonkman MF, Horváth B. Effectiveness and safety of rituximab in recalcitrant pemphigoid diseases. Front. Immunol. 2018;9:248.
7. Brunsting LA, Perry HO. Benign pemphigold; a report of seven cases with chronic, scarring, herpetiform plaques about the head and neck. AMA Arch Derm. 1957;75:489–501.
8. Lipozencic J, Ljubojevic S, Bukvic-Mokos Z. Pemphigoid gestationis. Clin Dermatol. 2012;30:51–5.
9. Zillikens D, Kawahara Y, Ishiko A, Shimizu H, Mayer J, Rank CV, Liu Z, Giudice GJ, Tran HH, Marinkovich MP, Brocker EB, Hashimoto T. A novel subepidermal blistering disease with autoantibodies to a 200-kDa antigen of the basement membrane zone. J Invest Dermatol. 1996;106:1333–8.
10. Meijer JM, Diercks GF, Schmidt E, Pas HH, Jonkman MF. Laboratory diagnosis and clinical profile of anti-p200 pemphigoid. JAMA Dermatol. 2016;152(8):897–904.

Mucous Membrane Pemphigoid

15

Joost M. Meijer, Hanan Rashid, and Jorrit B. Terra

Learning Objectives
After reading this chapter, you should be able to recognize the different clinical features of MMP, know the target antigens and IF findings. You should also know potential complications in MMP and should be able to practice general treatment strategies.

Mucous Membrane Pemphigoid

Short Definition in Layman Terms

Mucous membrane pemphigoid (MMP) is the name for the whole group of patients with pemphigoid mainly affecting the mucous membranes (Table 15.1). The autoimmune disease targets components of the epidermal basement membrane zone (EBMZ). In MMP the oral mucosa is mostly affected (85%), but all mucous membranes can be involved. In a minority of patients also the skin is affected. Patients clinically present with redness, erosions, vesicles or blisters or with redness of the gingiva. The intake of nutrition or fluids can be reduced because of pain. MMP with exclusively oral lesions is frequently unrecognized in the early stage and often misdiagnosed as oral lichen planus, oral aphthosis or other inflammatory oral diseases.

Table 15.1 Disease subtypes, target antigens and IF findings in mucous membrane pemphigoid

Disease type	Target antigens	IF findings DIF	IIF SSS
MMP	BP180, BP230, α6β4 integrin	Linear n-serrated EBMZ IgG ± IgA, C3c	Epidermal
	Type 7 collagen	Linear u-serrated IgG ± IgA, C3c	Dermal
Ocular MMP	BP180	Linear (n-serrated) EBMZ IgG ± IgA	Epidermal
Localized vulvar pemphigoid	BP180	Linear n-serrated EBMZ IgG ± IgA, C3c	Epidermal
Anti-laminin-332 MMP	Laminin-332	Linear n-serrated EBMZ IgG ± C3c	Dermal

J. M. Meijer (✉) · H. Rashid
Center for Blistering Diseases, Department of Dermatology, University Medical Center Groningen, University of Groningen,
Groningen, The Netherlands
e-mail: j.m.meijer@umcg.nl; h.rashid@umcg.nl

J. B. Terra
Department of Dermatology, Isala Hospital,
Zwolle, The Netherlands
e-mail: j.b.terra@isala.nl

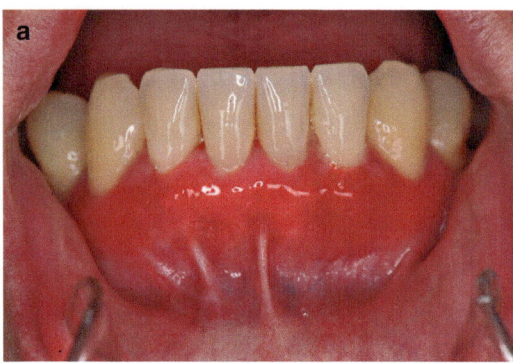 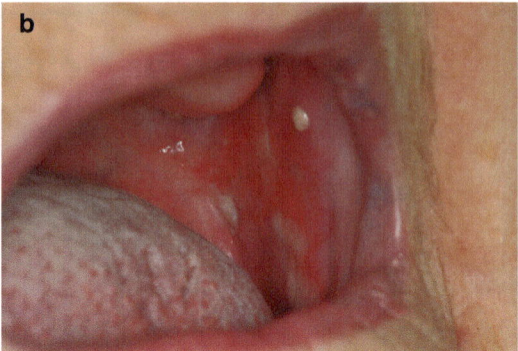

Fig. 15.1 (**a**) Clinical manifestations of a patient with monosite MMP limited to the oral mucosa with desquamative gingivitis, and (**b**) blistering on the buccal mucosa

Case Study: Part 1

A 62-year old man presents with desquamative gingivitis of the oral mucosa, diagnosed as oral lichen planus for several years (Fig. 15.1a). More recently, blisters developed on the buccal mucosa (Fig. 15.1b). His oral lesions were treated with superpotent topical corticosteroids, that did not relieve the symptoms. Because of failure of treatment he was referred to our clinic.

Didactical Questions: Cross Section of Questions to Prime the Readers Interest

What are clinical differences between MMP and pemphigus vulgaris oris? How can you clinically differentiate between oral lichen planus and oral MMP? On which criteria is the diagnosis MMP based and where should you take a biopsy for DIF?

Facts and Figures

MMP is a heterogeneous group of chronic subepidermal autoimmune blistering diseases (sAIBD) with predominantly mucosal involvement and is characterized by autoreactivity mostly to BP180 (Table 15.1). BP180 is a 180-kDa transmembrane glycoprotein that ultrastructurally spans the lamina lucida and curves back from the lamina densa into the lamina lucida. In MMP autoantibodies most often recognize the C-terminal epitopes of BP180. NC16A is the second immunodominant domain. In addition, autoantibodies may target BP230. Autoreactivity to the α6 and β4 integrin subunits have also been described. The main autoantibody isotype is IgG, predominantly of the IgG1 and IgG4 subclass, but deposits of IgA and complement C3 may be found [1, 2]. The incidence of MMP as a group has been estimated at 1.3–2.0 per million per year in France and Germany, respectively. MMP often occurs earlier in life than BP, with age of onset commonly observed between 60 and 70 years [2]. Women are affected almost two times more often than men. MMP is rare in children. No racial differences have been seen.

Diagnosis Paths

History and Physical Examination

Involvement of one or more mucosal sites may occur in MMP. Patients with involvement of only one mucosal site are termed monosite MMP (estimated 40%), such as monosite oral MMP or monosite ocular MMP, whereas patients with several affected mucosal sites are referred to as multisite MMP (estimated 60%). Patients with MMP clinically present with erosive or erythematous patches and small blisters of mucosa consisting of nonkeratinized stratified squamous

Table 15.2 Clinical symptoms of affected mucosal sites in mucous membrane pemphigoid

Affected mucosal site	Clinical features
Oral	Oral discomfort, burning sensation, gingival bleeding, mucosal peeling and difficulty in eating. Clinical features of erythematous patches, blisters and erosions/ulceration of the oral mucosa. Desquamative gingivitis
Nasal	Hemmorhagic nasal crusts, erosions and frequent nose bleeding
Ocular	Redness, tearing, burning, decreased vision, foreign body sensation or dry eyes. Clinical features of (chronic) conjunctivitis, trichiasis, fornix shortening, symblepharon, ankyloblepharon and blindness. Infrequently conjunctival ulceration
Genital and urological	Anogenital pain and/or pruritus, burning sensation, dyspareunia and dysuria. Clinical features of erythema, vesicles, blisters or erosions with potential mucosal adhesion and scarring or stenosis
Laryngeal/pharyngeal	Dyspnea and dysphonia, dysphagia, strictures or stenosis or laryngeal obstructions. Clinical features of erosions and ulcerations of the larynx, supraglottic area, potential esophageal involvement

epithelium (Table 15.2). Oral lesions occur most frequently (85%) and are mainly located on the gingival, buccal and palatal mucosa and less often on tongue or lip (Fig. 15.1). Other mucosa can be affected, such as the conjunctiva (30–60%), and less frequently the nasal mucosa (20–40%), esophagus (5–15%), pharynx (20%), larynx (5–10%) and genital mucosa (25%). MMP patients often present with complaints of bleeding, pain, dysphagia, and erosions or blister of the mucosa. Blisters of the mucosa are frequently seen, but often rupture rather quickly as a result of mechanical and traumatic forces. The majority of MMP patients with lesions limited to oral mucosa have gingival lesions resulting in desquamative gingivitis. The gingival erythema may be confused with non-specific gingivitis as part of chronic periodontal disease or oral lichen planus. The intake of nutrition or fluids can be reduced because of pain. In oral lesions re-epithelisation occurs without scarring, while in other forms of MMP lesions tend to heal with scar formation. The severity of MMP depends on the affected mucosal site. Patients with mild and moderate MMP often present with lesions limited to the oral mucosa, while patients with severe MMP usually have additional affected sites such as ocular, nasopharyngeal, laryngeal, esophageal, genital mucosa, or skin. An ophthalmologist or otolaryngologist should examine patients with ocular, nasal or laryngeal symptoms, whereas an oral and maxillofacial surgeon is expert on oral lesions. Furthermore, the extent of disease should be assessed, for example with the MMP Disease Area Index (MMPDAI, see Chap. 2).

Desquamative gingivitis in MMP may be seen as non-specific gingivitis

A multidisciplinary approach is recommended to prevent disease progression and complications

Diagnostics

MMP should be differentiated from other diseases with involvement of the (oral) mucosa, such as (erosive) oral lichen planus, pemphigus vulgaris, erythema multiforme, oral aphthosis, and dermatitis herpetiformis. Diagnosis of MMP is based on clinical presentation with predominant mucosal lesions and DIF of normal or perilesional buccal mucosa that shows a linear deposition of IgG and/or complement C3 and IgA along the EBMZ [3]. The n-serrated or u-serrated pattern is only observed in approximately 40% of mucosal biopsies. In case of negative DIF findings, a sequential biopsy from a different mucosal site may be performed if clinical suspicion of MMP persists. In addition, patients with MMP may show positive DIF findings of affected or unaffected skin. Therefore, an additional DIF skin biopsy of unaffected skin (for example on medial side of upper arm) or affected skin is recommended for diagnosis and serration pattern analysis. IIF performed on 1 M NaCl-split skin substrate shows binding of autoantibodies on the epidermal side of the artificial split. The titer of circulating autoantibodies in serum is frequently low and often not detectable. Immunoblot is of additional value in diagnostics of MMP. The IF findings of MMP are identical to

BP, the distinction should be made based on clinical symptoms of the predominant mucosal phenotype.

In case of initially negative DIF findings, it is recommended to take a sequential biopsy from mucosa and/or skin

> **Case Study: Part 2**
> A perilesional mucosal biopsy from buccal mucosa for DIF showed IgG 2+ and complement C3 1+ along the EBMZ, the serration pattern was undeterminable in this mucosal biopsy. Although skin was not affected, a simultaneously performed skin biopsy for DIF showed n-serrated IgG 2+ depositions along the EBMZ. Indirect IF on monkey-esophagus and salt-split skin was negative for IgG and IgA. Immunoblot showed positivity for BP180 IgG, but was negative for BP230. BP180 NC16A index was 39 (positive). The diagnosis of MMP was made, based on clinical symptoms of affected oral mucosa and a positive DIF.

Treatment Tricks

Initial Treatment and Treatment Ladder

Mild to moderate MMP can be treated effectively with moderate to superpotent topical corticosteroids, and/or dapsone (25–200 m/day), methotrexate (7.5–25 mg/week) or tetracyclines. In refractory cases systemic corticosteroids (0.5 mg/kg/day) may be added and/or treatment changed to azathioprine (100–150 mg/day) or mycophenolic acid (500–2000 mg/day). Another treatment option in severe MMP is dapsone or cyclophosphamide (50–200 mg/day) with systemic corticosteroids. Refractory cases may require treatment with anti-CD20 antibody rituximab, intravenous immunoglobulin (IVIG) or TNF-α inhibitor.

Follow-Up and Tapering

It has been suggested that MMP with lesions limited to the oral mucosa has a better prognosis compared to other subtypes of MMP. However, the clinical symptoms are highly variable and the number of reports in literature regarding follow-up and treatment is limited. Lesions on other mucosa may develop during follow-up, including ocular or largyngeal involvement. Therefore, the multidisciplinary approach is also advised during follow-up.

> **Case Study: Part 3**
> Treatment was started with dapsone 50 mg/day and, after a G6PD deficiency was excluded, increased to 100 mg/day. Because of increasing fatigueness and loss of appetite, treatment was switched oral corticosteroids and azathioprine up to 150 mg/day. Unfortunately, the disease was not controlled. Therefore, the patient received Rituximab treatment (see box # Chap. 8) which reduced the blister frequency and subjective complaints.

Ocular Mucous Membrane Pemphigoid

Short Definition in Layman Terms

Ocular mucous membrane pemphigoid, previously termed ocular cicatricial pemphigoid, is defined as MMP with lesions of the eyes. Ocular MMP may be present in monosite or multisite MMP. Clinical severity is variable and can range from burning sensation of the eyes to scarring resulting in blindness. Therefore, early recognition is important to prevent scarring.

Clinical Symptoms

Ocular MMP usually starts unilaterally with a recurrent inflammatory process resulting in clinical features of dry eye, conjunctivitis, trichiasis, fornix shortening, symblepharon and ankyloblepharon formation (Fig. 15.2). In the final stage of the disease pannus occurs: total keratinization of the entire ocular surface, resulting in blindness when not treated accurately. Although ocular

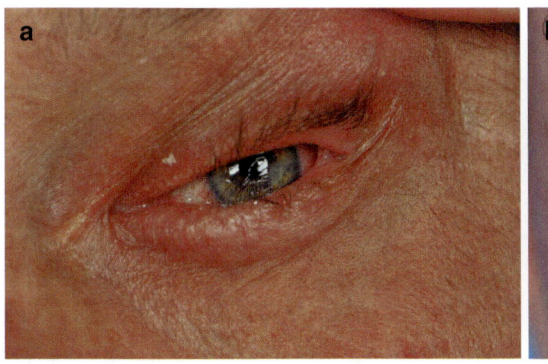 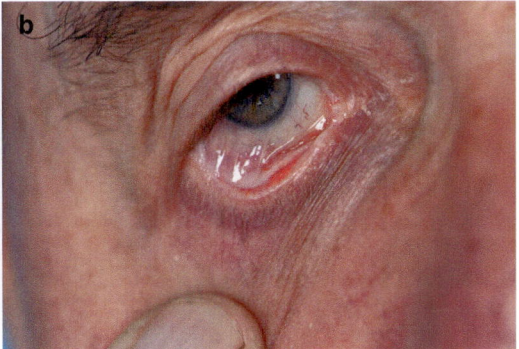

Fig. 15.2 Four clinical clues of ocular MMP: (**a**) conjunctivitis and trichiasis, (**b**) symblepharon and fornix shortening

MMP may initially start unilateral, in most cases the disease is bilateral within 2 years.

Diagnosis Paths

The target antigen in ocular MMP is the 180-kDa antigen (BP180). In patients with ocular MMP, a biopsy for DIF (of the conjunctiva) may show linear IgG and/or IgA depositions. These biopsies can be performed by the dermatologist or ophthalmologist (see Chap. 3 How to take a biopsy). However, up to 50% of ocular MMP patients show negative DIF and serology. With high suspicion of ocular MMP and negative DIF of the conjunctiva, repeated DIF of oral mucosa or skin and IIF are recommended for diagnosis. IIF performed on 1 M NaCl-split skin substrate showing binding of antibodies to the epidermal side (roof) of the blister and by immunoblot analysis revealing immunoglobulin binding to the 180-kDa antigen.

Treatment Tricks

Mild and moderate ocular MMP is treated with dapsone, methotrexate, azathioprine, mycophenolate mofetil or mycophenolic acid or cyclophosphamide. Blepharitis should be treated with eye lid hygiene and topical tetracycline cream. In rapidly progressive ocular MMP with impending blindness, methylprednisolone or systemic corticosteroids (1.0 mg/kg/day) in combination with cyclophoshamide is a recommended treatment. Consultation of the ophthalmologist is needed to evaluate the effect of treatment with slit-lamp examination. In refractory cases of ocular MMP rituximab treatment (see box # Chap. 8), intravenous immunoglobulin (IVIG) or TNF-α inhibitor may induce remission. Surgical intervention like eye lash ablation or amniotic membrane transplantation can be performed when ocular MMP is in clinical remission.

In rapidly progressive ocular MMP aggressive treatment is needed to prevent cicatrisation

Localized Vulvar Pemphigoid

Short Definition in Layman Terms

Localized vulvar pemphigoid (LVP) is a rare subtype of pemphigoid with solitary lesions in the genital region. Findings at vulva inspection can be very similar to lichen sclerosus and lichen planus. Full examination of skin, mouth, eyes and nasal mucosa is essential for adequate diagnosis.

Definitions and Classification

In classic MMP woman can present with erosions and blisters at any mucosal surfaces. LVP is

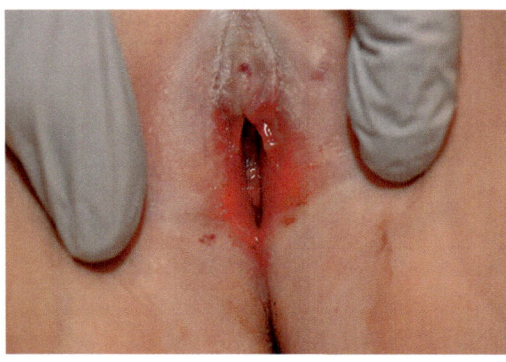

Fig. 15.3 A young girl with juvenile LVP, presenting with vulvar erosions, petechiae

defined as pemphigoid limited to the conified epithelium (skin) of the vulva and perineum. LVP can present at two different episodes in life: (1) in childhood, around 10 years, called juvenile or childhood LVP (Fig. 15.3) and (2) at postmenopausal age, called adult LVP. Because of the similarity with lichen sclerosus and lichen planus doctor's delay is frequently seen. On occasion the disease is erroneously confused with sexual abuse.

Clinical Symptoms

Patients may complain of vulvar itch, burning sensation, pain, dysuria, and in adults dyspareunia. Upon inspection of the vulva erosions and ulceration with structural architectural changes (scarring), labial fusion and clitoral burial can be seen. Vaginal involvement is unknown in LVP.

LVP clinically resembles lichen sclerosus and lichen planus

Diagnosis Paths

Histopathology in the early phase shows similarities with lichen sclerosus like subepidermal oedema. At a latter phase a subepidermal blister underneath with an infiltrate existing from lymphocytes eosinophils and / or neutrophils, with or without fibrosis is seen. DIF shows IgG, IgA and C3c depositions in the n-serrated pattern along the epidermal BMZ. IIF on monkey esophagus is often negative because the circulating autoantibodies usually have a low titre. IIF performed on 1 M NaCl-split skin substrate showing binding of antibodies to the epidermal side (roof) of the blister.

Treatment Tricks

Topical tetracycline cream is first-line therapy. Superpotent topical corticosteroids can be used after failure of treatment. Dapsone is treatment of choice when systemic treatment is needed. Refractory cases are treated following MMP recommendations.

Anti-laminin-332 Mucous Membrane Pemphigoid

Introduction

Short Definition in Layman Terms

Anti-laminin 332 MMP (anti-LN-332 MMP) is a rare subtype of MMP that is difficult to distinguish from other forms of MMP at first sight. It is known for scarring of the mucosal lesions. Furthermore patients have an increased relative risk for malignancy, especially adenocarcinoma. Because of this clinical aggressive behavior it is important to diagnose patients in an early phase of the disease.

Definitions and Classification

Anti-LN-332 MMP is previously known as anti-epiligrin cicatricial pemphigoid. Anti-epiligrin cicatricial pemphigoid with autoantibodies that bind epiligrin was first described in 2003. Epiligrin appeared to be a mixture of laminin 5, now named laminin 332 (LN-332), laminin-6 (LN-311), and laminin-7 (LN-321). LN-332 is a heterotrimeric protein consisting of α3, β3 and γ2 laminin subunits. Approximately 5–20% of all MMP patients show circulating IgG autoantibodies against LN-332.

Anti-laminin-332 MMP is previously known as anti-epiligrin cicatricial pemphigoid

Pathogenesis

Anti-LN-332 MMP is a form of MMP with circulating autoantibodies targeting LN-332. This protein is present in the lamina lucida of the basement membrane zone of keratinizing and nonkeratinizing stratified squamous epithelia, and connects hemidesmosomes to anchoring fibrils by interlinking integrin α6β4 and BP180 to type VII collagen. In most patients the IgG autoantibodies predominantly target the laminin α3 subunit, although IgG autoantibodies targeting the β3 or γ2 subunits have also been described.

Clinical Symptoms

Anti-LN-332 MMP mimics other forms of MMP and presents with involvement of the mucosal surfaces of the mouth, eyes, nasopharynx, oropharynx, larynx and anogenital region (Fig. 15.4). Complications of anti-LN-332 MMP are airway obstruction due to pharyngeal and laryngeal involvement or loss of vision because of subconjunctival fibrosis and cicatrisation. In most patients the skin is also involved, but usually less severe. In some cases the pharyngeal and laryngeal mucosa are the only regions involved (Fig. 15.5). Patients may present with aphonia (loss of voice) due to edema, erosions and ulcerations of the supraglottic area. This is followed by scarring of the larynx, and acute upper airway obstruction due to initial laryngeal edema may occur, necessitating tracheotomy. In these patients a diagnostic delay is frequently seen.

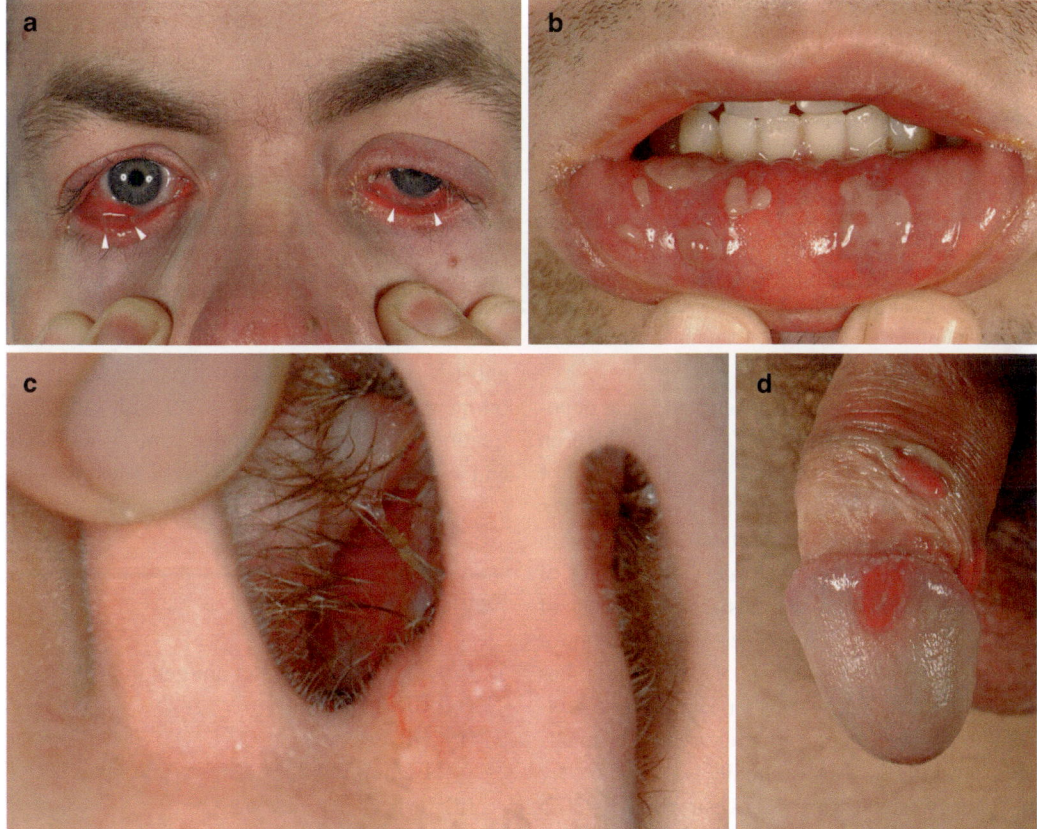

Fig. 15.4 Clinical features in a patient with anti-LN-332 MMP. (**a**) Conjunctivitis with symblepharon (arrow heads) and edema of the upper eyelid, (**b**) extensive blistering of the oral mucosa, (**c**) erosions on nasal mucosa, and (**d**) genital ulcers. (Reprinted from Terra et al. [4] with permission from Wiley)

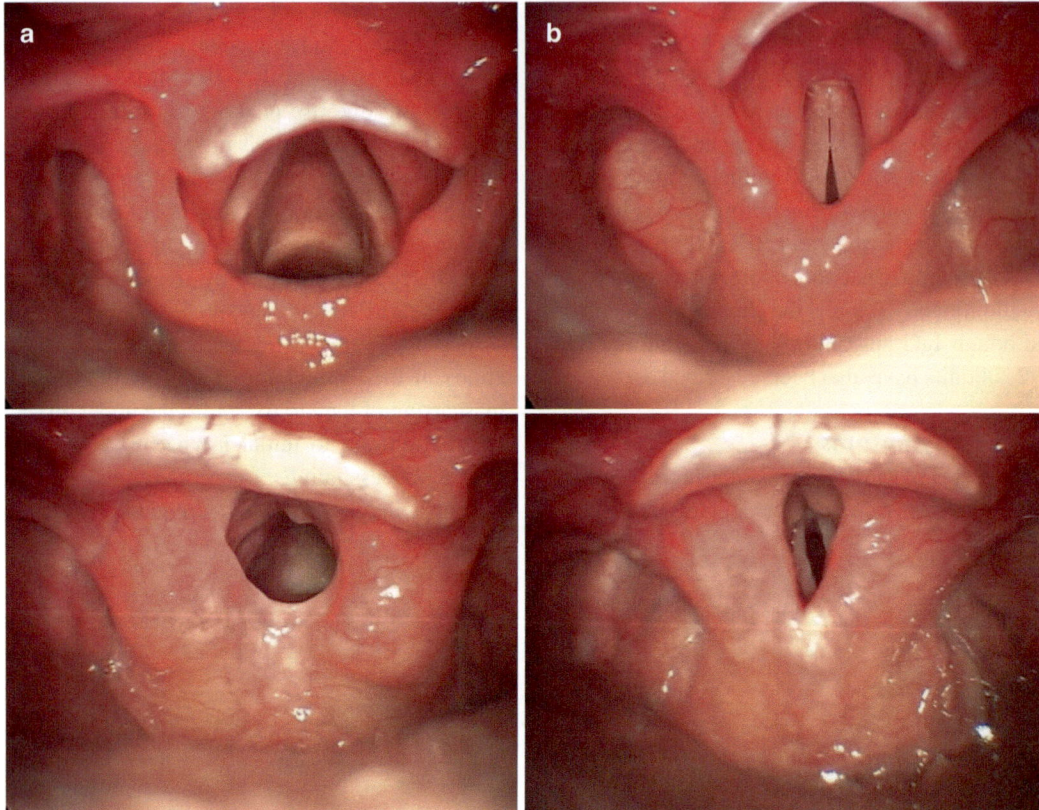

Fig. 15.5 Laryngeal cicatrisation of the ary-epiglottic folds with (**a**) supraglottic stenosis, and in healthy control. (**b**) Top is ventral side of patient. (Reprinted from Terra et al. [4] with permission from Wiley)

Diagnosis Paths

A biopsy for DIF shows an n-serrated linear deposition of IgG along the EBMZ. IIF performed on 1 M NaCl-split skin substrate reveals binding of antibodies to the dermal side (floor) of the blister in anti-LN-332 MMP, in contrast to MMP with BP180 reactivity and epidermal side staining of the blister. However, a substantial portion of patients require additional serological tests for antigen-specific detection of autoantibodies against laminin-332, such as the keratinocyte footprint assay (see Chap. 6 Immunoassays). Patients with anti-LN-332 MMP should be screened for malignancy, which is present in estimated 20–30% of the patients, mostly adenocarcinoma [1, 2, 5].

Because of the increased risk for malignancy, patients with anti-LN-332 MMP should be thoroughly screened

Treatment Tricks

Besides the screening and therapy of a potential underlying malignancy, treatment of patients with anti-LN-332 MMP follows the general MMP recommendations (see above). Prompt adequate treatment is advised to achieve control of disease and to delay disease progression of scarring.

Review Questions

1. What is the main target antigen in MMP?
   (a) BP180
   (b) BP230
   (c) Laminin 332
   (d) Type VII collagen
2. In rapidly progressive ocular MMP with impending blindness recommended treatment is:
   (a) Dapsone
   (b) Azathioprine
   (c) Cyclophosphamide and systemic corticosteroids
   (d) Mycophenolic acid

3. Specific diagnostics for anti-LN-332 MMP are:
   (a) DIF IgG u-serrated and SSS dermal binding
   (b) DIF IgG u-serrated and SSS epidermal binding
   (c) DIF IgG n-serrated and SSS dermal binding
   (d) DIF IgG n-serrated and SSS epidermal binding
4. First line therapy of juvenile LVP consists of:
   (a) Topical superpotent corticosteroids
   (b) Topical tetracycline cream
   (c) Oral corticosteroids (0.5 mg/kg/day)
   (d) Dapsone
5. Which statement about MMP is incorrect?
   (a) Oral mucosa is affected in the majority of the patients
   (b) Serration pattern analysis is less often possible on mucosal biopsies compared to skin biopsies
   (c) The titer of circulating autoantibodies in serum is frequently low and often not detectable
   (d) Patients with MMP do not have skin lesions, otherwise the diagnosis is bullous pemphigoid

Answers

1. (a)
2. (c)
3. (c)
4. (b)
5. (d)

References

1. Rashid H, Lamberts A, Borradori L, et al. S3 guideline on diagnosis and management of mucous membrane pemphigoid, initiated by the European Academy of Dermatology and Venereology (EADV)—part I: clinical presentation and outcome measurements for disease assessment. JEADV. 2021;35(9):1750–64.
2. Schmidt E, Rashid H, Marzano AV, et al. S3 guideline for diagnosis and management of mucous membrane pemphigoid, initiated by the European Academy of Dermatology and Venereology (EADV)—Part II. JEADV. 2021;35:1926–48.
3. Rashid H, Meijer JM, Diercks GFH, Sieben NE, Bolling MC, Pas HH, Horvath B. Assessment of diagnostic strategy for mucous membrane pemphigoid. JAMA Dermatol. 2021;157(7):780–7.
4. Terra JB, Pas HH, Hertl M, Dikkers FG, Kamminga N, Jonkman MF. Immunofluorescence serration pattern analysis as a diagnostic criterion in antilaminin-332 mucous membrane pemphigoid: immunopathological findings and clinical experience in 10 Dutch patients. Br J Dermatol. 2011;165:815–22.
5. Carey B, Joshi S, Abdelghani A, Mee J, Andiappan M, Setterfield J. The optimal oral biopsy site for diagnosis of mucous membrane pemphigoid and pemphigus vulgaris. Br J Dermatol. 2020;182(3):747–53. https://doi.org/10.1111/bjd.18032.

Epidermolysis Bullosa Acquisita

16

Joost M. Meijer and Marcel F. Jonkman

Introduction and AIMS

Short Definition in Layman Terms

Epidermolysis bullosa acquisita (EBA) means acquired, not inherited, bullous loosening of the skin. The autoimmune disease is caused by antibodies against a component of the skin that attaches the upper part to the bottom part. The original cause of this autoimmune disease is unknown. Patients with EBA complain of skin blisters after minor bumping or of red spots that may appear spontaneously. There is no cure, but the disease can be kept quit with medicine that alter immunity.

> **Learning Objectives**
> After reading this chapter you know the clinical subtypes of EBA, understand the pathogenesis, and are aware how to make the diagnosis. You also can make a treatment proposition that fits with the disease subtype and the patient needs.

J. M. Meijer (✉) · M. F. Jonkman (Deceased)
Center for Blistering Diseases, Department of Dermatology, University Medical Center Groningen, University of Groningen,
Groningen, The Netherlands
e-mail: j.m.meijer@umcg.nl

> **Case Study: Part 1**
> A 36-year-old woman noticed skin blisters on her feet after jogging. Later she also developed spontaneously blisters on the shoulders and abdomen. The lesions were painful and itchy. At physical examination tense blisters were seen on normal skin on both sites of the hands and feet, and on the extensor surface of the elbows.

Didactical Questions: Cross Section of Questions to Prime the Readers Interest

Why is EBA included in the pemphigoid spectrum? What determines the clinical subtype? What is the blister level considering that the immune deposits are so low in the basement membrane zone? How do you make the diagnosis? And what options do we have for this treatment refractory disease?

Facts and Figures

Definitions and Classification

Epidermolysis bullosa acquisita (EBA) is a subepidermal autoimmune blistering disease (sAIBD) characterized by autoreactivity to type

VII collagen located in the anchoring fibrils in the epidermal basement membrane zone (EBMZ) [1]. EBA is a clinically heterogeneous disease that may be characterized by either a mechanobullous or an inflammatory phenotype.

Epidemiology

The estimated EBA annual incidence in central European countries is about 0.25 new cases/million/year. The estimated frequency of EBA among patients with pemphigoid diseases is 5.5%. EBA may occur at any age, and occurs in both children and adults. A gender preference of females exists of 2.2. The ratio of the mechanobullous and inflammatory phenotypes of EBA is 1:2 [2].

Pathogenesis

The main autoantibody isotype in EBA is IgG, predominantly IgG1 and IgG4 subclass, but deposits of IgA, and complement may also be found along the epidermal BMZ. Most EBA patients' sera react with epitopes located within the non-collagenous (NC)-1 domain of human type VII collagen (Fig. 16.1). Binding of patient autoantibodies to the collagenous or the NC2 domain is rarely observed. No correlation is detected between antibody specificity to type VII collagen subdomains and clinical phenotype (mechanobullous/inflammatory).

Split formation is dependent on activation of neutrophils through the Fc domain of immunoglobulin. Split formation occurs in most cases at the level of the lamina lucida, and not at the level of the anchoring fibrils in the sublamina densa zone. These split formations within the lamina lucida most likely represent the intra-lamina lucida-separating effects of leukocyte-derived proteolytic enzymes, when those cells are chemoattracted to the dermo-epidermal junction by bound immunoreactants.

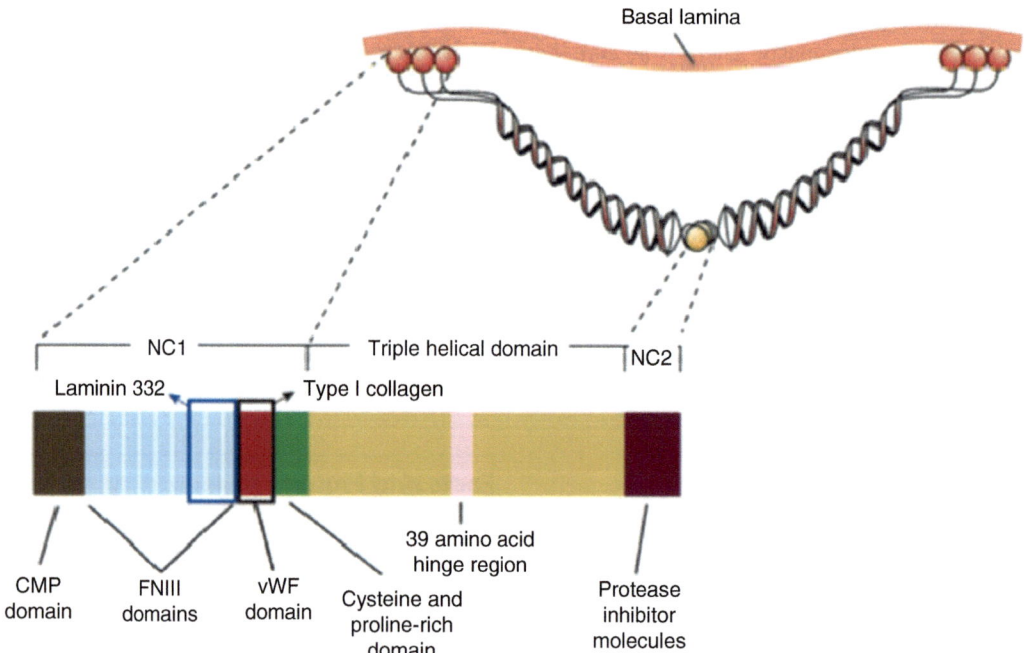

Fig. 16.1 Diagram of type VII collagen shows the immunodominant NC-1 domain. *N* aminoterminal, *C* carboxyterminal, *CMP* cartilage matrix protein, *FNIII* fibronectine-type III-like repeats, *VWFA* a domain of von Willebrand factor, *NC-1* non-collagenous aminoterminal domain, *NC-2* non-collagenous carboxy-terminal domain

Diagnosis Paths

History and Physical Examination

The classic mechanobullous phenotype mimics hereditary dystrophic epidermolysis bullosa, while mild cases may look like acral blistering of porphyria cutanea tarda that heal with atrophic scarring, milia and hypo- or hyperpigmentation (Fig. 16.2). Scalp, neck and shoulders involvement occurs in 20% and leads to extensive non-healing erosions with scarring, similar to clinical features of Brunsting-Perry pemphigoid (Fig. 16.3).

The inflammatory phenotype presents with widespread vesicles and bullae involving intertriginous and flexural areas, that heal with no or few milia without scarring (Fig. 16.4). This phenotype may appear similar to bullous pemphigoid or non-bullous pemphigoid, and a presentation with predominantly mucosal involvement similar to of mucous membrane pemphigoid with scarring on the mucosal surfaces (Fig. 16.5). EBA is associated with SLE and inflammatory bowel disease.

General Diagnostics

Transition from mechanobullous to inflammatory phenotype or vice versa is sometimes found. In a

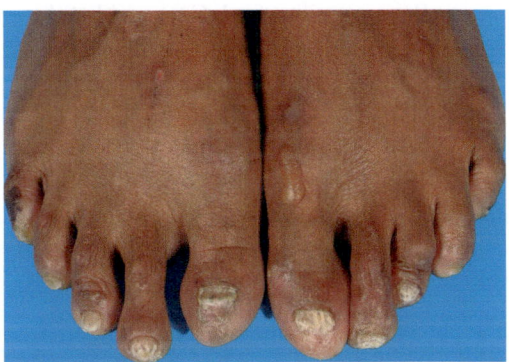

Fig. 16.2 Mechanobullous EBA in a young female showing bullae and crusts, and nail dystrophy on the feet

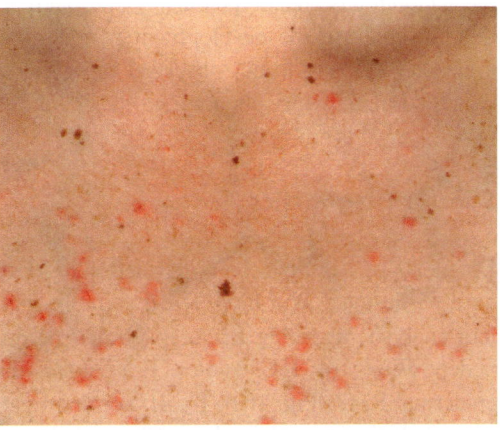

Fig. 16.4 Inflammatory EBA in a 37-y-old female showing lenticular erythematous papules with erosive top on the chest

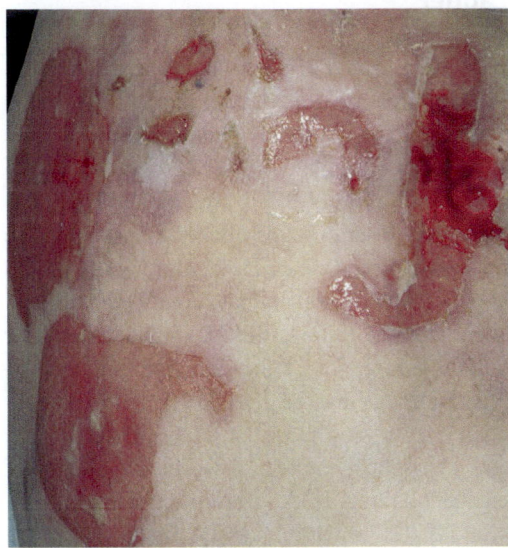

Fig. 16.3 Mechanobullous EBA similar to Brunsting-Perry pemphigoid in a female with scarring lesions affecting the neck and scalp

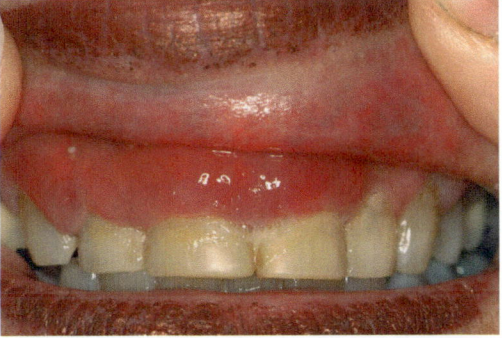

Fig. 16.5 Mucous membrane pemphigoid with antibodies against type VII collagen in a female with hypertrophic gingiva

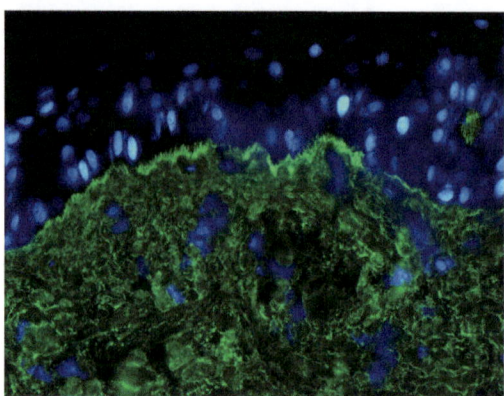

Fig. 16.6 U-serrated linear immunodeposition (IgG) along the EBMZ diagnostic for EBA or BSLE

minority of patients a temporary flare of widespread inflammatory bullae may occur in the mechanobullous phenotype during an exacerbation. In contrast, the development of extensive milia and scarring is not observed in patients with the inflammatory phenotype.

Specific Diagnostics

Diagnosis of EBA can be confirmed using DIF on a perilesional skin biopsy and serration pattern analysis, revealing linear u-serrated immunodepositions of IgG and/or IgA along the epidermal BMZ (Fig. 16.6) [3, 4]. Serration pattern analysis is explained in Chap. 4 Direct Immunofluorescence Microscopy. Only in approximately 50% of patients with EBA circulating autoantibodies can be detected, therefore DIF is essential for diagnosis of EBA. In serological negative cases direct immuno-electron microscopy, or DIF on sodium chloride-separated skin biopsy might reveal the diagnosis, but at risk of damaging the biopsy specimen [5]. Indirect immunofluorescence microscopy (IIF) performed on 1 M NaCl-split skin (SSS) substrate shows binding of antibodies to the dermal site (floor) of the blister, while immunoblot analysis may reveal immunoglobulin binding to the 290 kDa antigen. Autoantibody detection by type VII ELISA has a rather low sensitivity of 45%.

Combining IIF SSS and ELISA reaches a sensitivity of 50% [6]. Sophisticated serological methods may aid in diagnosis of EBA, such as IIF on skin deficient of type VII collagen of patients with hereditary dystrophic epidermolysis bullosa.

> **Case Study: Part 2**
>
> Skin biopsy for direct IF revealed linear depositions of IgG 4+, IgA 3+, and C3c 1+ in a u-serrated pattern along the EBMZ. Examination of the serum by indirect IF was positive for IgG 2+ and IgA 1+ in the floor of salt-split skin. IIF on knock-out skin was negative on type VII collagen deficient skin, whereas positive on laminin-332 deficient skin. The type VII collagen ELISA index of IgG was 137 (positive). A diagnosis was made of epidermolysis bullosa acquisita, mechanobullous type.

Treatment Tricks

Initial Treatment and Therapeutic Ladder

EBA is a chronic disease that is often refractory to many treatment modalities. The 1st line therapy for EBA is a combination of low dose corticosteroids, colchicine or dapsone. Colchicine is used at a dose of 0.5–1 mg/day and has a low incidence of serious side-effects. Dapsone can be prescribed at a dose of 25 mg/day that is gradually increased to 100 mg/day. Treatment with oral corticosteroid follows the recommendations for bullous pemphigoid. Other adjuvant immunosuppressive drugs may be considered; such as mycophenolate mofetil, azathioprine, methotrexate, and cyclophosphamide. In refractory cases of mechanobullous EBA intravenous immunoglobulin (IVIG) or rituximab treatment might be considered.

Follow-Up and Tapering

The median time to remission of patients with EBA is estimated 9 months. The long-term prognoses of patients with EBA has proven excellent, but continuous low-dose of immunosuppressive drugs can be necessary.

> **Case Study: Part 3**
> First line therapy with prednisolone 30 mg and azathioprine 150 mg was insufficient. Subsequently, she was treated with human intravenous immunoglobulin 2 g/kg/month for 1 year. The blister frequency reduced. A maintenance therapy consisted of prednisolone 7.5 mg and azathioprine 150 mg for several years.

Review Questions

1. The most frequent clinical phenotype of EBA is
   (a) Mechanobullous
   (b) Inflammatory
   (c) a and b are equally frequent
2. Which disease or syndrome is associated with EBA?
   (a) Atopic syndrome
   (b) Neoplasia
   (c) Inflammatory bowel disease
3. In which domain are the immunodominant epitopes of type VII collagen located?
   (a) NC1 domain
   (b) Collagenous domain
   (c) NC2 domain
4. What is the most essential routine diagnostic test for EBA?
   (a) Direct immune-electron microscopy
   (b) Type VII collagen ELISA
   (c) Direct immunofluorescence with u-serrated pattern
   (d) Histopathology
5. Treatment response of EBA compared to bullous pemphigoid is
   (a) Similar
   (b) Often more treatment refractory
   (c) More favourable

Answers

1. b
2. c
3. a
4. c
5. b

References

1. Woodley DT, Briggaman RA, O'Keefe EJ, Inman AO, Queen LL, Gammon WR. Identification of the skin basement-membrane autoantigen in epidermolysis bullosa acquisita. N Eng J Med. 1984;310:1007–13.
2. Buijsrogge JJ, Diercks GF, Pas HH, Jonkman MF. The many faces of epidermolysis bullosa acquisita after serration pattern analysis by direct immunofluorescence microscopy. Br J Dermatol. 2011;165:92–8.
3. Terra JB, Meijer JM, Jonkman MF, Diercks GF. The n- vs. u-serration is a learnable criterion to differentiate pemphigoid from epidermolysis bullosa acquisita in direct immunofluorescence serration pattern analysis. Br J Dermatol. 2013;169:100–5.
4. Meijer JM, Atefi I, Diercks GFH, Vorobyev A, Zuiderveen J, Meijer HJ, Pas HH, Zillikens D, Schmidt E, Jonkman MF. Serration pattern analysis for differentiating epidermolysis bullosa acquisita from other pemphigoid diseases. J Am Acad Dermatol. 2018;78(4):754–759.e6.
5. Prost-Squarcioni C, Caux F, Schmidt E, Jonkman MF, Vassileva S, Kim SC, Iranzo P, Daneshpazhooh M, Terra J, Bauer J, Fairley J, Hall R, Hertl M, Lehman JS, Marinovic B, Patsatsi A, Zillikens D, Werth V, Woodley DT, Murrell DF. International Bullous Diseases Group: consensus on diagnostic criteria for epidermolysis bullosa acquisita. Br J Dermatol. 2018;179(1):30–41.
6. Terra JB, Jonkman MF, Diercks GF, Pas HH. Low sensitivity of type VII collagen enzyme-linked immunosorbent assay in epidermolysis bullosa acquisita: serration pattern analysis on skin biopsy is required for diagnosis. Br J Dermatol. 2013;169:164–7.

Additional Reading

Fine J, Tyring S, Gammon W. The presence of intra-lamina lucida blister formation in epidermolysis acquisita: possible role of leukocytes. J Invest Dermatol. 1989;92:27–32.

Rusenko K, Gammon W, Fine J, Briggaman R. The carboxyl-terminal domain of type VII collagen is present at the basement membrane in recessive dystrophic epidermolysis bullosa. J Invest Dermatol. 1989;92:623–7.

Vorobyev A, Ludwig RJ, Schmidt E. Clinical features and diagnosis of epidermolysis bullosa acquisita. Expert Rev Clin Immunol. 2017;13(2):157–69.

Bullous Systemic Lupus Erythematosus

17

Marcel F. Jonkman and J. M. Meijer

Introduction and AIMS

Short Definition in Layman Terms

Bullous systemic lupus erythematosus (BSLE) is a condition when blisters occur in patients with SLE. Mostly it is an autoimmune disease against type VII collagen, and resembling epidermolysis bullosa acquista (EBA). Conversely, blistering may be caused by an acute, severe inflammatory skin reaction in patients with SLE.

Learning Objectives
After reading this chapter you understand the clinical presentations and the histological and immunelogical features, differential diagnosis, and treatment options of vesiculo-bullous eruptions in bullous systemic lupus erythematosus (BSLE).

Case Study: Part 1
A 22-year old female had an acute generalized vesiculo-bullous eruption that was controlled with systemic corticosteroids. One year before a vascular hemiplegia was reversed with aspirin. Two years later, she started having blisters on the extremities after trauma to the skin. Raynaud phenomenon was present. Blood tests revealed leucopenia, ANA positivity in 1:640 titer, and Coombs, nRNP, SSA, and lupus-anticoagulant all positive. A diagnosis of SLE was made, and she was initially treated with prednisolone 7.5 mg/day.

Didactical Questions; Cross Section of Questions to Prime the Readers Interest

What is the outcome of direct IF of a skin biopsy in BSLE? What autoantigen is involved in BSLE?

Facts and Figures

Definitions and Classification

Two immunologically distinct subtypes of BSLE are originally recognized in patients with con-

M. F. Jonkman (Deceased) · J. M. Meijer (✉)
Center for Blistering Diseases, Department of Dermatology, University Medical Center Groningen, University of Groningen,
Groningen, The Netherlands
e-mail: j.m.meijer@umcg.nl

firmed diagnosis of SLE, type I with type VII collagen autoantibodies, and type II without such autoantibodies (Table 17.1) [1, 2]. Blistering may also occur due to severe local inflammatory response in subacute cutaneous lupus erythematosus (SCLE) (Fig. 17.1).

Epidemiology

Cutaneous manifestations are not rare in SLE; more than 76% of the patient report cutaneous lesion during disease course. Only 1–5% of the patients with SLE are reported with bullous SLE [3, 4]. BSLE typically affects young adults and starts in the second or third decade of life.

Table 17.1 Diagnostic criteria for BSLE (adapted from [1] and revised [2])

1. A diagnosis of SLE based upon most recent diagnostic criteria (EULAR/ACR)
2. Vesicles and bullae arising upon but not limited to sunexposed skin
3. Histopathology compatible with dermatitis herpetiformis
4. Negative or positive indirect IF for circulating BMZ antibodies using separated human skin as substrate
5. DIF of lesional and nonlesional skin revealing linear or granular IgG and/or IgM and often IgA at the BMZ. Immunoelectron microscopy would demonstrate the immune reactants below the basal lamina

BSLE bullous systemic lupus erythematosus, *BMZ* basement membrane zone

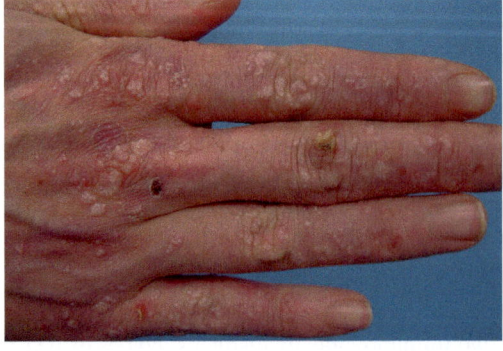

Fig. 17.1 Erosions and milia in an erythemato-squamous plaque on the hand in a patient with SLE

Pathogenesis

The pathogenesis of BSLE with autoantibodies against type VII collagen is similar to that of epidermolysis bullosa acquisita (EBA) (see Chap. 16). The typical histopathology is a subepidermal vesicle and neutrophil microabcesses papillary tips, indistinguishable from dermatitis herpetiformis.

BSLE without autoantibodies against type VII collagen is caused by a severe vacuolar alteration of the dermo-epidermal junction, dermal edema, and sometimes leucocytoclastic vasculitis. Blistering in SCLE is caused by apoptotic epidermal changes, that when fulminant may resemble toxic epidermal necrolysis.

Diagnosis Paths

History and Physical Examination

The clinical presentation of BSLE is generally that of an acute, generalized blistering eruption in patients with SLE. Patients may present with fever. Sun exposure may elicit the condition.

General Diagnostics

Patients with BSLE exhibit features of SLE including malar rash, cutaneous lupus erythematosus (LE), oral erosions, and photosensitivity. Serology reveals positive ANA, with Sm- and dsDNA-antibodies. Direct IF of unaffected skin might reveal a so-called lupus-band: granular or homogenous depositions of IgM, IgG, IgA or complement along the BMZ. In case of subacute cutaneous lupus erythematosus (SCLE) SSA antibodies can be detected, which are visible by direct IF of patient's skin as in-vivo ANA (Fig. 17.4).

At dermatological examination one may find a clinical presentation similar to chronic mechanobullous EBA (Fig. 17.2 and 17.3), or inflammatory EBA with a more acute, generalized blistering eruption with multiple vesicles on erythematous patches, and with a malar rash

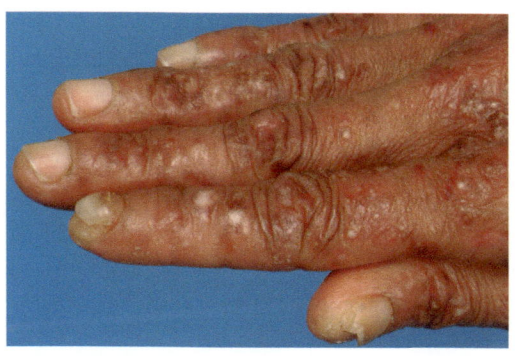

Fig. 17.2 Bullous systemic lupus erythematosus shows monomorphic blisters, skin atrophy, milia, and nail dystrophy of the dorsum of the hand resembling EBA

(Table 17.2). Mucous membranes may be involved. If the skin detaches in large sheets it may look like erythema multiforme (formerly known as Rowell syndrome) or toxic epidermolytic necrolysis (TEN).

Specific Diagnostics

The distinction between BSLE type I or type II in patients with SLE is based on presence of type VII collagen autoantibodies by DIF and serum [5, 6]. ANA is not a specific finding, since it may be pres-

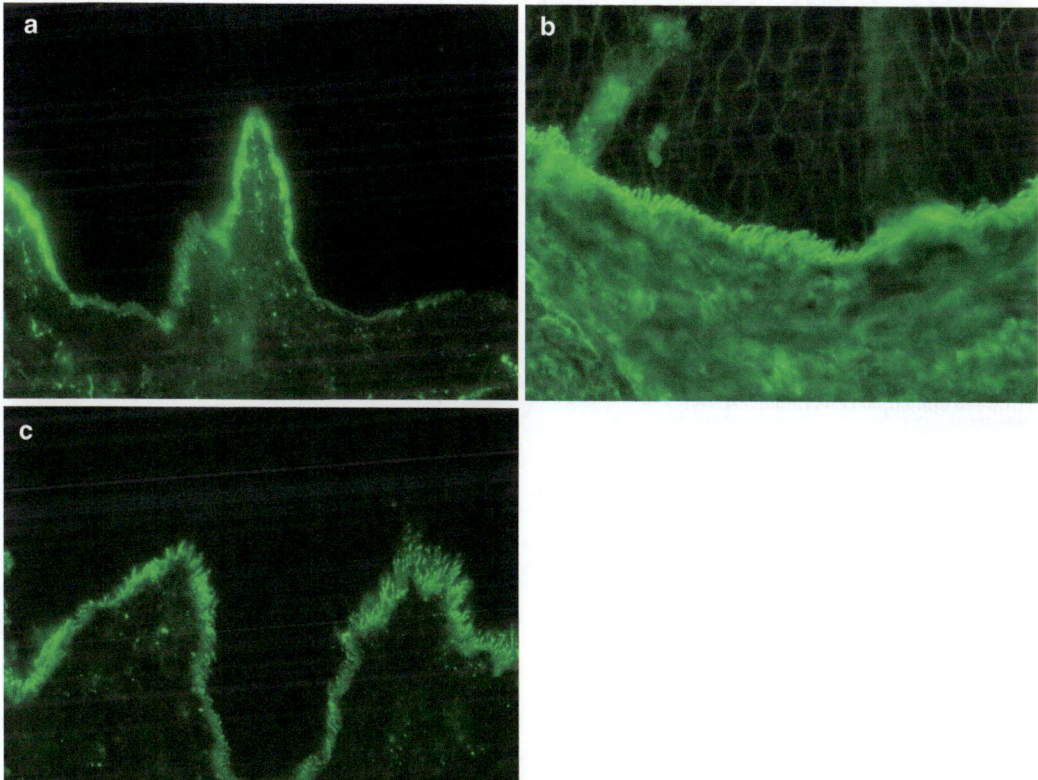

Fig. 17.3 DIF of sun exposed healthy skin (dorsum hand) in BSLE reveals fibrin in the high papillary blood vessels. Along the BMZ a broad homogenous and granular (**a**) IgM (2+) deposition and a linear deposition in u-serrated pattern is present of (**b**) IgG (3+) and (**c**) C3c (+)

Table 17.2 Classification of blistering in lupus erythematosus by immunofluorescence analysis

Type	DIF	IIF split human skin
BSLE, type I (a) EBA, mechanobullous (b) EBA, inflammatory	Linear, u-serrated, immunodepositions along BMZ	Dermal binding
BSLE, type II	Granular/homogeneous immunodepositions along BMZ	ANA
Bullous SCLE	Epidermal *in vivo* ANA	Negative
TEN-like (S)CLE	Epidermal *in vivo* ANA	Negative
TEN in SLE	Granular/homogeneous immunodepositions along BMZ	ANA

DIF direct immunofluorescence microscopy, *IIF* indirect immunofluorescence microscopy, *BSLE* bullous systemic lupus erythematosus (LE), *ANA* antinuclear antibodies, *SCLE* subacute LE, *SLE* systemic LE, *TEN* toxic epidermal necrolysis, *BMZ* epidermal basement membrane zone

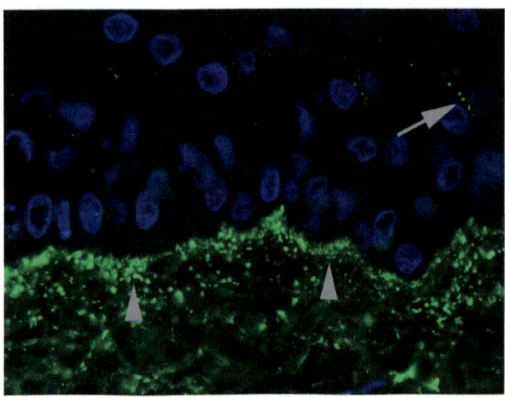

Fig. 17.4 DIF of bullous subacute cutaneous lupus erythematosus reveals granular deposition of IgG along the BMZ (arrow heads) and sparse intracellular antibodies (arrow) to epidermal cells (*in vivo* ANA)

ent in skin or serum in all SLE patients. Epidermal *in vivo* ANA is typically found in lesional and non-lesional SCLE skin (Fig. 17.4). A diagnosis of TEN is made by histopathology of erythematous skin showing transepidermal necrosis.

> **Case Study: Part 2**
>
> At age of 31 year, she was referred to our outpatient clinic. Dermatological examination is shown in Fig. 17.2. Direct IF is shown in Fig. 17.3. By indirect IF no binding of IgG and IgA was found to human split skin (IIF SSS), and immunoblot was negative for IgG and IgA. A diagnosis was made of BSLE type I based on the linear u-serrated pattern of IgG and C3c deposition.

Treatment Tricks

Initial Treatment and Therapeutic Ladder

The acute forms of BSLE may respond dramatically to dapsone. For acute cutaneous LE systemic corticosteroids might be necessary. Chronic forms of BSLE may better respond to systemic corticosteroids with an additional immunosuppressive agent, such as azathioprine (1–2 mg/kg) or mycophenolate mofetil (2 g). Rituximab is also a therapeutic option in EBA/BSLE.

Follow-Up and Tapering

Many patients with chronic BSLE need long-term low dose oral corticosteroids (<10 mg). Continuation of an alternative immunosuppressive agent is therefore advised. First line therapy for subacute and chronic cutaneous LE is topical potent corticosteroids and hydroxychloroquine (200 mg twice a day). Colchicine is a therapeutic option for treatment of neutrophil-mediated bullous diseases, and may be used in chronic BSLE.

> **Case Study: Part 3**
>
> The recurrent blistering improved by continuous daily medication of oral corticosteroids 7.5 mg, azathioprine 50 mg, and hydroxychloroquine 200 mg.

Review Questions

1. What is the most common location of acute BSLE?
   a. Cheeks and nose
   b. Dorsal side of the hands
   c. Feet
   d. Genitals
2. The immunodominant domain of type VII collagen in BSLE is the
   a. NC-1 domain
   b. Collagenous domain
   c. NC-2 domain
3. Which DIF deposition pattern at the BMZ can be seen in a patient with a diagnosis of BSLE without type VII collagen autoantibodies (type II)?
   a. Linear, n-serrated
   b. Homogenous
   c. Granular and linear, u-serrated
   d. None
4. First line treatment of acute BSLE is
   a. superpotent topical corticosteroids
   b. systemic corticosteroids
   c. azathioprine
   d. dapsone

Answers

1. b.
2. a.
3. b.
4. d.

References

1. Camisa C, Sharma HM. Vesiculobullous systemic lupus erythematosus. Report of two cases and a review of the literature. J Am Acad Dermatol. 1983;9:924–33.
2. Gammon WR, Briggaman RA. Bullous SLE: a phenotypically distinctive but immunologically heterogeneous bullous disorder. J Invest Dermatol. 1993;100:28S–34S.
3. Duan L, Chen L, Zhong S, Wang Y, Huang Y, He Y, Chen J, Shi G. Treatment of bullous systemic lupus erythematosus. J Immunol Res. 2015;2015:167064.
4. Contestable JJ, Edhegard KD, Meyerle JH. Bullous systemic lupus erythematosus: a review and update to diagnosis and treatment. Am J Clin Dermatol. 2014;15(6):517–24.
5. Camisa C, Grimwood RE. Indirect immunofluorescence in vesiculobullous eruption of systemic lupus erythematosus. J Invest Dermatol. 1986;86:606.
6. Buijsrogge JJ, Diercks GF, Pas HH, Jonkman MF. The many faces of epidermolysis bullosa acquisita after serration pattern analysis by direct immunofluorescence microscopy. Br J Dermatol. 2011;165:92–8.

Additional Reading

Vassileva S. Bullous systemic lupus erythematosus. Clin Dermatol. 2004;22:129–38.

Linear IgA Bullous Dermatosis

18

Barbara Horváth and Marcel F. Jonkman

Introduction and AIMS

Short Definition in Layman Terms

Linear IgA bullous dermatosis (LABD) is an itchy blistering skin disease with grouped vesicles on erythematous patches caused by linear IgA depositions in the epidermal basement membrane zone (EBMZ).

LABD is characterized by exclusively IgA autoantibodies targeting components of EBMZ

> **Learning Objectives**
>
> After reading this chapter you will be familiar with the clinical presentation of LABD, you will be able setup a diagnostic algorithm, and to propose a therapeutic plan.

> **Case Study: Part 1**
>
> A 44-year old female presented with itchy erythematous plaques with tense blisters, erosions and crusts at the periphery, on the head, trunk and extremities. She developed erosions at the vaginal mucosa, but other mucosal surfaces were spared. Previous medical history reported primary Sjögren's syndrome and idiopathic hyperhidrosis. There was no medication previously administered.

Didactical Questions; Cross Section of Questions to Prime the Readers Interest

How can you diagnose LABD? What would you see in the histopathological section? How can you make de difference between LABD and other autoimmune bullous diseases? What is the drug of choice for LABD?

Facts and Figures

Definitions and Classification

LABD is a heterogeneous group of subepidermal autoimmune blistering diseases characterized by

B. Horváth (✉) · M. F. Jonkman (Deceased)
Center for Blistering Diseases, Department of Dermatology, University Medical Center Groningen, University of Groningen,
Groningen, The Netherlands
e-mail: b.horvath@umcg.nl

autoantibodies exclusively from the IgA class targeting different antigens of the EBMZ. According to age LABD can be divided in juvenile and adult forms, which differ slightly in their clinical presentations but share common immunopathological features.

According to the splitting there are two different forms of LABD. In the lamina lucida-type LABD the two most common antigens are the 120 kDa molecular mass LAD-1 antigen, and the 97 kDa molecular mass LABD antigen 1 (LABD97) with BP180 being recognized by a minor subset. Laminin 332 and p200 are rare autoantigens in lamina lucida-type LABD [1]. In the sublamina densa-type LABD, also called IgA epidermolysis bullosa acquisita (EBA), the splitting level is deeper and the target antigen is type VII collagen (Chap. 16).

The LABD autoantigens are LAD-1, LABD97, BP180, laminin 332, p200 and type VII collagen

Epidemiology

LABD is a rare disease with an estimated incidence rate of 0.2–2.3/million/year depending of the geographical region [2]. The distribution in the population is biphasic affecting primarily young children at age of 4–5 years and adults in the fifth decade. The childhood form seems to be chronic but self-limiting with disease duration of 1–5 years [3]. The adult form is more chronic and recalcitrant to different treatments.

Although LABD is mostly idiopathic there are some known triggers such as drugs (mostly reported vancomycine), malignancies, UV-light and internal diseases (ulcerative colitis, collagen diseases). For drug-induced LABD we refer to Chap. 19.

LABD or chronic bullous dermatosis of childhood is the most common autoimmune blistering disease in children

Pathogenesis

The two most common LABD antigens are LAD-1 and LABD97 (Fig. 18.1). Both are cleaved from the extracellular domain of BP180 by ADAM9 and 10, and plasmin, respectively. The first cleavage is just in the NC16A domain of the BP180, and this explains that only 20% of the sera of LABD patients react with the NC16A domain [1]. IgA is a chemoattractant of neutrophilic granulocytes, leads to blister formation. In an animal model with passive transfer of murine IgA monoclonal antibodies against LABD autoantigens in a SCID mouse resulted in subepidermal vesicle formation with neutrophil influx [4].

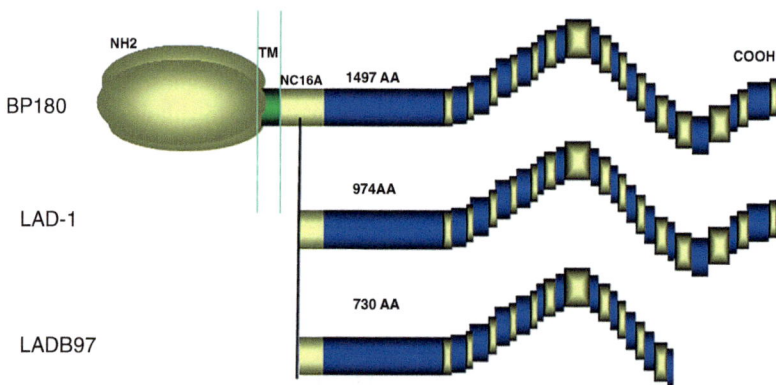

Fig. 18.1 Diagram of BP180 and shed derivates of its extracellular domain: LAD-1 and LABD97 proteins. BP180 is a transmembrane protein of the hemidesmosome containing an intracellular (N-terminus), transmembrane and extracellular (C-terminus) domain. The extracellular domain consists 15 collagenous domains (C1–15) at the C-terminus end and a non-collagenous NC16A domain downstream from the transmembrane domain (TM). LABD97 is a proteolytic product of the extracellular domain containing 1209 amino acids and the N-terminus is just within the domain 3 of the NC16A. The N-terminus of LAD-1 seems to be near the N-terminus of LABD97 but the C-terminus is the same as in the full BP180 protein (1497 amino acid)

Diagnosis Paths

History and Physical Examination

According to the biphasic population distribution, LABD has different phenotypes in adults and in children, the latter was previously called chronic bullous dermatosis of childhood (CBDC). In adults some cases resemble dermatitis herpetiformis (DH) with pruritic papulovesicular eruption on the extensor surfaces. The unique presentation of LABD are tense circinate vesicles and blisters on urticarial plaques on the trunk and limbs. The blistering in LABD is more grouped peripheral (circinate) to the plaques, and unlike BP where blistering is more to the spread over the urticarial plaque. The circinate configuration forms in a ring a "crown of jewels" (Fig. 18.2) or more serpenginous a "string of pearls" (Fig. 18.3b) [5]. In children the predilection sites are legs, lower arms and genitals (Fig. 18.3), or localized and exclusively on the lower eyelid (Fig. 18.4). Mucous membrane involvement occurs up to 80% of cases.

Moreover, drug induced cases are more atypical in the clinics with more severe course, especially cases mimicking toxic epidermal necrolysis (TEN) [6]. Careful medical history according medication in the last weeks is mandatory.

Several cases report associations with other diseases as hematological malignancies (Hodgkin's disease and B-cell lymphomas), different solid cancers (esophagus and bladder), other autoimmune diseases as SLE, multiple sclerosis, dermatomyositis, rheumatoid arthritis, Sjögren's syndrome and Crohn's disease. Whether these are true associations or co-incidences needs confirmation [5].

In juvenile LABD the skin lesions are located on the legs, lower arms and perineum in a configuration known as a "crown of jewels"

Another presentation with grouped vesicles in circinate configuration and arciform erythema resembles linear IgA bullous dermatosis, and is called IgA epidermolysis bullosa acquisita (IgA-EBA) with exclusively IgA deposits along the epidermal BMZ. IgA-EBA patients had widespread or localized vesicles, mostly without larger bullae formation (Fig. 18.5). Mucosal involvement is present in five out of eight patients with vesicular pemphigoid-like IgA-EBA but scarring of mucosal surfaces is absent.

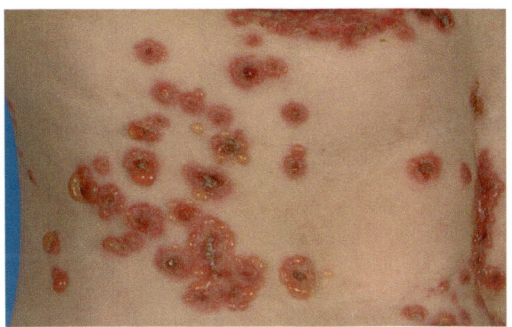

Fig. 18.2 Linear IgA bullous dermatosis in an adult presenting circinate grouped vesicles and bullae ('crown of jewels') on the abdomen

General Diagnostics

Histological examination of perilesional and lesional skin shows subepidermal blister formation with predominantly neutrophil infiltrate in the papillary dermis with occasionally some eosinophils or mononuclear cells.

Specific Diagnostics

The gold standard for the diagnostics of LABD is the linear deposition of IgA along the EBMZ by direct immunofluorescence (DIF) (Fig. 18.5). The autoantibodies are mainly from IgA1 class [7]. Indirect immunofluorescence (IIF) on monkey esophagus fails to detect autoantibodies in most cases due to the low circulating autoantibody titers. Using salt-split skin can raise the sensitivity of the serology, where the majority of the patients show epidermal bindings (lamina lucida-type LABD) and in a minority of the cases is the signal on the dermal side of the split (sublamina densa-type LABD). However some cases show a mixed pattern. Interestingly in drug-induced LABD circulating IgA against the EBMZ on salt-split skin is mostly not was detectable [8]. Western blotting seems to be more sensitive to detect circulating IgA autoantibodies against LABD97 and LAD-1.

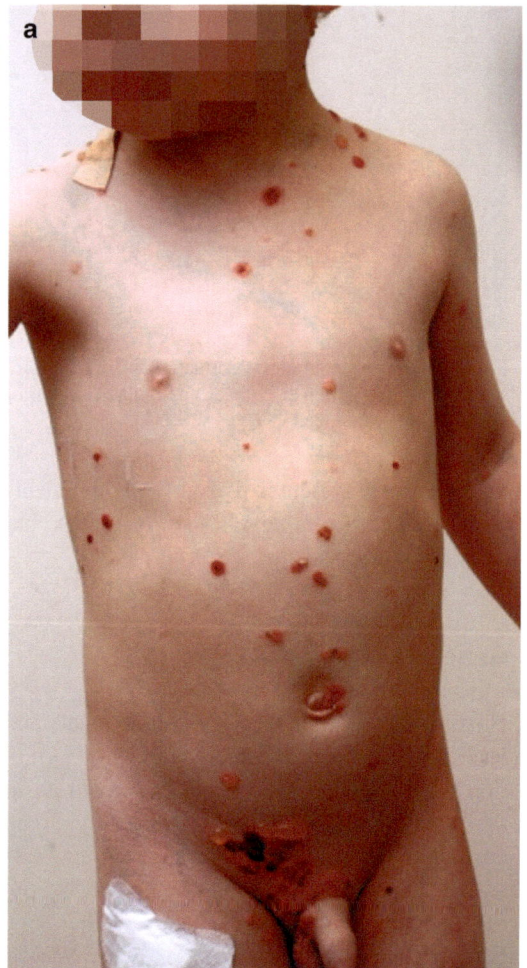
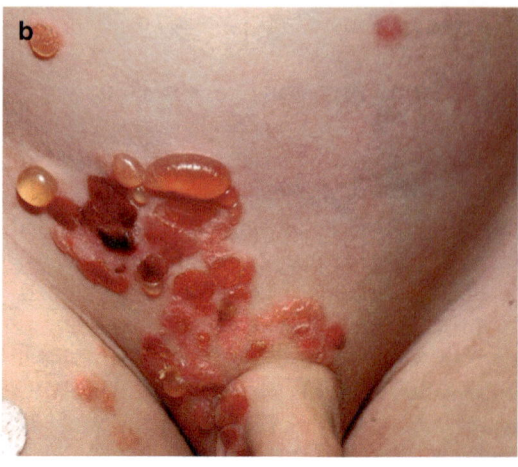

Fig. 18.3 (**a**) Juvenile linear IgA bullous dermatosis in a young boy presenting with serous bullae and hemorrhagic crusts on the trunk, and (**b**) a serpenginous configuration in pubic and genital area ('string of pearls')

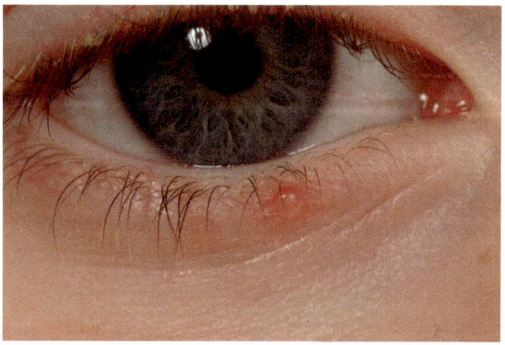

Fig. 18.4 Solitary vesicle on lower eye lid in a boy with localized linear IgA bullous dermatosis

It should be mentioned here, that in minority of the cases also IgG may be seen by DIF parallel to IgA, although in less intensity. These cases should be considered rather as overlap syndromes and designated mixed IgG/IgA bullous pemphigoid.

The linear deposition of IgA along the EBMZ in the lamina lucida-type of LABD has an n-serrated pattern (Fig. 18.6), whereas an u-serrated pattern in the sublamina densa-type LABD

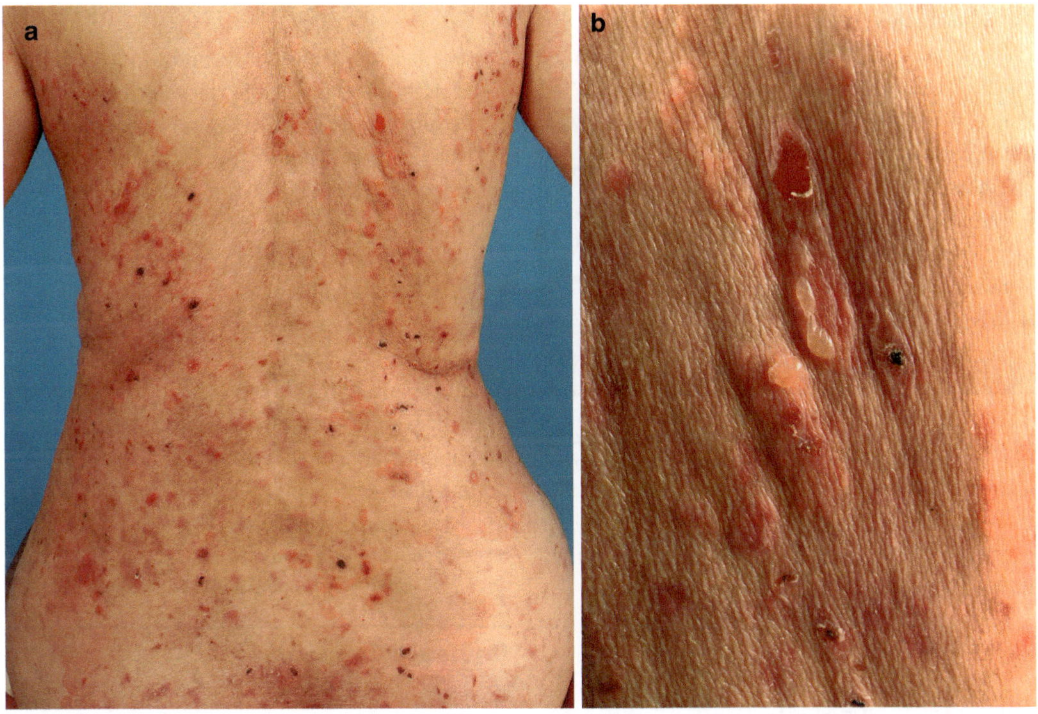

Fig. 18.5 Vesicular sublamina densa-type linear IgA bullous dermatosis (IgA-EBA) showing (**a**) multiple excoriated papules and macules on the trunk (**b**) with some small vesicles

Case Study: Part 2

Routine histopathology taken from the border of a blister showed subepidermal blister filled with almost neutrophils. DIF reveals exclusively IgA deposits in a linear n-serrated pattern along the EBMZ. IIF showed no binding of serum IgA to salt-split skin.

Treatment Tricks

Initial Treatment and Therapeutic Ladder

Dapsone is the first line treatment. Before starting glucose-6-phosphate dehydrogenase (G6-PD) deficiency should be excluded. Starting dose is 0.5 mg/kg daily slowly rising up to maximum 2.5–3.0 mg/kg until itch and blistering is controlled. The average dose to control the disease is about 100 mg daily, sometimes higher doses are needed, but hemolysis is obligate above doses of 100 mg [9]. The mechanism of dapsone to inhibit neutrophil chemotaxis on the site on IgA deposition is not well understood yet. It is known that dapsone inhibits neutrophil lysosomal activity and myeloperoxidase-mediated iodination, however it does not have any effect on antibody or complement deposition [4]. Further it was shown that dapsone inhibits neutrophil adherence to EBMZ antibodies on a dose dependent manner, which covers the pharmacological range of serum dapsone levels [4].

Alternatives are sulfonamides (sulfapyridine in a dose of 15–60 mg/kg/day) alone or in combination with dapsone. Combination of these two drugs has cumulative efficacy without additive toxicity [10]. In partial effect both can be combined with topical or oral corticosteroids [9]. There are several other treatment options reported as mycophenolate-mofetil, mycophenolic acid, colchicine, cyclosporine, methotrexate, HIVIG, cotrimoxa-

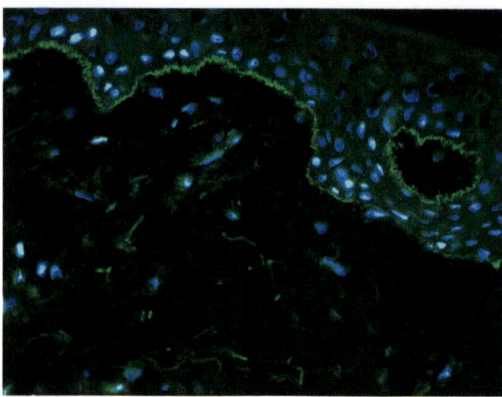

Fig. 18.6 Direct immunofluorescence in lamina lucida-type linear IgA bullous dermatosis shows linear, n-serrated, deposition of IgA along the EBMZ

zole, different antibiotics and immunoadsorption, most of them single or small case series [9].

First line treatment for LABD is dapsone

Follow-Up and Tapering

Patients on dapsone therapy should be carefully monitored for hemolysis and methemoglobinemia. Read more in Chap. 20. In cases with intolerance consider extreme low dapsone doses such as 12.5 mg daily (1/8 of tablet).

Case Study: Part 3

Patient was treated with dapsone climbing up to 200 mg daily without achieving remission. Later adalimumab and rituximab were tried in an off-label set-up without success. Systemic high dose corticosteroids and colchicine could not also book any success. Importantly patient developed several side effects from these systemic medications. From the chronic high dose dapsone usage she developed serious methemoglobinemia up to 21% MetHb in the peripheral arterial blood. Patient should receive several times methylene blue intervention to treat methemoglobinemia. Under adalimumab treatment patient developed an interstitial pneumonitis, which was considered as a side effect of the TNF-alpha blocker, however the underlying Sjögren disease could not be excluded. As a side effect of high dose steroid, patient developed Cushing syndrome with weight gain and diabetes. At the end patient was treated with mycophenolic acid in a dose of 360 mg QID, and she achieved at least partial remission.

Review Questions

1. What is the most common location of LABD in childhood?
   a. Perineum
   b. Head
   c. Pals and soles
2. The most important characteristics on DIF in LABD is
   a. IgA deposition in epithelial cell surface pattern
   b. Linear IgA deposition along the EBMZ
   c. Granular IgA deposition along the EBMZ
   d. Granular IgA deposition in dermal vessels
3. Mucosal involvement occurs in …% of the patients with LABD
   a. 10%
   b. 30%
   c. 80%
   d. 100%
4. First line treatment of LABD is
   a. superpotent topical corticosteroids
   b. systemic corticosteroids
   c. *dapsone*
   d. rituximab

Answers

1. a.
2. b.
3. c.
4. c.

On the Web

DermNet NZ: http://www.dermnetnz.org/immune/linear-iga.html

References

1. Kasperkiewicz M, Zillikens D, Schmidt E. Pemphigoid diseases: pathogenesis, diagnosis, and treatment. Autoimmunity. 2012;45:55–70.
2. Lings K, Bygum A. Linear IgA bullous dermatosis: a retrospective study of 23 patients in Denmark. Acta Derm Venereol. 2014. https://doi.org/10.1371/journal.pone.0112051
3. Jablonska S, Chorzelski TP, Rosinska D, Maciejowska E. Linear IgA bullous dermatosis of childhood (chronic bullous dermatosis of childhood). Clin Dermatol. 1991;9:393–401.
4. Zone JJ, Egan CA, Taylor TB, Meyer LJ. IgA autoimmune disorders: development of a passive transfer mouse model. J Invest Dermatol Symp Proc. 2004;9:47–51.
5. Egan CA, Zone JJ. Linear IgA bullous dermatosis. Int J Dermatol. 1999;38:818–27.
6. Chanal J, Ingen-Housz-Oro S, Ortonne N, Duong TA, Thomas M, Valeyrie-Allanore L, Lebrun-Vignes B, André C, Roujeau JC, Chosidow O, Wolkenstein P. Linear IgA bullous dermatosis: comparison between the drug-induced and spontaneous forms. Br J Dermatol. 2013;169:1041–8.
7. Wojnarowska F, Bhogal BS, Black MM. Chronic bullous disease of childhood and linear IgA disease of adults are IgA1-mediated diseases. Br J Dermatol. 1994;131:201–4.
8. Kuechle MK, Stegemeir E, Maynard B, Gibson LE, Leiferman KM, Peters MS. Drug-induced linear IgA bullous dermatosis: report of six cases and review of the literature. J Am Acad Dermatol. 1994;30:187–92.
9. Kasperkiewicz M, Schmidt E. Current treatment of autoimmune blistering diseases. Curr Drug Discov Technol. 2009;6:270–80.
10. Guide SV, Marinkovich MP. Linear IgA bullous dermatosis. Clin Dermatol. 2001;19:719–27.

Drug-Induced Pemphigoid and Linear IgA Disease

19

Sylvia H. Kardaun and Joost M. Meijer

Short Introduction in Layman Terms

Drug-induced bullous pemphigoid (DIBP) and drug-induced linear IgA disease (DILAD) are clinical variants that are caused or triggered by systemic or topical medication, and are identical or quite similar to idiopathic BP respectively LAD. The drug etiology and specific drug causality is mainly based on the time-relation between start of the suspected drug(s) and onset of the lesions. Key to diagnosis is awareness and recognition of the possibility of a drug etiology, followed by a thorough anamnesis, including an elaborate medication history. Recognition enables prompt withdrawal of the culprit drug and temporarily additional therapy, most often leading to reduced morbidity or a rapid and complete recovery.

- **Drug-induced pemphigoid**

Drugs may act as a trigger in patients with a (genetic) susceptibility, either by deregulating the immune response or by acting as haptens and changing the antigenic properties of proteins in the epidermal basement membrane zone (EBMZ) resulting in DIBP. However, the specific causal relationships in DIBP remain to be unraveled [1].

No more than 15% of BP was associated with inducing factors, including drugs [1]. Besides, DIBP has to be differentiated from several other (autoimmune) bullous diseases, including mucous membrane pemphigoid (MMP) [2]. Two types of DIBP have been described: an acute, self-limiting eruption, which responds rapidly after withdrawal of the causative drug (*drug-induced BP proper*); and a chronic eruption resembling BP, but with a more severe and persistent clinical course (*drug-triggered BP*) [3]. Finally, also cases with a drug associated exacerbation of BP have been described.

Polypharmacy and the presence of comorbidities, which are both regularly observed especially in the elderly, further complicate early recognition and establishment of the culprit.

Facts and Figures

After the first description in 1971, more than 90 different drugs have been associated with BP over the years. Originally, the associated drugs were classified in three pharmacological groups: the thiol-, the phenol-, and the non-thiol/

S. H. Kardaun (✉) · J. M. Meijer
Center for Blistering Diseases, Department of Dermatology, University Medical Center Groningen, University of Groningen, Groningen, The Netherlands
e-mail: j.m.meijer@umcg.nl

non-phenol group. Most commonly thiol compounds including D-penicillamine and furosemide and sulphonamide derivates were reported, followed by other loop diuretics, angiotensin-converting enzyme inhibitors, penicillins, neuroleptics, antidiabetics, and antiarrhythmics [3, 4]. Currently, an increasing number of reports of DIBP have been published related to the recent development of new types of drugs, some of which influence the immune system. Sufficient evidence supports a strong association of BP with dipeptidyl peptidase 4 (DPP-4) inhibitors (gliptins). The risk of BP in patients with type-2 diabetes, using gliptins, especially vildagliptin and to a lesser extent linagliptin and other gliptins (class effect) has significantly increased. The second group with an increased association consists of the immune checkpoint inhibitors PD-1/PD-L1 inhibitors (especially nivolumab and pembrolizumab). Furthermore, recent reports associate several other biologics or targeted therapies such as interleukins, cytokines, TNF-α antagonists, EGFR inhibitors and BRAF inhibitors [5].

In a systematic review including 170 studies, the strongest evidence for an association with DIBP was found for gliptins, in decreasing order followed by PD-1/PD-L1 inhibitors, loop diuretics, penicillins, NSAIDs, thiazides and PUVA [5]. Drugs associated with BP are shown in Table 19.1. At present it still remains uncertain whether BP is associated with neuroleptics or the underlying disorder, because several case-control studies revealed a higher risk of developing BP in this group of patients.

Contact Pemphigoid

In addition, external use of a number of preparations on the skin or mucous membranes has been documented to provoke cases of either local or generalized BP or mucous membrane pemphi-

> **Case Study: Part 1**
>
> A 47-year old man complained of tense blisters, erosions and itching on both upper legs, 6 days after start of flucloxacillin. Physical examination revealed localised tense blisters on normally appearing skin on the upper legs (Fig. 19.1). Mucous membranes were not involved.

goid (MMP), such as coal tar, 5-fluorouracil cream, benzyl benzoate or timolol (Table 19.1) [2].

Diagnosis Paths

DIBP is difficult to differentiate from idiopathic BP because differences in clinical presentation, histopathological and immunopathological findings are most often absent or only subtle. However, differentiation can be of major importance because of a different approach, prognosis, and treatment. DIBP tends to be more mild than idiopathic BP. Diagnosis of DIBP is mainly based on the (clear) time-relation between start of the suspected drug(s) and onset of the lesions. Drug-induced BP may arise up to 3 months and sometimes even longer after drug initiation. Moreover, DIBP should be distinguished from other (autoimmune) bullous diseases such as pemphigus, LAD, SJS/TEN and erythema multiforme. Features to suspect a drug-induced etiology in BP are more heterogeneous or atypical clinical manifestations opposed to idiopathic BP: a younger age at onset, tense bullae on healthy appearing skin (monomorphic blisters) (Fig. 19.1), mucous membrane involvement, erythema multiforme-like lesions, involvement of palms and soles, lesions resembling pemphigus or combined

19 Drug-Induced Pemphigoid and Linear IgA Disease

Table 19.1 Drugs associated with BP

Adalimumab	*Fluoxetine*	**Penicillamine**
Alogliptin	Flupenthixol	*Penicillin*
Amantadine	**Furosemide**	**Phenacetin**
Amlodipine	*Gabapentin*	Placental extracts
Amoxicillin	Galantamine hydrobromide	Potassium iodide
Ampicillin	Gold thiosulfate	Practolol
Anagliptin	*Griseofulvin*	**Psoralens**
Anti-influenza vaccine	Hydrochlorothiazide	**Rifampicin**
Aspirin	**Ibuprofen**	Risperidone
Arsenic	*Infliximab*	*Rosuvastatine*
Atezolizumab	Interleukin-2	Salicylazosulfapyridine
Azapropazone	*Ipilimumab*	**Serratiopeptidase**
Bumetanide	Levetiracetam	**Sirolimus**
Captopril	**Levofloxacin**	**Sitagliptin**
Celecoxib	**Linagliptin**	*Spironolactone*
Clonidine	*Lisinopril*	*Sulfasalazine*
Dabrafenib	*Losartan*	Sulfonamide
Dactinomycin (Actinomycin D)	*Mefenamic acid*	**Tenegliptin**
Diclofenac	Methyldopa	*Terbinafine*
Doxepin	Mesalazine	Thiopronin
Durvalumab	Metamizole	**Tiobutarit**
Efalizumab	Metronidazole	Tolbutamide
Enalapril	Nadolol	*Ustekinumab*
Enoxaparin	Nifedipine	**Vildagliptin**
Erlotinib	**Nivolumab**	Valsartan
Etanercept	Omeprazole	
Everolimus	**Pembrolizumab**	
Topical drugs:	*Vaccins:*	
5-Fluorouracil	*Hepatitis B vaccine*	
Anthralin (dithranol)	Herpes zoster vaccine	
Benzyl benzoate	*Hexavalent combined vaccine*	
Coal tar	Influenza vaccine	
Iodophor adhesive band	Rotavirus vaccine	
Photodynamic therapy	SARS-CoV-2 vaccine	
Timolol	Swine flue vaccine	
	Tetanus toxoid	

Bold: likely association, supported by recurrence or exacerbation with rechallenge or extensive evidence. *Italic*: probable association, with temporal relationship with initiation of drugs or resolution after cessation of culprit drug

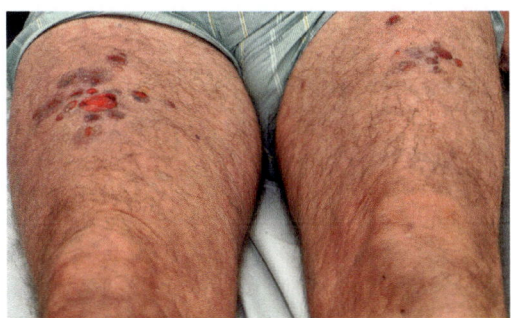

Fig. 19.1 Localized tense bullae and erosions on normal appearing skin on both upper legs in a patient with drug-induced BP

Case Study: Part 2

Histopathology showed a subepidermal blister with eosinophilic spongiosis and a dermal infiltrate with numerous eosinophils. DIF revealed linear n-serrated deposition of IgG (1+) and C3c (2+) along the EBMZ. IIF on monkey esophagus showed positive IgG along the EMBZ, and IIF on salt-split skin showed positive IgG (3+) epidermal binding. Further laboratory investigations revealed a mild peripheral blood eosinophilia (0.58×10^9/L).

clinical and histological features of pemphigus and BP.

The histopathological findings in drug-induced BP are mostly similar to idiopathic BP (see Chap. 15) and may additionally include intraepidermal vesicles and/or necrotic keratinocytes. The blister cavity and the dermis may contain numerous eosinophils and neutrophils. The findings in direct (DIF) and indirect immunofluorescence (IIF) microscopy are generally in accordance with BP. Laboratory studies may show marked blood eosinophilia [1, 3].

Dechallenge followed by rechallenge with the suspected culprit drug is the gold standard to establish drug causality, but often not ethical due to the potential severity of the reaction. In some cases, the culprit can be found by (stepwise) dechallenge.

Treatment Tricks

After withdrawal of the culprit most patients respond rapidly to treatment, generally without relapses, indicating that drug-induced BP should be considered. Treatment follows the guidelines for idiopathic BP, and usually consist of oral corticosteroids and/or potent topical corticosteroids, after which complete remission is most often achieved within 6 weeks. In cases of drug-triggered BP, additional maintenance therapy is needed and relapses may occur.

In DIBP associated with checkpoint inhibitors, flare-ups may occur at repeated treatment. However, high-dosed oral corticosteroids are associated with reduced overall survival, introducing a dilemma to maintain the anticancer regimen. Continuation of immune checkpoint inhibitor therapy is to be considered when <10% body surface area (BSA) is involved or discontinuation when >30% BSA is affected. Moreover, it is advised to minimize (long-term) broad immunosuppression and to preferentially optimize treatment with superpotent topical corticosteroids.

> **Case Study: Part 3**
> Laboratory investigations confirmed BP. An association with flucloxacillin was suspected. After withdrawal of flucloxacillin and therapy with daily lesional superpotent topical corticosteroids (clobetasol 0.05% cream) and zincoxide oil, the lesions healed within 4 weeks, without relapse. The time relation with flucloxacillin, the quick response after its withdrawal and the presentation with bullae on normal appearing skin made drug-induced BP the preferred diagnosis.

- **Drug-induced Linear IgA Disease**

Most reported cases of LAD have been classified as idiopathic; drug-induced cases have been estimated ranging from only 2.3% of LAD up to 37.5% of LAD in adults [6, 7]. After the first report of DILAD in 1981, approximately 100 cases have been associated with medication. Although the mucocutaneous manifestations are rather similar to idiopathic LAD, DILAD tends to be more atypical and severe. Next to medication, an association of LAD is demonstrated with several auto-immune diseases or infections and their subsequent treatment, and malignancies [7, 8]. Drug-associated case reports may suffer from lack of a reliable causality in absence of a dechallenge-rechallenge procedure, because of multiple drug use and confounding comorbidity [9, 10]. Typically, causative medication is initiated <4 weeks before disease onset [10].

Facts and Figures

Various drugs have been associated with LAD, of which vancomycin has been reported most frequently. A (not comprehensive) list of drugs associated with LAD is shown in Table 19.2. According to a recent review of the literature,

Table 19.2 Drugs associated with LAD

Acetaminophen	Ketoprofen
Amiodarone	Lithium carbonate
Amoxicillin	Metronidazole
Ampicillin-sulbactam	Moxifloxacin
Atorvastatin	Naproxen
Captopril	Penicillin G
Cefamandole	**Phenytoin**
Ceftriaxone	Piperacillin-tazobactam
Diclofenac	Piroxicam
Furosemide	**Sulfamethoxazole-trimethoprim**
Gemcitabine	**Vancomycin**
Infliximab	Verapamil
Interferon-γ/Interleukin-2	Vigabatrin
Iminipem	5-fluorouracil (cream)
Iodine	

Bold: top-3 most frequently associated drugs

vancomycin is the leading drug (56%), followed by phenytoin 6%, and trimethoprim-sulfamethoxazole 3%, whereas all other drugs are only occasionally reported. Recently the anti-TNF α antibody infliximab has also been implicated [8]. The onset of symptoms ranges from 1 to 21 days after initiation of vancomycin and probably longer for other drugs [9, 10]. Pathogenesis of DILAD is not yet fully elucidated. Drug-specific T cells and their cytokines such as several interleukins and transforming growth factor β may play an important role in increasing IgA synthesis [8]. Drugs may cause the reaction by cross reacting with target epitopes, by altering the confirmation of epitope, or by exposing previously sequestered antigens.

Diagnosis Paths

Diagnosing DILAD is similar to idiopathic LAD (see Chap. 18), while other autoimmune bullous diseases should be considered. A clear time-relation of start of the suspected medication and onset of the reaction is needed to differentiate DILAD from LAD, followed by full recovery after its withdrawal. Clinically, the mean age at disease onset is higher of DILAD (66.5 years vs 51 years), lesions tends to be more severe, extensive, and atypical with larger erosions that may clinically resemble toxic epidermal necrolysis (TEN) or SJS/TEN overlap [7, 8, 10]. Histopathology and DIF are essential to differentiate from SJS/TEN at an early stage, especially in severe cases. No significant difference has been demonstrated in histopathology and DIF between idiopathic and DILAD, although focal necrotic keratinocytes arranged near the EBMZ are more frequent in DILAD. The rate of positive IIF reactivity in drug-induced LABD is rather low, probably due to the heterogeneity of target antigens or incapacity of binding the antigens in native form [8, 10].

Treatment Tricks

After withdrawal of the suspected culprit (dechallenge), symptoms of DILAD usually resolve within weeks to several months after withdrawal and maintenance therapy is not necessary [7, 9, 10]. Up to 50% of patients may require additional therapy for several weeks to months. Recommended first-line treatment includes moisturizing ointments, dapsone, topical or oral corticosteroids [10]. Because of the severity of the reaction, a dechallenge-rechallenge procedure to identify the potential culprit is complicated due to ethical problems. Stepwise dechallenge may provide a solution in cases of polypharmacy.

Review Questions

1. Which clinical symptoms could differentiate drug-induced BP?
    a. tense bullae on healthy appearing skin (monomorphic blisters)
    b. young age of onset
    c. erythema multiforme-like lesions
    d. all of mentioned above
2. Which drug is most often associated with drug-induced BP?
    a. DPP-4 inhibitors
    b. enalapril
    c. furosemide
    d. ibuprofen

3. Which drug is most often associated with drug-induced LAD?
   a. captopril
   b. naproxen
   c. vancomycin
   d. trimethoprim-sulfamethoxazole
4. Onset of symptoms in vancomycine-induced LABD ranges from:
   a. <3 days
   b. 1–21 days
   c. 1–2 months
   d. >6 months

Answers:

1. d.
2. a.
3. c.
4. b.

References

1. Lo Schiavo A, Ruocco E, Brancaccio G, Caccavale S, Ruocco V, Wolf R. Bullous pemphigoid: etiology, pathogenesis, and inducing factors: facts and controversies. Clin Dermatol. 2013;31(4):391–9.
2. Vassileva S. Drug-induced pemphigoid: bullous and cicatricial. Clin Dermatol. 1998;16(3):379–87.
3. Stavropoulos PG, Soura E, Antoniou C. Drug-induced pemphigoid: a review of the literature. J Eur Acad Dermatol Venereol. 2014;28(9):1133–40.
4. Bastuji-Garin S, Joly P, Picard-Dahan C, Bernard P, Vaillant L, Pauwels C, et al. Drugs associated with bullous pemphigoid. A case-control study. Arch Dermatol. 1996;132(3):272–6.
5. Verheyden MJ, Bilgic A, Murrell DF. A systematic review of drug-associated bullous pemphigoid. Acta Derm Venereol. 2020;100:adv00224.
6. Yamagami J, Nakamura Y, Nagao K, Funakoshi T, Takahashi H, Tanikawa A, et al. Vancomycin mediates IgA autoreactivity in drug-induced linear IgA bullous dermatosis. J Invest Dermatol. 2018;138:1473–80.
7. Lings K, Bygum A. Linear IgA bullous dermatosis: a retrospective study of 23 patients in Denmark. Acta Derm Venereol. 2015;95:466–71.
8. Lammer J, Hein R, Roenneberg S, Biedermann T, Volz T. Drug-induced linear IgA bullous dermatosis: a case report and review of the literature. Acta Derm Venereol. 2019;99:508–15.
9. Fortuna G, Salas-Alanis JC, Guidetti E, Marinkovich MP. A critical reappraisal of the current data on drug-induced linear immunoglobulin A bullous dermatosis: a real and separate nosological entity? J Am Acad Dermatol. 2012;66(6):988–94.
10. Chanal J, Ingen-Housz-Oro S, Ortonne N, Duong TA, Thomas M, Valeyrie-Allanore L, et al. Linear IgA bullous dermatosis: comparison between the drug-induced and spontaneous forms. Br J Dermatol. 2013;169(5):1041–8.

Dermatitis Herpetiformis

Barbara Horváth and Marcel F. Jonkman

Introduction and AIMS

Short Definition in Layman Terms

Dermatitis herpetiformis is the skin manifestation of coeliac disease. The trigger of both diseases is known; ingestion of gluten in certain HLA phenotypes (HLA-DQ8 or HLA-DQ2) leading to an autoimmune reaction characterized by IgA autoantibodies against tissue transglutaminase (tTG) and later in DH patient against the epidermal transglutaminase (eTG).

Dermatitis herpetiformis (DH) is the specific skin manifestation of coeliac disease (CD) caused by the digestion of gluten in HLA-DQ2 or HLA-DQ8 individuals

Didactical Questions; Cross Section of Questions to Prime the Readers' Interest

How can you diagnose DH? What would you see in the histopathological section? How can you make de difference between other autoimmune and immunological diseases? In this section the focus is on the clinical differential diagnostics and work up of patients suspected for DH.

> **Learning Objectives**
> After reading this chapter you will be able to differentiate dermatitis herpetiformis from other pruritic dermatoses and to recognize the classic clinics of DH. You will be able to perform and interpret the immunological tests, to make a treatment algorithm and to manage patients with DH.

> **Case Study: Part 1**
> 41-year-old male patient presented with itchy papules, blisters on knees, elbows, shoulders and lower back for 3 years. He had no mucosal involvement, nor digestive tract symptoms. He was non-atopic, family history reported no skin disease or other problems. There was no medicine administered before.

B. Horváth (✉) · M. F. Jonkman (Deceased)
Center for Blistering Diseases, Department of Dermatology, University Medical Center Groningen, University of Groningen,
Groningen, The Netherlands
e-mail: b.horvath@umcg.nl

Facts and Figures

Definitions and Classification

Dermatitis herpetiformis is the cutaneous manifestation of coeliac disease, both disease are the different phenotype of glutens sensitive disease (GSD). This means that in both diseases gluten is the trigger that in certain susceptible HLA phenotypes provokes autoimmune reaction. An autoantibody population against tTG characterizes CD. As gluten sensitivity is obligate to develop in DH, also DH patients have tTG autoantibodies, however with low affinity. Moreover patient with DH develop another autoantibody population against the eTG [1].

Epidemiology

Due to its genetic background DH has a different prevalence geographically. DH is most common in patients with North-European origin. Studies report a prevalence of 1.2 to 39.2 per 100,000 people, with an incidence range of 0.4 to 2.6 per 100,000 people per year. DH is rare in the Asian population and even more rare in African Americans. Familial cases were reported. Male female ratio is 1.5:1 to 2:1. Interestingly an opposite female predominance is known in CD. The onset of the disease is variable; mostly in the fourth decade, but childhood and geriatric cases are not rarity. The childhood onset is more reported in the Mediterranean area [2].

DH is most common in patients with North-European origin

Pathogenesis

There is a strong genetic predisposition for DH. In patients with HLA-DQ2 and/or HLA-DQ8 phenotype an autoimmune reaction develops after the ingestion of gluten (Fig. 20.1). First, tTG modifies gliadine, the alcohol-soluble fraction of gluten to an antigen, which binds to the HLA-DQ2/HLA-DQ8 molecule to evoke cellular and humoral (anti-gliadine antibodies) immune reactions. Moreover the tTG-bound gliadine serves also as a strong antigen producing excessive autoantibody production against the enzyme complex (tTG antibodies). This humoral and cellular immune reaction leads to inflammation and damaging of the gut mucosa, resembling changes seen in CD [2].

The subclinical gluten sensitivity is obligate to develop DH. eTG and tTG share common epitopes within the enzymatically active domain. It is hypothesized, that epitope spreading is the suspected mechanism after the development of the new autoantibody population targeting the eTG. This is supported by the facts that children have mainly CD with high levels anti-tTG and low levels of anti-eTG compared with adults. Moreover CD mainly develops in childhood whereas DH is the disease of adults. Suggesting that the epitopes spreading needs time to take place [2].

The circulating IgA autoantibodies against eTG in DH target epidermal transglutaminase, a protein playing role in the formation of the cornified envelop of the epidermis. In DH skin eTG is co-localized with IgA at the BMZ in the papilla tips supporting that eTG is the autoantigen of DH [1]. However it remains to be elucidated whether there are true circulating IgA-eTG immune complexes in DH, since deposits of IgA and eTG in the dermal vessel are seen frequently (Fig. 20.2) [3] clinically corresponding with the digital purpura in DH (Fig. 20.3) [4].

In DH skin eTG is co-localized with IgA at the EBMZ in the papillary tips supporting that eTG is the autoantigen of DH

Diagnosis Paths

History and Physical Examination

The classic clinical presentation of DH is a very itchy polymorphous skin eruption comprising erythema, urticarial plaques, papules, vesicles, excoriations and purpura sometimes in herpetiform configuration. The lesions are distributed typically on the extensor surfaces of the body; knees, elbows (Fig. 20.4), shoulders, in the so-called vertical distribution (Fig. 20.5). Large blister are rarely seen. The disease has a fluctuating course driven mostly but not always by gluten ingestion, improves under UV light (seasonal flare-ups). There are known associations with autoimmune thyroid disease and other autoimmune diseases [4].

Fig. 20.1 Diagram of the hypothetical pathogenesis of DH. Incomplete metabolized gluten peptides are deaminated in the gut and covalent crosslinked with TGc (=tTG). The gluten peptide TGc-complex induces a anti-TGc, and anti-TGe autoimmune response by glutenpeptide specific T-cells, which activate a TGc-specific B-cells. The subsequently produced IgA autoantibodies, which crossreact with TGe, are deposited as TGe-immune complexes in the dermis. *TZR* T-cell receptor. Reprinted from Sardy and Tieze with permission from Springer Science and Buisness Media

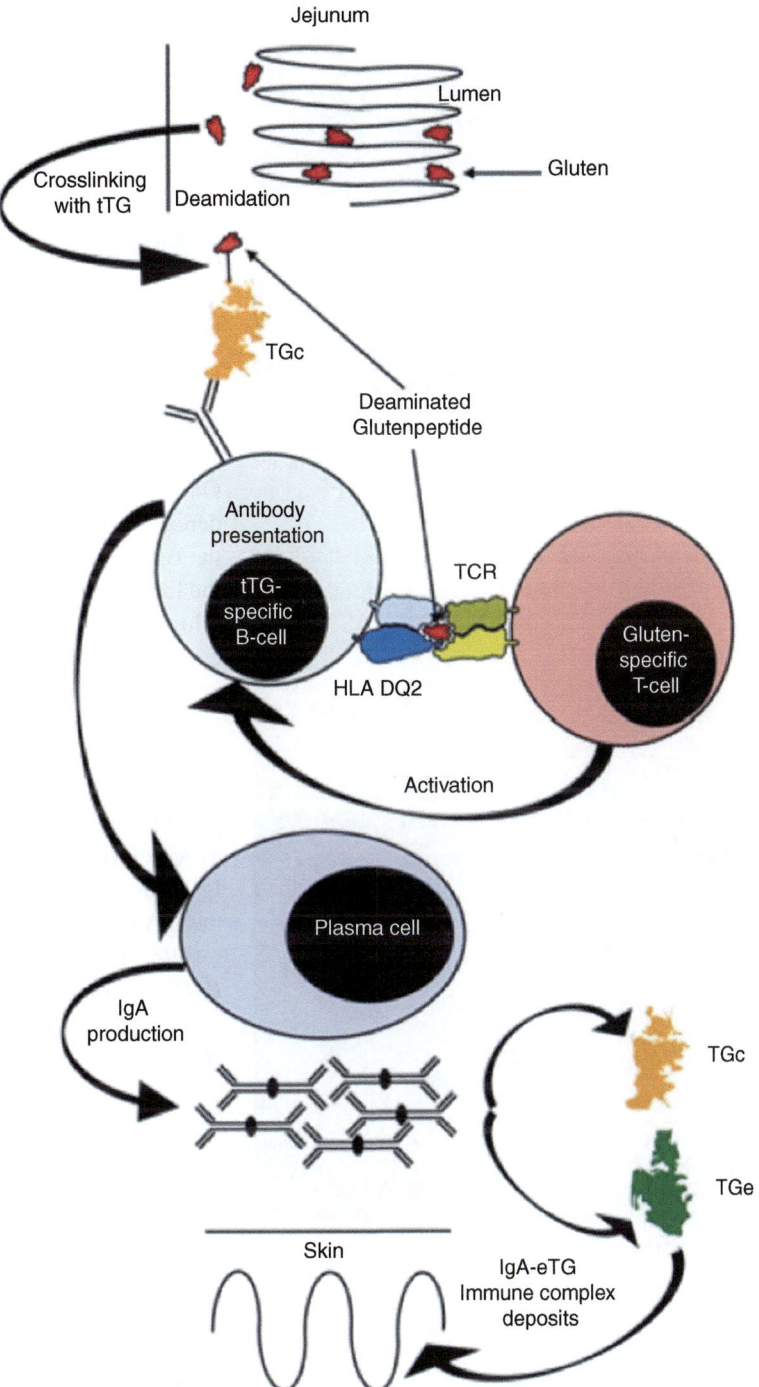

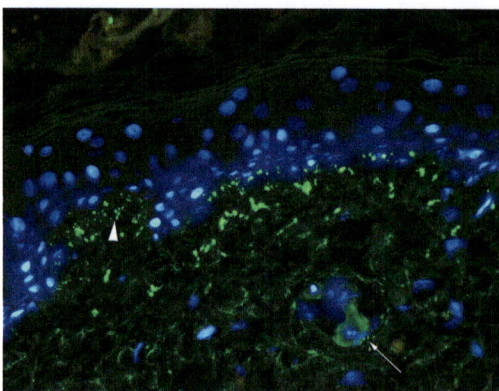

Fig. 20.2 DIF of DH shows granular depositions below the basement membrane zone (arrowhead) and in the walls of dermal blood vessels (arrow)

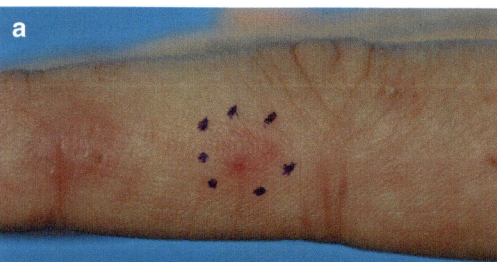

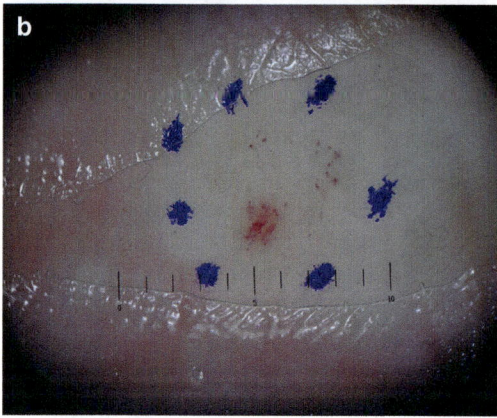

Fig. 20.3 (a) Digital purpura in dermatitis herpetiformis. (b) Dermoscopy reveals coagulated capillaries

General Diagnostics

The histological picture is unique in DH. Routine histology in DH shows infiltration of neutrophils at the dermo-epidermal junction just above the papilla tips, called microabscesses (Fig. 20.6).

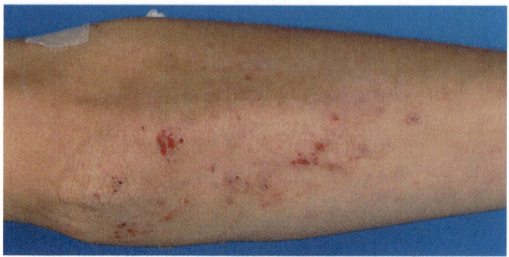

Fig. 20.4 The extensor surface of the elbow is a predilection place in DH, and preferable side for IF biopsy

Specific Diagnostics

On direct immunofluorescence (DIF) granular deposits of IgA at the dermal papilla tips or along the BMZ is seen (Fig. 20.2), mostly representing the location of the neutrophils on the routine histology (Fig. 20.6). On indirect immunofluorescence (IIF) on monkey oesophagus IgA binding is seen on the smooth muscle layer corresponding with the endomysium (EMA positivity, Fig. 5.3a). The major antigen of EMA is tTG [4]. In the blood IgA anti-tTG is positive. However patients with IgA deficiency can also develop CD as well DH resulting in autoantibodies from the IgG class. Therefore simultaneous measurement the IgA levels is mandatory for diagnostics.

DIF shows granular IgA deposits along the BMZ. On monkey esophagus EMA positivity is seen representing autoantibodies against tTG

> **Case Study: Part 2**
> Routine laboratory examination showed no abnormality. On histopathological examination subepidermal blister forming with neutrophil microabcesses at the dermal papilla tips were seen. On direct immunofluorescence granulair deposits of IgA (2+) and complement (C3C 1+) were seen at the BMZ. On indirect immunofluorescence on monkey esophagus anti-EMA positivity (1+) was seen.

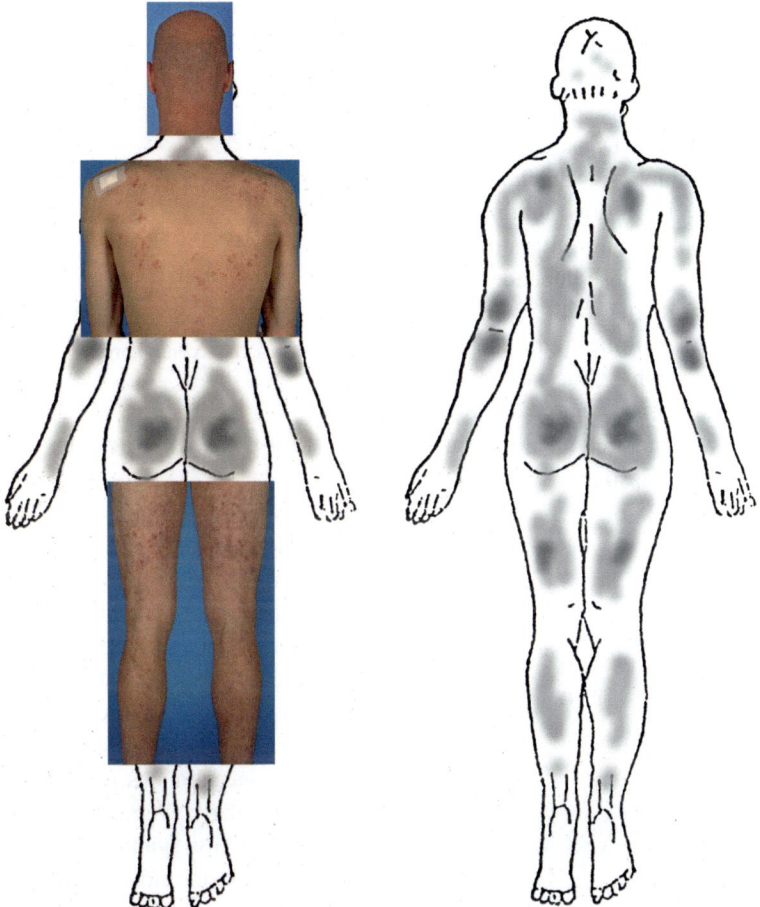

Fig. 20.5 The vertical distribution of skin lesions at the backside of the body typical for DH

Treatment Tricks

Initial Treatment and Escalator

Gluten free diet (GFD) is the first choice of treatment (Table 20.1). Every patient with DH should be informed about this, however consistent adherence on GFD is difficult. Patient with symptoms of celiac disease should be referred to gastroenterologists. Patient without gut symptoms can be managed primary at dermatologists. Since most patients with DH have mild CD, denying of GFD is acceptable as long as they are carefully monitored for sign of malabsorption, anemia, vitamin B12-deficiency, osteoporosis, and thyroid dysfunction.

Patients with severe CD may develop enteropathy associated T-cell lymphoma (EATL). Since patients with DH—per definition—do not develop severe CD, they do not develop EATL, and therefore do not have to be warned for the possibility of developing intestinal lymphoma.

Unfortunately the effect of GFD takes time. The skin rash disappears in months after the cessation of gluten, and gluten re-challenge causes flare-up of the disease within days.

To achieve quick improvement of itch, patients need dapsone as medication at the beginning of the therapy. Dapsone, a member of the sulfonamide antibiotics, is the first line medical treatment for DH. Dapsone inhibits the diapedesis of neutrophils and migration to the EBMZ bound IgA in a dose dependent manner [5]. Dapsone can be started with 50 mg per day. Administration of dapsone reduces the itch promptly within 48 h. Glucose-6-phosphate dehydrogenase deficiency should be excluded within the first week of treatment and prior to raising the dosage of dapsone.

Table 20.1 Gluten free diet

Foods to avoid	Foods allowed
Grains and starches	Grains and starches
• Wheat	• Tapioca
• Kamut	• Soybean
• Rye	• Potato
• Barley	• Buckwheat
• Oats	• Quinoa
• Many cereals	• Rice
	• Corn
	• Coconut flour
	• Almond meal flour

http://www.celiaccentral.org

Follow-Up and Tapering

Hemolysis is obligate during dapsone treatment, and is dose dependent. It is compensated by reticulocytosis. During the dapsone treatment patient should be carefully monitored for excessive hemolysis: drop in the hemoglobin concentration with 1g/dL, insufficient elevation of reticulocytes, lactate dehydrogenase above 225 U/L and total bilirubin above 17 µmol/mL For methemoglobinaemia arterial concentrations of metHb should be measured regularly. Agranulocytosis and dapsone hypersensitivity syndrome are the most feared idiosyncratic side effects of dapsone. When remission is achieved, dapsone can be tapered to the minimal effective dose. If the patient constantly adheres to GFD the dosage of dapsone can be further reduced or even stopped (see box below).

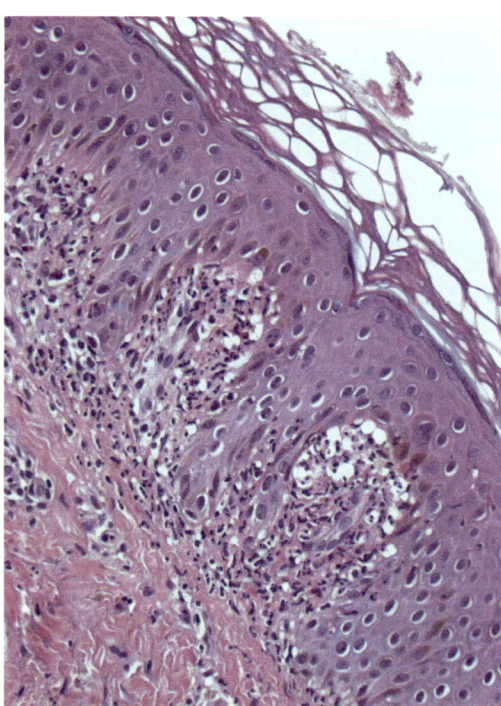

Fig. 20.6 Histopathology of DH shows neutrophil microabcesses in the dermal papillae

> **Case Study: Part 3**
>
> After excluding glucose-6-phosphat dehydrogenase (G6PD) deficiency patient received dapsone orally. The initial dose was 50 mg per day, which was increased up to 75mg daily after one week under blood controls. Follow-up and tapering

Pharmacology of Dapson [6]

Oral availability is as high as 86%, so it is administered exclusively orally. During its metabolisms in the liver two metabolites are produced: via acetylation the non-toxic metabolites acetyl and diacetyl dapsone and via N-hydroxylation the potentially toxic hydroxylamine. The latter reaction occurs on the cytochrome P450 enzyme-complex (CYP450), so medicines competing these enzymes can influence the production of the toxic metabolites [6]. Table 20.2 shows the medicines influencing the CYP450.

The side effects of dapsone are either dose-dependent or dose-independent.

- Dose-dependent side effects:
  - **Methemoglobinemia.** The development of methemoglobinemia is the direct effect of the toxic metabolite hydroxylamine, which transforms the hemoglobin to MetHB, which binds and release less oxygen. Clinical symptoms of methemoglobinemia are due to the lack of oxygen in the tissues (Table 20.3).
  - **Hemolysis.** It is an indirect effect of hydroxylamine and related on oxygen free radicals. Moreover addition of cimetidine can reduce the concentration of hydroxylamine. Interestingly G6PD-deficient patients are less susceptible to methemoglobinemia, and more susceptible to hemolysis due to decrease in NAPDH formation in the erythrocytes.
- Dose-independent side effects.

  - **Agranulocytosis** is idiosyncratic, thought that hydroxylamine binds in the bone marrow to the myeloprecursor cell to inhibit their maturation. Typically fever with neutropenia appears 1 to 3 months after the first dose of dapsone.
  - **Dapsone hypersensitivity syndrome (DHS)** with fever, rash and organomegaly (lymphadenopathy, hepato-splenomegaly) with elevated erythrocyte sedimentation rate and liver enzymes. The interval is much shorter 1 up to 6 weeks after the first dose.

Table 20.2 Medications inducting and inhibiting cytochrome P450 (CYP450) [7]

Inhibitors of CYP450	Inductors of CYP450
• Diltiazem	• Glucocorticosteroids
• Itraconazol	• Rifampycine
• Ketoconazol	• Carbamazepine
• Metronidazole	• Phenobarbital
• Omeprazol	• Phenytoine
• Paroxetine	
• Fluoxetine	
• Amitryptilline	
• Cimetidine	
• Haloperodol	
• Eryhtromycine	
• Clarythromycine	
• Ritonavir	

Table 20.3 Clinical symptoms of methemoglobinemia [8]

% of total hemoglobin[a]	Symptoms
<10%	None
10–20%	Cyanotic discoloration of the skin
20–30%	Anxiety, headache, tachycardia, lightheadedness
30–50%	Fatique, confusion, dizziness, tachypnea, tachycardia
50–70%	Coma, seizures, arrhythmias, acidosis
>70%	Death

[a]Assumes hemoglobin = 15 g/dL. Patients with lower hemoglobin concentrations may experience more severe symptoms for a given percentage of metHb level

Review Questions

1. What is the trigger of DH?
   a. Gluten
   b. Gliadin
   c. Reticulin
   d. Drugs
2. Which HLA loci are associated with DH and CD?
   a. HLA-DQ8
   b. HLA-B51
   c. HLA-DQ2
   d. a+c are correct
3. Which are the typically involved areas on the body in DH?
   a. Backside of body
   b. Mucosal surfaces
   c. Palms and soles
   d. Front side of body
4. First line medication of DH is
   a. Systemic corticosteroids
   b. Gluten free diet
   c. Doxycycline
   d. Dapsone
5. Which is allowed in the gluten free diet?
   a. Wheat
   b. Potato
   c. Rye
   d. Barley

Answers

1. a.
2. d.
3. a.
4. d.
5. b.

References

1. Sardy M, Karpati S, Merkl B, Paulsson M, Smyth N. Epidermal transglutaminase (TGase 3) is the autoantigen of dermatitis herpetiformis. J Exp Med. 2002;195:747–57.
2. Bolotin D, Petronic-Rosic V. Dermatitis herpetiformis. Part I. Epidemiology, pathogenesis, and clinical presentation. J Am Acad Dermatol. 2011;64:1017–24.
3. Preisz K, Sardy M, Horvath A, Karpati S. Immunoglobulin, complement and epidermal transglutaminase deposition in the cutaneous vessels in dermatitis herpetiformis. J Eur Acad Dermatol Venereol. 2005;19:74–9.
4. Karpati S. Dermatitis herpetiformis: close to unravelling a disease. J Dermatol Sci. 2004;34:83–90.
5. Thuong-Nguyen V, Kaduce DP, Hendrix JD, Gammon WR, Zone JJ. Inhibition of neutrophil adherence to antibody by dapsone: a possible therapeutic mechanism of dapsone in the treatment of IgA dermatoses. J Invest Dermatol. 1993;100:349–55.
6. Zhu YI, Stiller MJ. Dapsone and sulfones in dermatology: overview and update. J Am Acad Dermatol. 2001;45:420–34.
7. Kempeneers D, De Haes P. Dapsone, nog steeds nuttig in de dermatologie? (article in Dutch). Ned Tijdschr Dermatol Venereol. 2011;21:362–7.
8. Wright RO, Lewander WJ, Woolf AD. Methemoglobinemia: etiology, pharmacology, and clinical management. Ann Emerg Med. 1999;34:646–56.

21. Stevens Johnson Syndrome/Toxic Epidermal Necrolysis and Erythema Exsudativum Multiforme

Sylvia H. Kardaun

Introduction and Aims

Short Introduction in Layman Terms

Stevens Johnson syndrome (SJS) and toxic epidermal necrolysis (TEN) are the most severe, mainly drug induced reactions with widespread skin and mucous membrane involvement, characterised by massive epidermal necrosis, and associated with significant morbidity, mortality, and long-lasting sequelae. Erythema exsudativum multiforme (EEM) presents an acute, most often acrofacial eruption characterised by target lesions. Although generally relatively mild and self-limiting, EEM can be recurrent and is generally triggered by infections.

Learning Objectives

After reading this chapter you are able to distinguish SJS/TEN from EEM and other (autoimmune) blistering diseases. You understand that SJS/TEN presents a spectrum that can be divided in three subtypes, predominantly based on the percentage of the detached and detachable body surface area (BSA), and is most often caused by drugs. Besides, you are able to identify the associated medication. Moreover, you will know that EEM, although not an infection by itself, is most often caused by various infections, with herpes simplex virus (HSV) as the most important, while drugs are rarely the cause.

Didactical Questions; Cross Sections to Prime the Readers Interest

What are typical and atypical targets and what is their importance? Can EEM evolve to SJS or TEN? Which drugs are notorious for inducing SJS/TEN and should patients avoid all of these after having experienced SJS/TEN? What are long-lasting sequelae of SJS/TEN? What special care should be taken for patients, suffering from eye involvement?

S. H. Kardaun (✉)
Center for Blistering Diseases, Department of Dermatology, University Medical Center Groningen, University of Groningen,
Groningen, The Netherlands
e-mail: s.h.kardaun@gmail.com

Case Study: Part 1

A 46-year old man complained of a painful throat and subfebrile temperature starting 2 weeks after neurosurgery. Because 2 days later a skin rash and stinging eyes develop, he decides to consult his GP. What is your differential diagnosis? What further info do you need to come to a diagnosis?

Definitions and Classification

SJS/TEN are severe, potentially fatal, mucocutaneous adverse drug reactions, characterised by massive epidermal necrolysis. EEM has been reported under a variety of labels and eponyms, and up to now is still surrounded by some confusion. It can be divided in two main types: EEM minus, characterised by the sudden onset of red papules or plaques, some of which develop to "target" or "iris" lesions, and EEM majus, showing in addition haemorrhagic mucosal involvement as can be seen in SJS/TEN. In particular EEM majus and SJS are still often erroneously used as synonyms. However, EEM is an entity different from SJS/TEN with a different course, prognosis, and aetiology. In 1993, consensus was reached on case definition, classification and nosology, recognising four main categories varying from EEM majus to TEN (Table 21.1) [1]. Within this classification, SJS and TEN are considered to represent two ends of a spectrum of a single disease in which TEN is the maximal variant, mainly differing by the extent of skin detachment, but based on similar pathogenesis, risk factors and causality, whereas EEM majus is regarded a distinct entity. In contrast to SJS/TEN, there is no risk for skin failure or visceral involvement in EEM.

The classification is based on three clinical criteria: the morphology of the individual lesions, their distribution, and the maximal extent of epidermal detachment. Typical target lesions have regular round and well-defined borders with at least three different concentric zones: a purpuric central disk with or without a blister, a raised oedematous, pale intermediate ring, and an erythematous outer ring (bull's eye or iris lesion) (Fig. 21.1). By contrast, atypical target lesions, which can be raised or flat, have an appearance reminiscent of targets, but present with only 2 zones and/or poorly defined borders, while the centre can also be vesicular or bullous (Fig. 21.2). Detachment of skin and mucosae can present as blistering or erosions.

EEM majus is characterised by mainly acrofacial raised typical or atypical targets and epidermal detachment <10% of the BSA. In the spectrum of SJS/TEN on the other hand, skin

Table 21.1 Differences between erythema exsudativum multiforme majus (EEM majus), Stevens Johnson syndrome (SJS), toxic epidermal necrolysis (TEN) and SJS/TEN overlap syndrome

Clinical entity	EEM majus	SJS	SJS/TEN overlap	[a]TEN
Primary lesions	Raised typical or atypical target lesions	Flat atypical target lesions, erythematous/purpuric maculae	Flat atypical target lesions, ill-defined erythematous/purpuric maculae	Ill-defined (dusky) erythema and maculae, flat atypical target lesions
Distribution	Mainly acrofacial	Isolated lesions, partly confluent on the face and trunk	Isolated lesions, partly confluent on the face and trunk	Isolated lesions, partly confluent on the face, trunk, and elsewhere
Intensity	+	+	++	+++
Mucosae	Involved	Involved	Involved	Involved
Systemic symptoms	Minimal/absent	Usual	Always	Always
Detached body surface area (BSA)	<10%	<10%	10–30%	>30%[a]

+ mild, ++ moderate, +++ severe
[a]NB: including TEN with large confluent erythema without discrete lesions with a detached BSA ≥10%

21 Stevens Johnson Syndrome/Toxic Epidermal Necrolysis and Erythema Exsudativum Multiforme

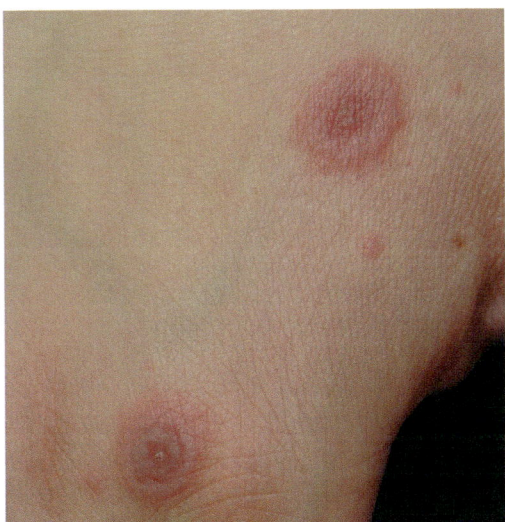

Fig. 21.1 Typical target lesions in EEM minor showing three well-defined color zones and borders

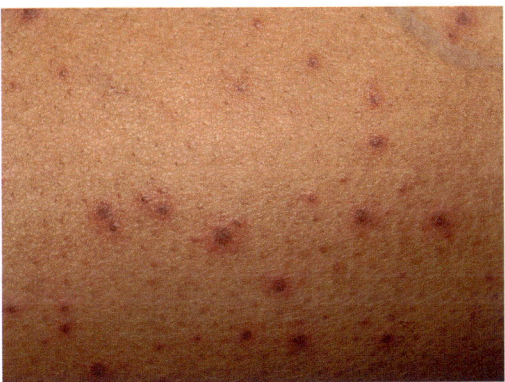

Fig. 21.2 Flat atypical target lesions in SJS with poorly defined borders and two color zones

associated with infections, SJS/TEN is most often drug induced. However, especially at their early stages, differential diagnosis can be challenging. Moreover, SJS can progress into TEN.

Stevens Johnson Syndrome/Toxic Epidermal Necrolysis (SJS/TEN)

Facts and Figures

The onset of SJS/TEN is abrupt. It can be preceded by prodromes, usually starting as flu-like symptoms such as fever, sore throat, anorexia and malaise, often followed by erosive stomatitis and eye involvement. Next, burning, painful, and often ill-defined erythematous and/or purpuric maculae (spots), flat atypical target lesions, and photophobia occur. Maculae most often start in a symmetrical distribution on the face, neck, and upper trunk, extending distally with a tendency to rapid coalescence. Generally, within hours extensive mucocutaneous blistering and detachment on an erythematous base develop within 1 week up to 10 days. Blisters are flaccid and can become confluent, while large sheets of epidermis slough off, leaving an exposed, weeping dermis and large areas of detachment. At gentle pressure, blisters can often be moved laterally due to detachment (positive Asboe Hansen sign, Fig. 2.3). Also pressure on erythematous skin may cause detachment (pseudo-Nikolsky's sign, Fig. 2.2). Target lesions in SJS/TEN reminiscent of the target lesions in EEM, however, are flat and atypical.

In SJS, maculae, atypical target lesions, blisters and areas of detachment are most often prominent on the upper chest and face. Although boundaries are rather artificial, total detached and detachable skin at the maximum stage in SJS is <10% of the BSA, between 10 and 30% in SJS/TEN overlap, and over 30% in TEN (Figs. 21.3, 21.4, and 21.5).

Generally, multiple mucosal membranes, including oral, ocular, nasal, urethral, vaginal, anal, tracheobronchial, and gastrointestinal mucosae can be affected in SJS/TEN, with haemorrhagic blistering and erosions. Visceral involvement (liver) may occur; anaemia and lym-

lesions are widespread with blisters arising on erythematous or purpuric macules and/or flat atypical targets. In EEM, lesions usually appear symmetrically on the distal extremities and may progress proximally, while in SJS/TEN the reaction often starts on the upper trunk and face and evolves distally. Mucous membrane involvement, present in both SJS/TEN and EEM majus, tends to be more severe in SJS/TEN. EEM majus differs from SJS/TEN by occurrence in younger males, frequent recurrences, less fever, milder mucosal lesions and lack of risk factors associated with SJS/TEN [2]. Where EEM is mainly

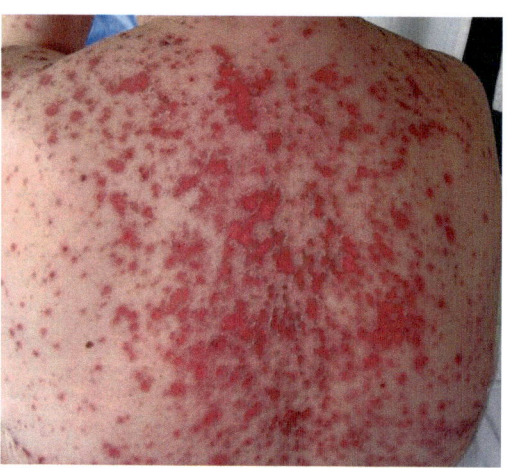

Fig. 21.3 SJS showing wide-spread small erythematous macules. Mainly on the central part of the thorax the lesions are partly confluent with small areas of detachment

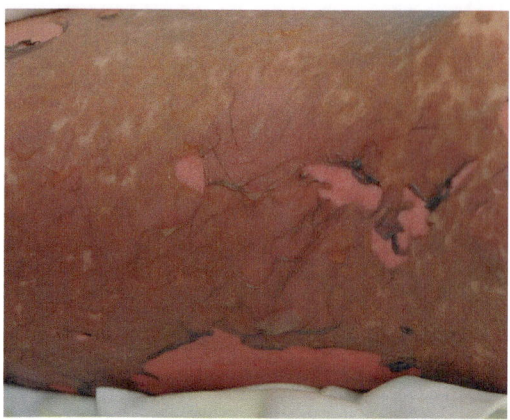

Fig. 21.5 TEN with large areas of necrotic epidermis and large sheets of sloughed-off moist, erosive erythematous skin

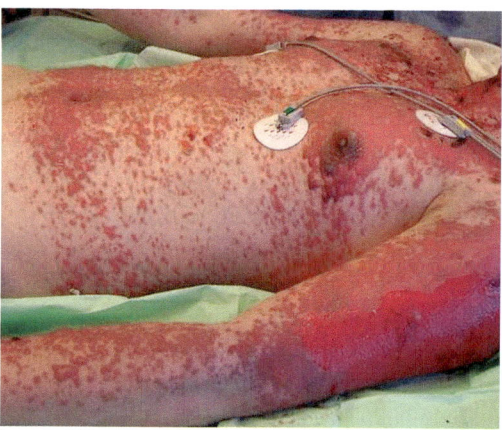

Fig. 21.4 SJS/TEN-overlap with widespread maculopapular lesions on the face, neck, arms and thorax and hemorrhagic mucosal involvement. Lesions are confluent on the neck, arms and central thorax and in addition show bullae and extensive erosive areas

phopenia are frequent, while neutropenia often predicts bad prognosis. Pneumonitis or even acute respiratory distress syndrome may occur. Complete healing, especially in TEN, can last 3–6 weeks, while especially erosions on the back, buttocks and mucosae may take longer.

SJS/TEN presents a severe, life-threatening disease. The overall mortality rate, mainly caused by sepsis or multiorgan failure, is on average about 25%, ranging from 12% in SJS to 46% in TEN [3]. Over 90% of survivors suffer from variable long-term sequelae, and/or long-lasting, often underrecognized psychosocial problems, strongly affecting the quality of life. Frequent, often ongoing ocular complications, not rarely leading to impaired vision and even blindness, are most feared. Over 50% of survivors are afraid of taking drugs or avoid taking them. Other sequelae include lung function impairment, symblepharon, conjunctival synechiae, dry eyes, entropion, ingrowing eyelashes, cutaneous scarring, altered pigmentation, eruptive nevi, dental problems, persistent erosions/strictures of the mucous membranes (especially genital), nail changes and post-traumatic stress disorders [4].

Epidemiology

In Europeans, the incidence of SJS is estimated at 1.2–6.0 and that of TEN at 0.4–1.2 per million per year. The mean age for SJS/TEN ranks between 48.2 and 53.4 years (range 1–98 years), with a slight female preponderance in TEN [2]. In HIV the incidence was approximately 1000-fold higher than in the general population.

Pathogenesis

Although pathogenesis is not yet fully elucidated, several mechanisms have been postulated. Nowadays it is believed that SJS/TEN is a process in which an inappropriate immune activation is triggered in response to certain drugs or their (toxic) metabolites. Massive keratinocyte apoptosis is the main feature and drug-specific cytotoxic CD8+ T cells (CTLs) and NK-cells are the main effector cells. CTLs can activate the caspase cascade, including apoptosis either through Fas-Fas ligand binding or the perforin/granzyme B pathway, TNF-α and annexin A1 release, responsible for keratinocyte death in SJS/TEN [5]. Blister T cells from patients exert drug specific cytotoxic activity against both autologous B-lymphocyte cell lines and keratinocytes, and is mediated by granzyme B. The discrepancy between the paucity of the infiltration of immune cells in the skin of patients with SJS/TEN and the overwhelming keratinocyte apoptosis has led to the search for cytotoxic proteins and/or cytokines that may "amplify" the extent of keratinocyte apoptosis that CTLs alone could induce upon cell-cell contact. Recent findings suggest that especially granulysin, a powerful pro-inflammatory cytotoxic cationic protein released from CTLs and NK-cells, turns on extensive keratinocyte apoptosis [5]. Serum levels of granulysin and IL-15 are associated with severity and mortality in SJS/TEN.

Risk factors include immune dysregulation (HIV, SLE), active malignancy and genetic predisposition. A strong association has been found between SJS/TEN and specific drugs in ethnicity specific populations with some genes coding for specific HLA or drug metabolizing enzymes: HLA-B*1502 for instance, is strongly associated with the use of carbamazepine in SJS/TEN patients of Southeast Asian ancestry, especially in Han Chinese [5]. Genetic pretesting has since then significantly reduced the prevalence in at-risk populations for carbamazepine.

Aetiology

SJS/TEN nearly always represents an idiosyncratic reaction to medication. Although about 200 drugs have been reported to cause SJS/TEN, only a limited number of drugs is responsible for the majority of the reactions. In absolute case numbers, allopurinol is the most common cause of SJS/TEN in Europe. The highest risk occurs during the first 2 months of first treatment with a sharp drop of incidence thereafter. However, although some drugs have a high relative risk compared to other drugs, the actual risk remains low. Drugs with a significantly raised risk are allopurinol, carbamazepine, phenytoin, phenobarbital, lamotrigine, sulfamethoxazole-trimethoprim and other sulphonamide antibiotics such as sulfasalazine, NSAID's of the oxicam-type, and nevirapine [6].

Targeted drugs and immunotherapy that have revolutionized cancer therapy and are increasingly used, have also been implicated. Amongst them are PD-1 (e.g. nivolumab and pembrolizumab), PD-L1, and CTLA-4 (e.g. ipilimumab) checkpoint inhibitors, but also EGFR-inhibitors, and combinations of BRAF (e.g. vemurafenib) and MEK inhibitors. However, these reports, especially those implicating checkpoint inhibitors, often relate to atypical, SJS/TEN-like bullous lichenoid reactions, regularly in patients on polypharmacy (including high-risk drugs for SJS/TEN) and/or (pre)treated with another immunomodulating agent. Of note, these reactions regularly only occur after prolonged drug use and show a mild initial presentation and slowly evolving course, followed by a rapid progression.

The ALDEN score, an SJS/TEN-specific drug-causality score, can be helpful to identify the culprit drug, especially in cases with polypharmacy. It is based on the time latency between start of drug use and onset of the adverse reaction, drug presence in the body at onset (drug's half-life and liver- and kidney function), drug notoriety, prechallenge, rechallenge and dechallenge, and exclusion of alternative causes.

However, some cases are of infectious origin (e.g. Mycoplasma pneumonia in SJS) or are without any plausible identifiable cause (especially in the under-18-year-olds). Confounding non-drug risk factors are HIV, other infections, recent cancer, recent radiotherapy, and collagen vascular disease [6].

Diagnosis Paths

History and Physical Examination

Most important is the acute onset of extensive painful mucocutaneous blistering with the typical clinical presentation and systemic symptoms, often preceded by a prodromal stage. At suspicion of SJS/TEN, an early accurate medication history is essential to detect a possible association, with special attention to drugs, introduced 4–28 days before onset of the reaction.

General Diagnostics

Diagnosis mainly relies on the clinical picture, confirmed by histopathology (clinicopathological correlation) and negative immunofluorescence investigations. Typical clinical signs initially include painful erythematous and violaceous purpuric macules on the skin with progressive coalescence on which a positive pseudo-Nikolsky's sign (Fig. 2.2) can be induced. This is often followed by blistering and epidermal detachment within hours. Involvement of two or more mucosae develops shortly before or simultaneously with skin signs in almost all cases.

Work up of immediate cryosections or conventional formalin-fixed sections of the skin, preferentially taken from a blister edge, should confirm diagnosis. Histopathology of SJS, SJS/TEN overlap and TEN essentially shows the same picture, featuring widespread keratinocyte apoptosis scattered throughout the epidermis with subepidermal blistering secondary to extensive presence of necrotic keratinocytes, resulting in (almost) full-thickness epidermal necrosis. The dermis may show slight perivascular lymphocytic infiltrates (Fig. 21.6).

Specific Diagnostics

To distinguish SJS from SJS/TEN-overlap or TEN the total maximum detached BSA is the predominant discriminating factor (Figs. 21.3, 21.4, and 21.5).

The main differential diagnoses of SJS/TEN are acute generalized exanthematous pustulosis (AGEP), generalized bullous fixed drug eruption (GBFDE), staphylococcal scalded skin syndrome (SSSS), graft versus host disease (GvHD) and autoimmune blistering diseases, including linear IgA bullous dermatosis and paraneoplastic pemphigus, but also pemphigus vulgaris, bullous pemphigoid, and (sub)acute lupus erythema-

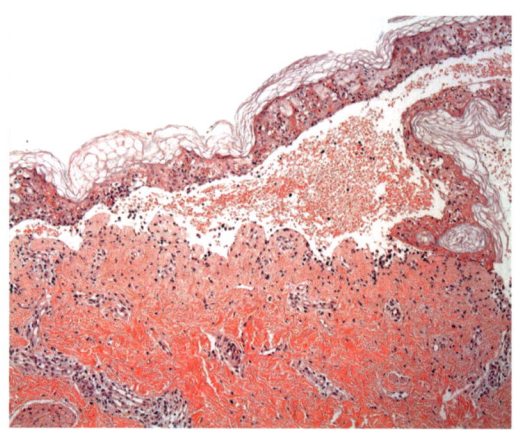

Fig. 21.6 Histopathology of SJS/TEN showing many apoptotic cells resulting in almost total necrotic epidermis and subepidermal splitting. The dermis shows very sparse lymphocytic infiltrates

Table 21.2 SCORTEN criteria and mortality

Independent prognosis factors	Weight
Age ≥ 40 years	1 point
Malignancy present	1 point
Detached body surface area ≥ 10%	1 point
Heart rate ≥ 120/min	1 point
Serum urea >10 mmol/l	1 point
Serum glucose >14 mmol/l	1 point
Serum bicarbonate <20 mmol/l	1 point
Total score	**Mortality (%)**
0–1 points	3.2
2 points	12.1
3 points	35.3
4 points	58.3
≥5 points	90.0

todes. Differentiation of AGEP and SSSS can be made by histopathology, while autoimmune blistering diseases can be ruled out by (in)direct immunofluorescence investigations. Differentiation of GBFDE is difficult and can be made on subtle differences in the clinical presentation and on history.

Within the first 3 days of admission SCORTEN, a severity-of-illness score for TEN predicting prognosis, should be performed (Table 21.2). Although in vivo or in vitro testing (patch test or lymphocyte transformation test) may confirm the suspected culprit drug, the sensitivity of these tests is rather limited in SJS/TEN.

> **Case Study: Part 2**
>
> History reveals that carbamazepine was taken since 2 weeks. Two days later body temperature is 38.9 C. The skin eruption has meanwhile extended and is very painful, with many erythematopapular lesions mainly on the upper torso, face, arms and legs, some with blistering. Severe conjunctivitis is observed, while lips, mouth and genital area show extensive blistering and erosions. Pseudo-Nikolsky's sign is positive (Fig. 21.7). What is your differential diagnosis now?

Treatment Tricks

Initial Treatment and Therapeutic Ladder

Treatment requires specific expertise and facilities: early admission to a referral centre reduces the risk of infection, mortality and length of hospitalisation. Management in the acute stage should be multidisciplinary and includes supportive care and evaluation of the severity and prognosis by means of SCORTEN. With a score of ≥3 or when ≥20% of the BSA is detached or detachable, transfer to an intensive care unit should be considered. Restoring the barrier function of skin and mucosae as quickly as possible and in the meantime preventing the negative effects of its loss is of eminent importance [7]. Because of massive loss of body temperature and fluid, the patient is preferentially treated on an "air-fluidized" bed in a temperature and moisture regulated room with, for aseptic reasons, a laminar down flow stream. To protect patients from infection, nursing has to be barrier protected.

First line of treatment is cessation of the suspected culprit. For drugs with short half-lives, prompt withdrawal on the first day of blistering/erosions has a positive effect on the outcome and lowers mortality.

Apart from withdrawal of the culprit and intensive, multidisciplinary, supportive care, various options for immunomodulating treatment have been suggested. However, results are variable and generally accepted guidelines are still lacking. Corticosteroids, especially a short course of high dosed pulse therapy, e.g. 1.5 mg/kg bodyweight dexamethasone on 3 consecutive days, early in the process, might positively influence the immune mediated cascade leading to apoptosis [7]. The supposed rationale that intravenous immunoglobulins (IVIG) inhibit activation of the death receptor by Fas-inhibiting antibodies is questioned and the reported results are inconsistent. More recently, also TNF-α blockers, espe-

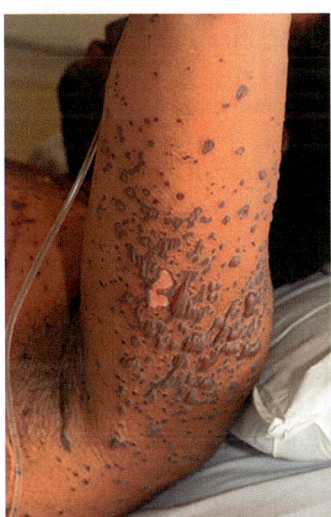 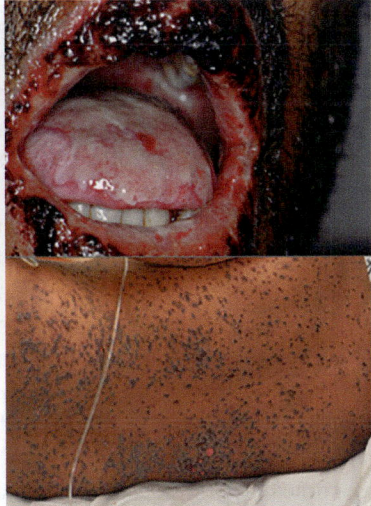 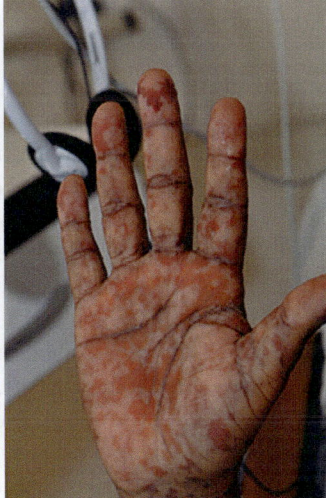

Fig. 21.7 Describe what you observe. What is your diagnosis?

cially etanercept have been suggested and a favourable outcome has been reported for treatment with ciclosporin [8, 9].

Follow-Up and Tapering

Intensive monitoring includes vital parameters, laboratory investigations (blood count, electrolytes, renal-, liver function, blood gases, bicarbonate, glucose, blood culture, urine analysis, etc.) mucocutaneous cultures, and BSA involvement.

The hypercatabolic state and mucosal involvement induced by SJS/TEN often demands nutritional correction by nasogastric feeding. A critical element of supportive care is the management of fluid and electrolyte requirements. Hyponatremia, hypokalaemia or hypophosphatemia, which quite frequently do occur, necessitate appropriate early and aggressive replacement therapy.

Blisters should be treated conservatively because blistered skin acts as a natural biological dressing, likely favouring re-epithelialization. Removing only epidermis that is curled up is preferred over debridement, which is still regularly performed in burn units. Extensive wound care includes emollients (petrolatum gauzes), local antiseptics, and non-adhesive dressings. Central lines should be avoided while antibiotics are only given if needed. Pain and anxiety control are essential; systemic corticosteroids should be avoided late in the process [7, 9].

Because of the combined involvement of skin, eyes and other mucous membranes, interdisciplinary follow up and treatment of sequelae is recommended. Special attention should be given to the prevention of genital and ocular complications. Daily examination by an ophthalmologist can help to diminish the risk for permanent visual loss due to corneal scarring or neovascularisation. Preservative-free eye drops including saline, topical steroids or antibiotics should be installed every two hours; developing synechiae should be disrupted. In the early phase of corneal defects, amniotic membranes covering the ocular surface decrease pain, preserve visual acuity, and protect against scarring [9]. Scleral contact lenses may promote corneal healing. Prolonged ophthalmologic follow up is recommended because corneal involvement may progress for months to years.

Survivors should be educated on the cause of the reaction and future drug use, and not be re-exposed to the suspected or chemically related drugs.

> **Case Study: Part 3**
> Histology of the edge of a blister reveals nearly full thickness epidermal necrosis, subepidermal splitting and sparse dermal lymphocytic infiltrates. Together with the clinical picture the diagnosis fits within the spectrum of SJS/TEN. The total detached BSA that will ultimately be reached, determines the final diagnosis. Carbamazepine is immediately stopped and treatment is started with dexamethason pulse therapy 1.5 mg/kg for 3 days intravenously. Patient is nursed barrier protected in a laminar down flow room on an "air-fluidized" bed and intensively monitored e.g. including SCORTEN and vital parameters and received extensive wound care.

Erythema Exsudativum Multiforme (EEM)

Facts and Figures

Definitions and Classification

EEM is an acute, often symmetrical, mucocutaneous, polymorphous eruption, with a diversity of lesions: erythema, papules or plaques, vesiculo-bullae, and purpura. It may present with only few lesions, but can also be rather extensive. Characteristic is the acrofacial distribution, which may spread centripetal. Most lesions develop within 24–72 hrs as small wheal-like erythematous lesions, which may become papular and individual lesions may persist for over a week; lesions however, may also appear in serial crops. Some are highly regular and circular, measuring a few millimetres to three centimetres and may become livid. Bullae or purpura may develop in the center, creating the so-called target or iris lesions. Target lesions in EEM are raised and can be typical (Fig. 21.1) and/or atypical (Fig. 21.2).

EEM varies from mild (EEM minus, the most common form with symmetrical distributed, most often mildly itching or burning classical "target lesions" on the extensor sides of the extremities, face, and neck), to a more severe form (EEM majus). The difference is based on the presence and severity of systemic symptoms (e.g. fever and malaise) and involvement of mucosae, which is absent or minor and often restricted to the lips in the minus, and more pronounced in the majus form.

EEM majus may be preceded by influenza-like prodromes with a classic time course, usually starting 1–14 days before lesions appear, while prodromal symptoms are mostly absent or mild in EEM minus. Lesions evolve over 1–2 weeks. Mucosal involvement often presents with clearly haemorrhagic crustae and erosions including on lips, mouth, eyes, nose, genitals, urethra and/or anus. In children and adolescents, the mucosae can be severely affected in cases caused by Mycoplasma pneumoniae (M. pneumoniae) or respiratory infections, sometimes even extending into the throat, larynx and bronchi [10]. Whatever the clinical relevance, further subtypes have been identified, e.g. atypical EEM majus (with giant targets located on the trunk) and the recently introduced qualification "M. pneumoniae-induced rash and mucositis" (MIRM). In all subtypes, infections have been found the most common aetiology.

Resolution normally results within 2–3 weeks; EEM majus may have a more protracted course: mucosal lesions generally heal without sequelae within 3–6 weeks, except in severe eye involvement. Skin lesions may heal with hyper- and/or hypopigmentation, scarring is usually absent. Most patients have an uncomplicated course, with exception of the immunocompromised and those with secondary bacterial infections. Although generally self-limiting, recurrences are common and are most often preceded by or occur with an overt or subclinical HSV infection.

Mortality in EEM minus is virtually absent and approximately 1% in EEM majus, mainly concerning patients of older age and with underlying conditions; sepsis secondary to loss of the cutaneous barrier is the principle cause [2].

Epidemiology

The exact incidence of EEM is not known, but is estimated at somewhere between 0.01% and 1% of the population, with the minus variant as the most prevalent. EEM occurs in patients of all ages, but is predominantly observed in adolescents and young adults with a peak incidence in the second and third decades of life. It is rare during early childhood and in adults older than 50 years, EEM majus has a slight male preponderance, but no racial bias. Recurrences occur in 30% of EEM minus and of 10% of EEM majus [10].

Pathogenesis

Pathophysiology of EEM is still not fully understood. Most likely it is a distinct hyperergic mucocutaneous immune reaction, triggered by a variety of stimuli, in particular various infections (about 90%) or chemical products in certain "predisposed" individuals. Although, predisposing genes have been associated (HLA-DQB1*0301), its predictive value is too low to have clinical relevance. Otherwise, a clear genetic predisposition for EEM is still to be defined. Of note, several physical agents such as trauma, cold, and ultraviolet radiation have been described as triggers for outbreaks of EEM related to infectious agents, drugs or systemic disease.

HSV is clearly most commonly associated with EEM minus and in the majority of adults with EEM majus. M. pneumoniae is the second cause of EEM overall and the first in children. In cases related to mycoplasma, the target lesions are usually atypical and appear predominantly on the trunk [10]. Rarely, EEM has been associated with drugs or systemic disease. The majority of children and adults where the disease is precipitated by HSV types 1 and 2 have a normal immunity to HSV, but they possibly have difficulty in clearing the virus. HSV suppression and prophylaxis with antiviral therapy (e.g. valacyclovir) has been shown to prevent recurrent EEM.

Diagnosis Paths

History and Physical Examination

The most important differential diagnosis is SJS, because of its possible life-threatening complications and the need of timely withdrawal of a suspected drug. Diagnosis relies on the clinical picture: typically, it presents as an acute mucocutaneous eruption in an adolescent or young adult, suffering or recovering from herpes, or having a history of recurrent, similar attacks. Characteristic is the presence of typical target lesions and the acral predilection on the back of the hands and feet (sometimes palmoplantar), and extensor sites of the elbows, knees, neck, face, mouth, eyes and genitals. History should document recent constitutional symptoms, previous or current HSV, M. pneumoniae or other infections, and all use of medication, in particular started in the previous 2 months.

General Diagnostics

Besides SJS/TEN, several other diseases may be considered including urticaria, (urticarial)vasculitis, toxic/viral exanthema, serum sickness-like eruption, annular/gyrated erythemas, and M. Sweet; while e.g. herpes stomatitis, aphtosis, auto-immune bullous diseases, including (sub) acute cutaneous lupus erythematodes, and SJS should be considered in cases with mucosal involvement. The possibility of SJS, GBFDE, polymorphous maculopapular eruption or urticaria should be strongly considered if the presumed aetiology is drug-induced. The most important differential diagnosis however is urticaria, especially in its early acute stage. The main difference is that in EEM the centre of the lesions may show a darker, dull, purple aspect, blisters, erosions or crusts, versus normal skin in urticaria. Moreover, in EEM lesions are not transient, but will remain during a period of several days, while oedema is not a prominent feature.

Specific Diagnostics

Histopathology typically reveals an acute interface dermatitis with apoptotic epidermal keratinocytes, especially at the interface, sometimes resulting in more widespread epidermal necrosis, and in addition a moderate lymphocytic, sometimes mixed superficial perivascular infiltrate. Differentiation from SJS/TEN just on histopathology can be problematic and should be based on the clinicopathological correlation. Most important clues for SJS/TEN are a severely painful skin, rapid progression with dark violaceous, often confluent macules and blisters, constitutional symptoms, and recent drug use. In urticaria, histopathology shows some perivascular mixed infiltrates, while an interface dermatitis or apoptotic epidermal cells, characteristic for EEM, are lacking. Immunofluorescence findings can help to exclude autoimmune bullous disorders. HSV can be confirmed by PCR. Chest radiography, PCR-assay and/or serology, especially in cases with respiratory symptoms, may help to detect M. pneumonia,

Treatment Tricks

Most often, EEM is self-limiting. However, it is essential to potentially identify and treat the eliciting factor. Admission should be considered for patients with severe oral involvement, impairing feeding and drinking, or presenting with severe constitutional symptoms.

Otherwise, treatment is usually symptomatic, including oral antihistamines, analgesics, local skin and mucosal care. Liquid antiseptics, such as 0.05% chlorhexidine, help to prevent superinfection. Patients feeling ill and having extensive lesions can be treated with corticosteroid creams against pruritus and anti-inflammatory drugs and/or xylocaine for pain management. For oral lesions antiseptics can be useful, as are local corticosteroids and/or painkilling preparations. For eye involvement an ophthalmologist should be consulted, especially in the acute phase to prevent infection and scarring. Topical treatment, including for genital lesions, can be performed with gauze dressings or a hydrocolloid. In more severe cases, meticulous wound care is needed. Infections should be appropriately treated after cultures/PCR and/or serologic tests have been performed. Suppression of HSV can prevent HSV-associated recurrent EEM, but antiviral treatment after the eruption of EEM has started, is without effect on the course of EEM. Treatment of M. pneumonia can be useful in case of respiratory symptoms, but does not result in a more rapid healing of the associated EEM. Although systemic corticosteroids are often given in severe cases, their beneficial use has not been evidenced; they should be restricted to the very early stage of the disease. Azathioprine, thalidomide, and mycophenolate mofetil have been suggested for recurrent or therapy resistant cases [10].

Review Questions

1. Which drug is most often associated with SJS/TEN?
   a. Allopurinol
   b. Penicillin and its derivates
   c. NSAIDs
   d. Quinolones
2. The following clinical symptoms differentiate SJS from EEM majus:
   a. Typical target lesions
   b. Detached and detachable BSA > 10%
   c. Fever
   d. All of mentioned above
3. Regular observed long-lasting sequelae in SJS/TEN are:
   a. Impaired vision
   b. Disturbed liver function
   c. Disturbed kidney function
   d. Cutaneous scarring
4. SCORTEN indicates:
   a. The severity of SJS/TEN
   b. The total detached and detachable BSA
   c. The prognosis in TEN
   d. The severity and prognosis in EEM/SJS/TEN
5. Regarding medication in SJS/TEN:
   a. SJS and TEN can be elicited by identical medication
   b. In SJS/TEN the half-life of a culprit medication that has been withdrawn is decisive for its course
   c. In SJS/TEN all medication should be stopped
   d. A relatively limited number of drugs has been associated with SJS/TEN

Answers

1. a.
2. a.
3. a.
4. c.
5. a.

References

1. Bastuji-Garin S, Rzany B, Stern RS, Shear NH, Naldi L, Roujeau JC. Clinical classification of cases of toxic epidermal necrolysis, Stevens-Johnson syndrome, and erythema multiforme. Arch Dermatol. 1993;129:92–6.
2. Auquier-Dunant A, Mockenhaupt M, Naldi L, Correia O, Schröder W, Roujeau JC, SCAR Study Group. Severe cutaneous adverse reactions. Correlations between clinical patterns and causes of erythema multiforme majus, Stevens-Johnson syndrome, and toxic epidermal necrolysis: results of an international prospective study. Arch Dermatol. 2002;138:1019–24.
3. Sekula P, Dunant A, Mockenhaupt M, Naldi L, Bouwes Bavinck JN, Halevy S, Kardaun S, Sidoroff A, Liss Y, Schumacher M, Roujeau JC. Comprehensive survival analysis of a cohort of patients with Stevens-Johnson syndrome and toxic epidermal necrolysis. J Invest Dermatol. 2013;133:1197–204.
4. Paulmann M, Kremler C, Sekula P, Valeyrie-Allanore L, Naldi L, Kardaun SH, Mockenhaupt M. Stevens-Johnson syndrome and toxic epidermal necrolysis: long-term sequelae based on a 5-year follow-up analysis. Pharmacoepidemiol Drug Saf. 2016;25(Suppl.3):118–9.
5. Chung WH, Hung SI. Genetic markers and danger signals in Stevens-Johnson syndrome and toxic epidermal necrolysis. Allergol Int. 2010;59:325–32.
6. Mockenhaupt M, Viboud C, Dunant A, Naldi L, Halevy S, Bouwes Bavinck JN, Sidoroff A, Schneck J, Roujeau JC, Flahault A. Stevens-Johnson syndrome and toxic epidermal necrolysis: assessment of medication risks with emphasis on recently marketed drugs. The EuroSCAR-study. J Invest Dermatol. 2008;128:35–44.
7. Kardaun SH, Jonkman MF. Dexamethasone pulse therapy for Stevens-Johnson syndrome/toxic epidermal necrolysis. Acta Derm Venereol. 2007;87:144–8.
8. Valeyrie-Allanore L, Wolkenstein P, Brochard L, Ortonne N, Maître B, Revuz J, Bagot M, Roujeau JC. Open trial of ciclosporin treatment for Stevens-Johnson syndrome and toxic epidermal necrolysis. Br J Dermatol. 2010;163:847–53.
9. Torres-Navarro I, Briz-Redón Á, Botella-Estrada R. Systemic therapies for Stevens-Johnson syndrome and toxic epidermal necrolysis: a SCORTEN-based systematic review and meta-analysis. J Eur Acad Dermatol Venereol. 2021;35:159–71.
10. Roujeau JC, Mockenhaupt M. Erythema multiforme. In: Kang S, Amagai M, Bruckner AL, et al., edi-

tors. Fitzpatrick's dermathology. 9th ed. New York: McGraw-Hill Education; 2019.

Additional Reading

Bastuji-Garin S, Fouchard N, Bertocchi M, Roujeau JC, Revuz J, Wolkenstein P. SCORTEN: a severity-of-illness score for toxic epidermal necrolysis. J Invest Dermatol. 2000;115:149–53.

Sassolas B, Haddad C, Mockenhaupt M, Dunant A, Liss Y, Bork K, Haustein UF, Vieluf D, Roujeau JC, Le Louet H. ALDEN, an algorithm for assessment of drug causality in Stevens-Johnson Syndrome and toxic epidermal necrolysis: comparison with case-control analysis. Clin Pharmacol Ther. 2010;88:60–8.

Shear NH. Litt's drug eruption and reaction manual. 27th ed. CRC Press ISBN 9780367649531.

Porphyria Cutanea Tarda and Pseudoporphyria

Marjolein S. Bruijn and Jorrit B. Terra

Introduction and AIMS

Short Definition in Layman Terms

Porphyria cutanea tarda (PCT) is a metabolic disorder in which porphyrins accumulate in the skin. Skin fragility and blistering arise after UVA light exposition. Pseudoporphyria mimics PCT, but not due to underlying porphyrin disorder, but due to abnormal drug metabolism.

> **Learning Objectives**
> After reading this chapter, you should be able to recognize the typical clinical presentation of PCT, and know the triggering factors for PCT and pseudoporphyria.

> **Case Study:**
> A 39-year old woman presented with complaints of skin fragility and bullae on the dorsum of the hands (Fig. 22.1), and bullae and hemorrhagic crusts and erosions on her face and neck. She noticed hypertrichosis on her face (Fig. 22.2). The skin lesions gave burning sensation, especially after sun exposure. Mucosae were not involved.

Didactical Questions; Cross Section of Questions to Prime the Readers Interest

What could have made you think of PCT and what is your strategy to confirm diagnosis? What do you see in the histopathology and direct immunofluorescence.

(DIF) when you take a biopsy of a fresh blister? What are the risk factors for PCT and pseudoporphyria?

Facts and Figures

Definitions and Classification

PCT is a bullous photosensitivity disorder. Partial deficiencies in the heme biosynthesis pathway

M. S. Bruijn
Department of Dermatology, Ommelander Hospital Groningen, Scheemda, The Netherlands
e-mail: m.s.bruijn@umcg.nl

J. B. Terra (✉)
Department of Dermatology, Isala Hospital, Zwolle, The Netherlands
e-mail: j.b.terra@umcg.nl

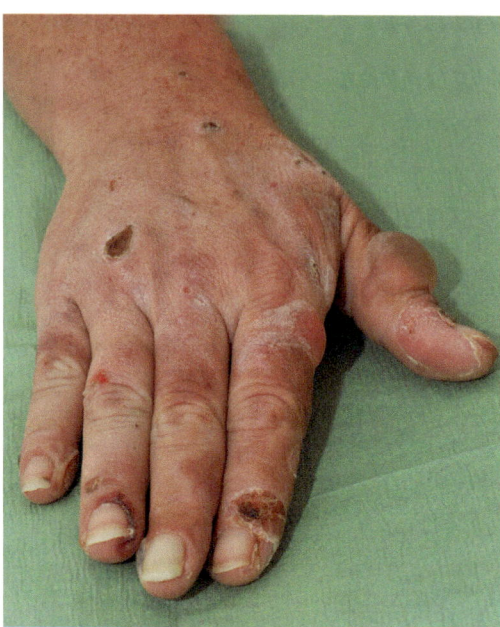

Fig. 22.1 PCT with bullae, hemorrhagic crusts and erosions on the dorsum of the hand

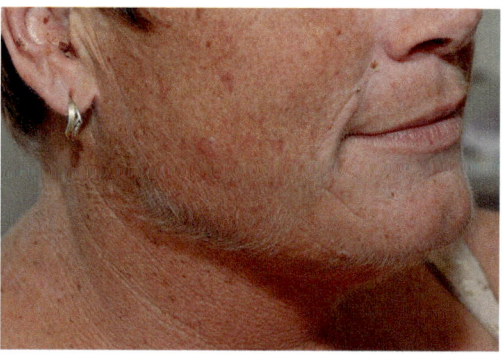

Fig. 22.2 PCT with lanugo-like hypertrichosis on the face

lead to accumulation of porphyrins. PCT can be subdivided in an acquired and a familial form. The familial form is not very penetrant and therefore triggering factors are crucial to create clinical findings.

Pseudoporphyria mimics PCT. The clinical, histological and immunofluorescent characteristics are similar but there are no accompanying biochemical porphyrin abnormalities.

Epidemiology

PCT is worldwide the most common porphyria and typically presents in the fourth decade of life. PCT overall affects males and females equally, with some studies suggesting male predominance in the acquired form [1]. The epidemiology of pseudoporphyria differs depending on the etiologic agent.

Pathogenesis

PCT is the result of inhibition of uroporphyrinogen decarboxylase (UROD) in the liver, which causes accumulation of mainly uroporphyrins. This inhibition is established in the presence of iron, reactive oxygen species and activation of cytochrome P450 [2]. Alcoholism, estrogens, iron overload and liver related diseases like hepatitis C and hemochromatosis are therefore risk factors. HIV is also reported as a predisposed factor for PCT [2]. Uroporphyrin diffuse into the dermal epidermal junction where they interact with UVA light, of approximately 400 nm wavelength radiant energy [2, 3]. As a result, reactive oxygen species are formed which produce the main symptoms of PCT.

The precise pathophysiologic mechanism of pseudoporphyria is not fully understood yet. Pseudoporphyria is a photosensitive disorder caused by abnormal drug metabolites that act as photoactive substances. Medication particularly nonsteroidal anti-inflammatory drugs (NSAIDs) like naproxen can cause pseudoporphyria. Other suspected medications are antibiotics, diuretics and retinoids [4]. Other causes of pseudoporphyria are excessive exposure to UVA light by tanning beds and chronic renal failure or dialysis (Table 22.1).

Diagnosis Paths

History and Physical Examination

Cutaneous findings exclusively involve sun-exposed areas of the body like the dorsum of the hands, forearms, upper chest and face. Patients complain of photosensitivity and skin fragility. Cutaneous findings include hemorrhagic crusts, vesicles, bullae and superficial scars or milia. The bullae are tense and filled with clear fluid (Fig. 22.1). Additional hypo- and hyperpigmentation,

Table 22.1 Causes of pseudoporphyria [4]

Ultraviolet light
UVA tanning beds
PUVA
Excessive sun exposure

NSAIDs
Naproxen
Nabumetone
Oxaprozin
Ketoprofen
Mefenamic acid
Diflunisal

Chronic renal failure/dialysis

Antibiotics
Nalidixic acid
Tetracyline

Diuretics
Chlorthalidone
Bumetanide
Furosemide
Hydrochlorothiazide/ triamterene

Retinoids
Isotretinoin
Etretinate

Miscellaneous
Cyclosporine
Fluorouracil
Carisoprodol/aspirin
Pyridoxine
Amiodarone
Flutamide
Dapsone
Coca-cola

Reprinted from Ref. [4] © 2001, with permission from Elsevier

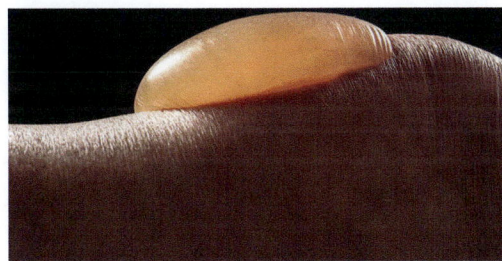

Fig. 22.3 Pseudoporphyria in a paraplegic wheelchair patient showing a tense monomorphic bulla filled with clear fluid on the sun-exposed knee. The culprit drug was tolterodine [5]

hypertrichosis, sclerodermoid plaques, scarring alopecia, onycholysis and dystrophic nails may be present. Patients, particularly females, may have lanugo-like hypertrichosis on the peri-orbital and temporal regions of the face (Fig. 22.2). Although most clinical features in PCT and pseudoporphyria are similar, features as hypertrichosis, hyperpigmentation and sclerodermoid plaques are rarely present in pseudoporphyria [4]. The clinical presentation of PCT and pseudoporphyria is subacute and the relationship with sun exposure may therefore be missed (Fig. 22.3).

General Diagnostics

The diagnosis PCT is made with urine test demonstrating increased uroporphyrin levels, but also increased levels of precursors like penta-, hexa-, hepta-carboxylated porphyrins and coproporphyrins can be detected in the urine. Also plasma and feces porphyrin levels are increased. Screening of urine on uroporphyrins is however sufficient for PCT diagnosis. Almost all patients have elevated serum iron and ferritin levels. A biopsy of a fresh blister for histology shows a subepidermal cell-poor blister with 'festooning' of dermal papillae, PAS positive glycoproteins at the basement membrane zone and around blood vessels. DIF shows homogeneous immunoglobulin, mainly IgG, and complement deposition at the basement membrane zone and around blood vessels (Fig. 4.8).

Specific Diagnostics

Exclude risk factors like hemochromatosis, hepatitis C and HIV infections.

Treatment Tricks

Initial Treatment and Therapeutic Ladder

Sunlight avoidance is the first step in the treatment of PCT and pseudoporphyria. Besides sun protection, treatment entails discontinuation of suspected risk factors. Other measures include iron depletion by regular phlebotomy or low dose chloroquine. Chloroquine is capable of binding porphyrins, forming water-soluble complexes readily excreted in the urine [3]. Higher doses of chloroquine can cause liver toxicity and should be avoided. In pseudoporphyria the culprit drug should be stopped for at least three months before evaluation.

Follow-Up and Tapering

Once a biochemical remission in PCT is instigated, there is a high chance of relapse even if the underlying cause has been treated. Additionally potential development of hepatocellular carcinoma is possible and therefore follow up is advised.

Review Questions

1. How can you differentiate between PCT and mechanobullous EBA?
   a. Clinical symptoms
   b. Histological findings
   c. DIF serration pattern analysis
2. What is the main treatment of PCT?
   a. Phlebotomy
   b. Low dose chloroquine
   c. Sun protection
3. What is the most frequent cause of pseudoporphyria?
   a. Tetracycline
   b. Naproxen
   c. Excessive use of Coca-Cola

Answers

1. c.
2. c.
3. b.

Acknowledgement We would thank M. Gyldenløve for providing Fig. 22.3.

References

1. Frank J, Poblete-Gutierrez P. Porphyria cutanea tarda--when skin meets liver. Best Pract Res Clin Gastroenterol. 2010;24:735–45.
2. Ryan Caballes F, Sendi H, Bonkovsky HL. Hepatitis C, porphyria cutanea tarda and liver iron: an update. Liver Int. 2012;32:880–93.
3. Sarkany RP. The management of porphyria cutanea tarda. Clin Exp Dermatol. 2001;26:225–32.
4. Green JJ, Manders SM. Pseudoporphyria. J Am Acad Dermatol. 2001;44:100–8.
5. Gyldenløve M, Due E, Jonkman MF, Faurschou A. Pseudoporphyria - a case report. J Eur Acad Dermatol Venereol. 2014; https://doi.org/10.1111/jdv.12433.

Additional Reading

Horner ME, Alikhan A, Tintle S, Tortorelli S, Davis DM, Hand JL. Cutaneous porphyrias part I: epidemiology, pathogenesis, presentation, diagnosis, and histopathology. Int J Dermatol. 2013;52:1464–80.

Tintle S, Alikhan A, Horner ME, Hand JL, Davis DM. Cutaneous porphyrias part II: treatment strategies. Int J Dermatol. 2014;53:3–24.

Bullous Dermatitis Artefacta

23

Marcel F. Jonkman, Wianda A. Christoffers, and Barbara Horváth

Introduction and AIMS

Short Definition in Layman Terms

Bullous dermatitis artefacta is a mental abnormality in patients who mimic skin disease by inflicting themselves blisters. The diagnosis is immediately apparent to the doctor at first visit. The patient should be approached in such a way that the he is not losing face. Premature confrontation or embarrassing accusations should be avoided. Treatment strategy is narrow escape: the patient is almost confronted while he gets the chance to opt out by avoiding any scapegoat (coffee) or taking any rescue (vitamin C) that cleared the skin. In difficult cases the patient has to be confronted with the diagnosis by a psychiatrist.

Despite the spot diagnosis, DA needs a serious workup.

M. F. Jonkman (Deceased) · B. Horváth (✉)
Center for Blistering Diseases, Department of Dermatology, University Medical Center Groningen, University of Groningen, Groningen, The Netherlands
e-mail: b.horvath@umcg.nl

W. A. Christoffers
Isala Klinieken, AB, Zwolle, The Netherlands
e-mail: w.a.christoffers@isala.nl

Learning Objectives
After reading this chapter you understand the clinical presentation, histopathology, differential diagnosis, and treatment approaches of bullous vesiculo-bullous eruptions in bullous dermatitis artefacta (DA).

Case Study: Part 1
A mother with child consulted the Center for Blistering Diseases after visiting three dermatologists before in the last year because of episodes of erosions in the face of the 12-year-old daughter. All dermatologists came to a prompt diagnosis of dermatitis artefacta, and ask the girl if she did it herself. She denied. The episodes persisted.

At dermatological examination I saw a shy but cooperative girl with linear erosions in the face with erythematous border. The mother was receptive for advice.

A skin biopsy for direct IF was negative.

Didactical Questions; Cross Section of Questions to Prime the Readers Interest

What is the presentation of DA? What is the approach to avoid frustration of the doctor?

Facts and Figures

Definitions and Classification

Bullous dermatitis artefacta (DA) is a psychiatric factitious disorder in which the patient intentionally evokes blisters or erosions but denies self-infliction (Fig. 23.1). The synonym bullous pathomimia [1] is not used anymore, since not all patients are fully aware of their self-inflicting behavior that mimics bullous disease (Table 23.1). In automutilation (non-suicidal self-injury, DSM V) the patient also purposely wounds its own skin, but in contrast to DA admits self-infliction, such as cutting with a knife that does not mimic other skin disease. Neurotic excoriations are due to excessive compulsory scratching because of perceived itch.

Epidemiology

The patient with DA is predominantly female, and the bullous subtype mostly teenager. One of the parents, mostly the mother, is present at first consultation. The prognosis improves with younger patient, and shorter history of DA.

Pathogenesis

The patient keeps the secret of self-infliction or shares it with a relative ('folie à deux') or is the victim of a parent (Munchausen-by-proxy syndrome). The loneliness of the secret is compensated by the attention that the skin disease evokes in others. The patient may also not be fully conscious of the self-harm by dissociation. The psychopathology of this behavior is associated with border line personality disorder, multiple personality disorder, posttraumatic stress syndrome, anorexia and bulimia. Simply said: the patient dies for attention, but shows indifference for pain ('la belle indifference').

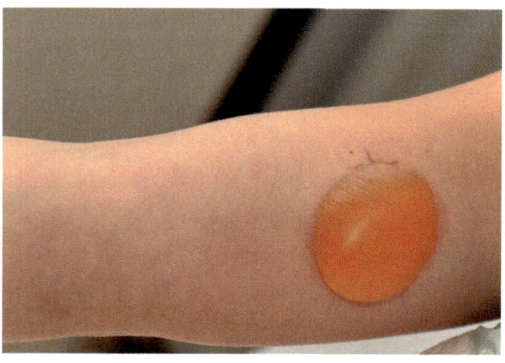

Fig. 23.1 Solitary monomorphic bulla on the arm of a teenager with bullous dermatitis artefacta. The level of blistering was subepidermal, and probably due thermally induced

Table 23.1 Diagnostic criteria for factitious disorders [3]

#	Criteria
1	Intensional production of physical or psychological signs or symptoms
2	Motivation for the behavior is to assume the sick role
3	Absence of external incentives for the behaviour (e.g., economic gain, avoiding legal responsibility, or improving physical well-being, as in malingering

Diagnosis Paths

History and Physical Examination

Bullous DA is a spot diagnosis (Fig. 23.1): the physician immediately recognizes the bizarre pattern of the skin lesions, and considers artefacts. New lesions have developed "spontaneously" days before the first visit. The medical history is hollow with no timeline or evolution pattern. The patient appeals the competence of the doctor by questioning how these lesions suddenly can develop (Table 23.2).

General Diagnostics

Despite the spot diagnosis, DA needs a serious workup. This is important for a trustful patient-physician relation, but may also prevents to step into the pitfall of missing DA-like autoimmune blistering disease. I remember the case of a 58-year old female with a 10-year history of crusted erosions on arms and neck that healed with scars. She had visited three dermatologists, a rheumatologist and a psychologist who all presumed the diagnosis bullous DA. Taking a DIF biopsy turned out to be linear IgA bullous dermatosis. Treatment with dapsone cleared the lesions within weeks and saved her marriage.

The most important differential diagnosis of bullous DA is porphyria cutanea tarda and pseudoporphyria (Chap. 22). Therefore, take a biopsy, examine urine for uroporphyrines, and check history for culprit drugs. Limit the investigations and visits however, since that keeps the doctor to remain expert in the eyes of the patient.

The physician should take all efforts at the first visit to develop a trustful relation with the patient. Show genuine personal interest and ask the patient questions about social setting (home, school, sports). Address the accompanying person separately in the conversation. Do not let the patient loose face in anyway.

Specific Diagnostics

Histopathology of the edge of a blister may reveal the factitious nature. The level of blistering depends on the type of trauma (Table 23.2 and Table 23.3).

The weakest spot (locus minoris resistence) in the skin may divert due to skin disease. For instance, repeated friction by handling a gardening tool (Fig. 23.2) results in a *physiological* friction blister in the granular layer (interface between living and dead epidermis, Figs. 23.3 and 23.4). However, in patients with hereditary epidermolysis bullosa the *pathological* friction blister is intrabasal or subepidermal at the site of the affected adhesion molecule.

> **Case Study: Part 2**
>
> My spot diagnosis was dermatitis artefacta. The patient with the nurse were sent away for drinking thee, and I took the opportunity to confront the mother with the diagnosis in an empathetic yet definite way. She initially could not believe my conclusion. The patient and her mother agreed to keep a skin diary.

Table 23.2 Signs of bullous dermatitis artefacta

Type	Example
Bizar or regular distribution of lesions	Bullae at regular distance (like wallpaper), symmetrical, on arms
Does not fit in known disease	Solitary blister without primary erythema
Medical shopping	Visited several dermatologists including a rheumatologist
'La belle indifference'	Looking untouched while presenting with several painful erosions
Improves under zinc oxide plaster	Healed lesions on lower legs, except at edge of the plaster

Table 23.3 Level of blistering in artificial bullae

Level of blistering	Trauma
Intracorneal	Plucking
Subcorneal of granular	Rubbing
Intrabasal or intraspinal	Electric
Subepidermal	Suction, thermal, acids
Deep cutaneous	Alkalines

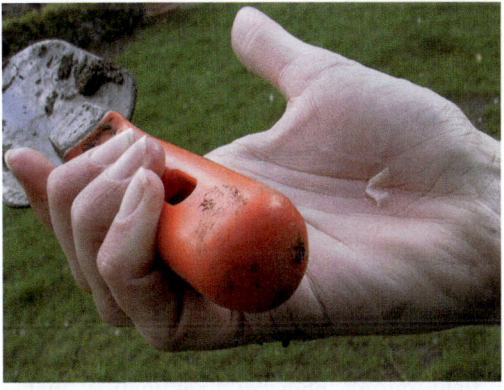

Fig. 23.2 Physiological friction blister in normal individual due to repeated trauma with shovel during gardening

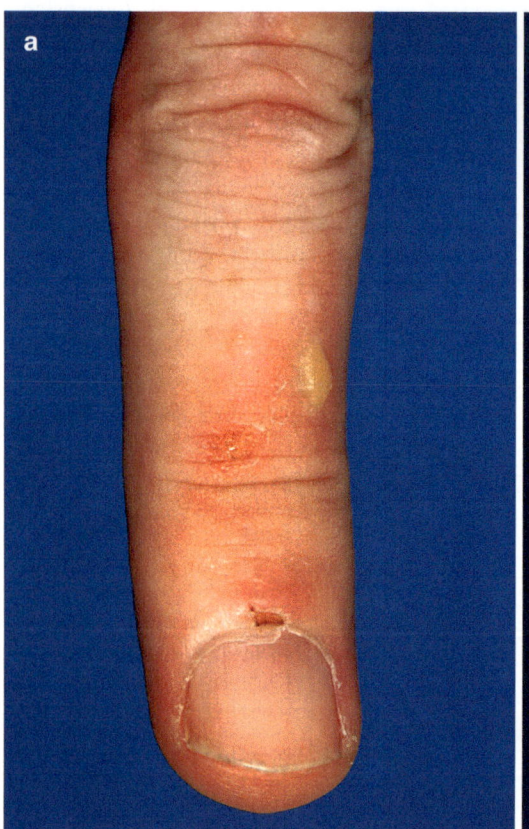

Fig. 23.3 (a) Vesicle on the digit in a patient with factitious disorder. (b) Patient in (a) was able to induce a vesicle in 30 s on the digit of his doctor by friction with his thumbnail (reprinted with permission Ned. Tijdschrift Geneeskd. 2000; 144(31): 1465–9)

Treatment Tricks

Narrow Escape

Tell your patient which diagnoses have been excluded with certainty. Take skin complains seriously and treat symptomatically. Build a safe environment.

First step in treatment is "narrow escape" thus avoiding loss of face of the patient [2]. Create a narrow escape by giving the patient the feeling you know that it self-inflicted, but never directly question it, nor accuse the patient. For instance, at first visit I told a patient during physical examination that I have seen this before, and it remarkably looks like a burn blister. At the end of the consultation I promise the patient to tell what it is at next visit after finishing all examinations. In the meanwhile I ask the patient to keep a dairy of new blisters. Keeping a diary provides extra attention. At second visit the lesions may have cleared. I have heard because the patient stopped drinking coffee, took vitamin C, or confessed to mother when brought to bed. Show happiness and agree with the conclusion of the patient. If the problem persists then introduce the psychiatrist.

The first line management of DA is narrow escape, the second is confrontation

Dual Approach

DA that is not responding to narrow-escape is generally managed by dual (or holistic) approach by dermatologist as the skin expert and the psy-

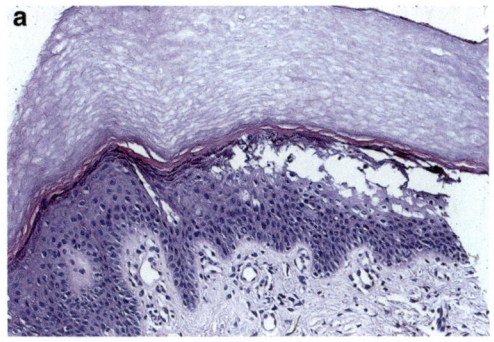

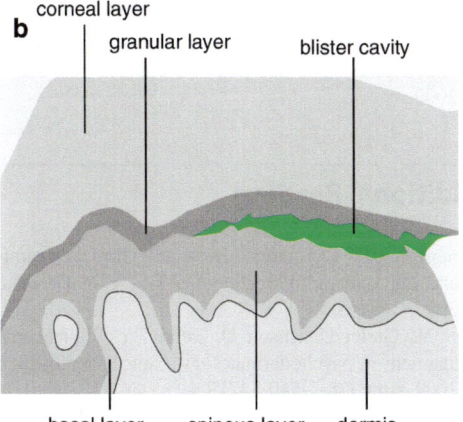

Fig. 23.4 (a) Histopathology of physiological friction blister in patient with dermatitis artefacta reveals split level beneath granular layer. (b) Diagram depicting (a). (Reprinted with permission Ned. Tijdschrift Geneeskd. 2000; 144(31): 1465–9)

chiatrist/psychologist for mental exploration. Offer psychological help by explaining that such as chronic skin disorder will have serious impact on the patient's mental well-being. The psychiatrist may be introduced after the second visit, or be present from the start in special clinics for psychodermatology.

The aim is not to elicit a confession. Patient sins against the ground rule, that he or she is dedicated to be cured. The dual approach also protects the dermatologist from incompetent feelings, elicited by patient demands when relapse occurs. Aggressive emotions in physician may lead to aim of unmasking the patient. Be conscious of this countertransference.

At some stage, in refractory cases, there is no other option than to confront the patient with the self-inflicted nature of the skin problem. This should be done without moral judgment preferable by or in the presence of the psychiatrist. If the patient-doctor relation developed in trust, the patient will not walk away, and let her lesions be treated symptomatically. After all, they also deserve compassion as sufferers of a chronic skin disorder.

> **Case Study: Part 3**
>
> The parents supported her in keeping a skin diary. They noticed repeated rubbing of the face. One night before bed the daughter confessed to her mother that she was nervous at school before math and then rubbed her face. The mother suggested to take a different doll to school every week, and every time she felt nervous cuddle the doll instead of rubbing her face. Complete remission was reached! The doll was the narrow escape introduced by the mother. Other scholars now also took a doll to school to desensitize themselves when nervous. As follow-up, I advised consultation by a pediatric psychiatrist to screen for anxiety disorders in her child.

Review Questions

1. What is most typical of the distribution of DA lesions?
   a. multiple
   b. asymmetrical
   c. trunk
   d. regular
2. The blister level of a thermal blister is
   a. subgranular layer
   b. spinous
   c. intrabasal
   d. subepidermal
3. First approach to a patient with DA is
   a. confrontation
   b. supportive empathy and serious investigation
   c. narrow escape
   d. referral to psychiatrist
4. What examples are NOT a narrow escape

a. starting a food supplement
   b. stopping certain food
   c. zinc plaster
   d. placebo

Answers

1. d.
2. c.
3. b.
4. c.

On the Web

Wikipedia: http://en.wikipedia.org/wiki/Factitious_disorder

Psycho-dermatology, British Association of Dermatology: http://www.bad.org.uk/healthcare-professionals/clinical-services/service-standards/psycho-dermatology

Merck Manuals: http://www.merckmanuals.com/professional/psychiatric_disorders/somatic_symptom_and_related_disorders/factitious_disorder_imposed_on_self.html

NYU Langone: http://www.med.nyu.edu/content?ChunkIID=165426

References

1. Brehmer-Andersson E, Goransson K. Friction blisters as a manifestation of pathomimia. Acta Derm Venereol. 1975;55:65–71.
2. van Rijssen A, Molier L, Vrijlandt AJ, Jonkman MF. Bullous dermatitis self-induced. Ned Tijdschr Geneeskd. 2000;144:1465–9.
3. American Psychiatric Association. Diagnostic and Statistical Manual of Mental Disorders. 4th text rev ed. Washington, DC: American Psychiatric Association; 2000.

Additional Reading

Koblenzer CS. Dermatitis artefacta. Clinical features and approaches to treatment. Am J Clin Dermatol. 2000;1:47–55.

Harth W, Gieler U, Kusnir D, Tausk FA. Clinical management in psychodermatology. New York: Springer; 2009. isbn:978-3-540-34719-4.

Harth W, Taube K-M, Gieler U. Facticious disorders in dermatology. J Dtsch Dermatol Ges. 2010;8:361–72.

Autoimmune Bullous Diseases in Childhood

24

Maria C. Bolling and Joost M. Meijer

Introduction and Aims

Short Definition in Layman Terms

Autoimmune bullous diseases (AIBDs) in childhood encompass the same spectrum of subtypes as the group of AIBDs in adults, both from the pemphigoid group, the pemphigus group and dermatitis herpetiformis (DH). Linear IgA disease (LAD) is the most common AIBD in children, followed by DH and bullous pemphigoid (BP). Neonatal AIBD variants exist, in which passive transfer of autoantibodies from the mother to the child has occurred. These types are usually self-limiting in a few weeks.

> **Learning Objectives**
> After reading this chapter, you will be able to recognize clinical features of different AIBDs in childhood and know the differential diagnosis of bullous diseases in childhood. You will also be aware of differences between childhood and adult AIBDs, treatment options and prognosis.

M. C. Bolling · J. M. Meijer (✉)
Center for Blistering Diseases, Department of Dermatology, University Medical Center Groningen, University of Groningen,
Groningen, The Netherlands
e-mail: m.c.bolling@umcg.nl; j.m.meijer@umcg.nl

> **Case Study: Part 1**
> A 3-month-old girl was referred by a pediatrician because of vesicles evolving to blisters on the feet and hands and spreading to the trunk (Fig. 24.1). The mucosal surfaces were unaffected. The girl was the first child of non-consanguineous parents. Pregnancy and childbirth were uneventful. No exogeneous factors were involved. Family history was negative for skin fragility disorders. The lesions started several days after vaccination (diphtheria, tetanus, pertussis, polio, hepatitis B, haemophilus influenza type b, pneumococcal vaccine). Because PCR for coxsackievirus and enteroviruses were negative, the working diagnosis of hand-foot-mouth disease was discarded, and the girl was referred to our dermatology clinic.

Didactical Questions

Are there specific clinical features in the different AIBDs in childhood? What is the most frequent AIBD in children? How are AIBDs in children diagnosed? What is the course and long-term prognosis of the different forms of AIBDs in childhood? Does therapy in AIBDs in children differ from that in adults? Are comorbidities associated with AIBDs in children?

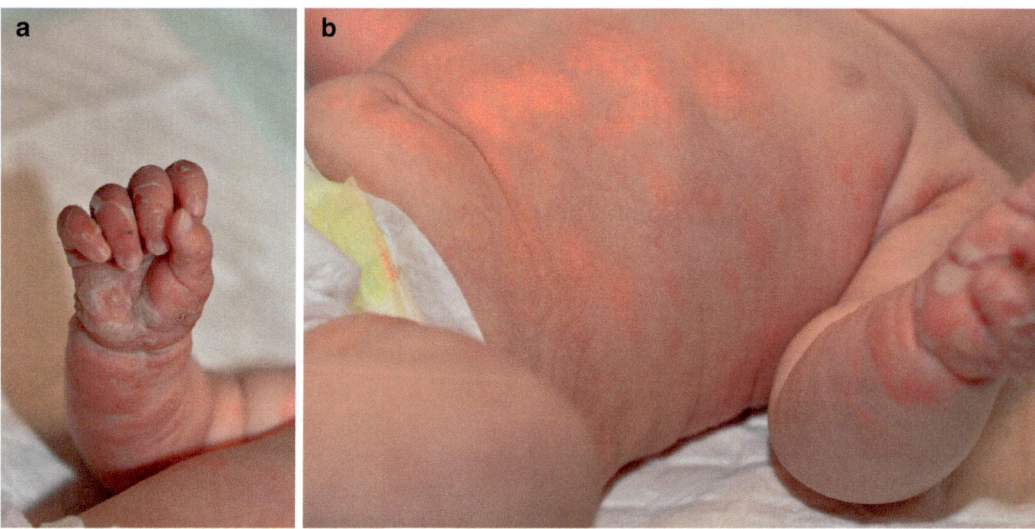

Fig. 24.1 A 3-month-old with tense blisters, vesicles, crusts and erythematous plaques on the hand and lower arm (**a**), and erythematous papules and plaques on the trunk (**b**)

Facts and Figures

The spectrum of AIBDs in children comprises the same subtypes as in adults, as also the recognized autoantigens in the different forms of AIBDs in children (see also the respective chapters of the different AIBDs). AIBDs in childhood are very rare. The prevalence in the German population was estimated to be around 100 cases per million children [1]. In most of the reported pediatric AIBD populations LAD was reported to be the most frequent AIBD in childhood followed by DH and BP [2, 3]. Neonatal forms of LAD, BP, pemphigus vulgaris (PV) and pemphigus foliaceus (PF) due to transplacental maternal antibodies have been reported with the majority having a self-limiting course in several weeks when maternal antibodies subside, or only minor treatment [4]. A few neonatal LAD cases have been reported with a more severe and prolonged course requiring systemic immunosuppressive therapy.

Vaccinations and antibiotics have been reported in several cases as eliciting factors for LAD and BP in children, although the exact correlation remains difficult to establish [5]. Epidermolysis bullosa acquisita (EBA) in children has been associated with inflammatory bowel disease [6]. The underlying neoplasm in paraneoplastic pemphigus (PNP) in children is most often Castleman's disease.

LAD is the the most frequent childhood AIBD

Diagnosis Paths

History and Physical Examination

The presenting clinical features of AIBDs in childhood may vary from the adult variants [7]. The clinical features of the different AIBD types in children are summarized here.

Clinical features of LAD in childhood include pruritus and annular configuration of blisters on the skin in a "crown of jewels" or "string of pearls" pattern. Primary lesions are clear and/or hemorrhagic firm vesicles and bullae on normal or erythematous maculae or plaques. New lesions are formed at the edges of the older lesions (Fig. 24.2a). They typically appear on the abdomen, groin and thighs, the anogenital skin, feet, hands, face and perioral area. The mean age of onset of childhood LAD is around 5–6 years.

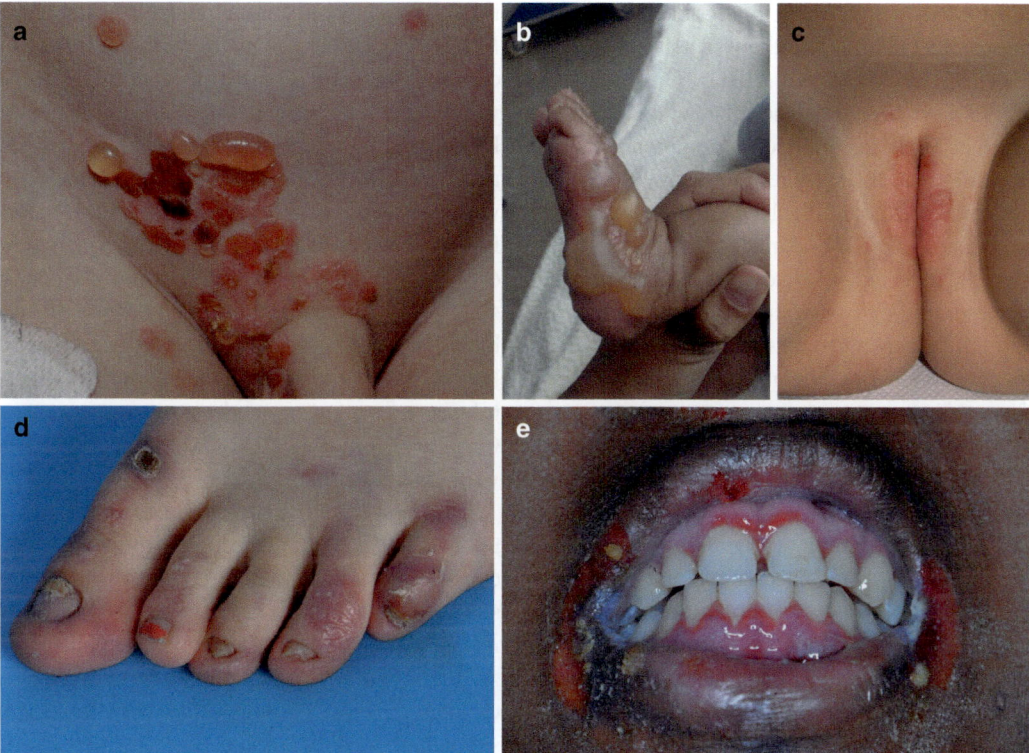

Fig. 24.2 LAD in a young boy presenting with serous bullae and hemorrhagic crusts in a serpiginous configuration in the pubis/genital area (**a**). BP in an infant with multiple tense, serous blisters and vesicles on the foot (**b**). LVP in a young girl, presenting with vulvar erythema and erosions (**c**). EBA in a 12-year-old girl with scars, milia and crusts on the dorsum of the foot and toes, and partly absent, partly dystrophic toenails (**d**). Pemphigus vulgaris in a 10-year-old girl with a desquamative gingivitis and erosions peri-oral and on the lips and (**e**)

The clinical manifestations of DH are similar in children and adults, classically presenting as intensely pruritic polymorphous eruption favoring extensor surfaces (see also Chap. 20).

BP in childhood may present at different ages. Commonly involved body site in infantile BP (<1 year of age) are the palms, soles and head (Figs. 24.1 and 24.2b) [8]. Childhood BP (>1 year of age) has a more diffuse distribution of lesions, including the mucosae. The vulvar area is often involved as well. Firm vesicles and blisters on erythematous or normal-appearing skin can be seen. In addition, pruritic, erythematous papules and plaques with irregular, annular and polycyclic configurations are usually present, and may precede or coexist with blisters. Blisters may vary in size, are usually symmetrical and ungrouped with serous and/or hemorrhagic contents. Lesions of childhood BP are non-scarring and usually pruritic.

EBA can be divided in two clinical variants: a classic mechanobullous phenotype (more common in adults and older children) which has clinical similarities with hereditary dystrophic epidermolysis bullosa, and an inflammatory phenotype which shows similarities in presentation to bullous pemphigoid (more common in children younger than 5 years of age). In mechanobullous EBA clinical characteristics include clear or hemorrhagic blisters on extensor surfaces of extremities at sites of trauma that heal with scarring (Fig. 24.2d). Mucosa (oral and genital) are often affected in childhood EBA. Furthermore, nail dystrophy, milia, and alopecia may be seen. The lesions of EBA may heal with scarring.

Mucous membrane pemphigoid (MMP) may present in childhood, although it is one of the least frequent childhood AIBDs. Only few case reports have been published. The clinical presentation of MMP in childhood is comparable to that in adulthood. It may likewise vary in presentation, mucosal sites involved, and severity (see also Chap. 15). The oral mucosa is the most common site involved, with a desquamative gingivitis as presenting sign. Affection of the vulvar mucosa and skin may be the only site involved in juvenile localized vulvar pemphigoid, Fig. 24.2c and see Chap. 15).

The clinical presentation of PV usually starts with painful mucosal blisters and erosions. Oral mucosal lesions, most often the gingiva, occur in 50–70% of childhood patients (Fig. 24.2e). Mainly non-pruritic flaccid blisters that easily erode on skin will develop after a period of weeks to months. Preferred locations of PV in both adults and children are the mucous membranes, upper torso (in a V-shape), the face including the eyelids, the scalp and the flexural areas. PF presents similar in children as in adults, with erythematosquamous plaques with a predilection for the scalp, face and upper trunk (see also Chap. 9). It may mimic seborrheic dermatitis. A clue to the diagnosis (also tor pemphigus vulgaris) is the positive Nikolsky sign. Pemphigus variants may present at any age in childhood.

PNP in children has a severe stomatitis as its most frequent clinical presentation. In addition, erythematosquamous papules and plaques with lichenoid appearance are observed. In children, PNP is often accompanied by pulmonary involvement leading to bronchiolitis obliterans and subsequent high morbidity.

A baby with acral vesicles and blisters with negative skin swabs should be suspected of infantile BP

Diagnostics

The differential diagnosis of blistering in children may differ per age group and depending on the localization (mucosa, skin) and distribution. Most often AIBDs in children are confused with infectious causes like impetigo bullosa and hand-foot-mouth disease. The differential diagnosis comprises genetic diseases (forms of epidermolysis bullosa and related skin fragility disorders, keratinopathic ichthyoses, bullous mastocytosis, acrodermatitis enteropathica (may be acquired as well), autoinflammatory syndromes, m. Behcet), infectious diseases (like candida, herpes, varicella, impetigo bullosa, staphylococcal scalded skin syndrome, hand-foot-mouth disease ad scabies), inflammatory diseases (lichen planus, lichen sclerosus, erythema multiforme), acropustulosis of infancy, and exogenous causes. Childhood vulvar pemphigoid may be confused with sexual abuse.

Diagnosis of AIBDs in children is made based upon clinical features, direct immunofluorescence (DIF) microscopy of perilesional skin and serology screening for tissue bound and circulating autoantibodies respectively, similar as in AIBD in adults (see the respective chapters). In childhood BP the serology seems to be more sensitive than in adults. In neonates with a suspicion for an AIBD it is important to pay attention to skin complaints of the mother during pregnancy and right afterwards that may point to an AIBD in the mother and the possibility of transplacental transfer of autoantibodies. Bacterial and yeast swabs, and PCR swabs of affected/eroded skin may help in differentiating with infectious causes. In case PNP is diagnosed, screening for underlying neoplasms should initiated. Careful history should be taken for bowel complaints, and, if indicated, the child should be referred for screening for inflammatory bowel diseases.

Childhood AIBD is diagnosed with DIF of perilesional skin for tissue bound autoantibodies and serology for circulating autoantibodies

> **Case Study: Part 2**
> Physical examination revealed multiple vesicles and bullae on erythematous and urticarial plaques, mainly on hands and feet, but also on proximal extremities and trunk (Fig. 24.1). Mucosal surfaces were unaffected. No scars or milia were

seen. A differential diagnosis was considered of acropustulosis of infancy, viral infection (herpes simplex/zoster), bacterial infection (impetigo bullosa), bullous scabies, linear IgA disease, neonatal bullous pemphigoid or epidermolysis bullosa acquisita, epidermolysis bullosa (simplex) or diffuse cutaneous mastocytosis.

Skin swabs were negative. A skin biopsy for histopathology showed an eosinophilic spongiotic dermatitis and subepidermal blister formation. A skin biopsy for DIF showed IgG 3+, IgA 1+ and complement C3 3+ along the EBMZ in a linear n-serratted pattern. Indirect IF on salt-split skin showed positive IgG 2+ roof staining, with also a positive BP180 NC16A ELISA (titer 116 U/ml). The diagnosis of **neonatal bullous pemphigoid** was made, possibly triggered by vaccination. The positive DIF biopsy with IgG, IgA and C3c depositions in an n-serrated pattern and findings of indirect IF on salt-split skin exclude linear IgA disease and epidermolysis bullosa acquisita.

Treatment Tricks

Initial Treatment and Therapeutic Ladder

No treatment guideline is available specific for AIBDs in childhood, the treatment and medication is similar to adults, but dosages taken into account. The various AIBDs in childhood may require specific treatments, such as dapsone in LAD, a gluten-free diet combined with dapsone in DH, topical tetracycline cream in juvenile LVP and treatment with topical and/or oral corticosteroids with potential adjuvant immunosuppressive agents in subtypes of pemphigoid and pemphigus. In general, topical corticosteroids (class III–IV) alone is a first step in treatment and often sufficient in milder forms of AIBD. The use of oral corticosteroids remains a treatment for moderate and severe forms of bullous pemphigoid, mucous membrane pemphigoid, epidermolysis bullosa or pemphigus. Especially in recalcitrant cases, adjuvant immunosuppressive agents may be considered, such as mycofenolate mofetil, colchicine or rituximab. Colchicine is a treatment option for childhood EBA with relative mild side effects, and suitable for mild cases or when other immunosuppressive agents fail.

Follow-Up and Long-Term Prognosis

AIBDs in childhood in general have a milder course, a good treatment response and a better long-term prognosis than AIBD in adults [2, 7]. Nevertheless, large areas of eroded skin always pose a threat for superinfection, and loss of fluid and electrolytes. Therefore, AIBDs in children should be considered a serious condition that requires fast treatment and adequate and hygienic skin care (see also Chap. 25). Long term follow-up of our own cohort of childhood AIBD (44 patients) did not reveal any associated diseases in a mean time of follow-up of almost 9 years.

EBA and MMP may have a more prolonged and therapy resistant course, similar as in adults. PNP in children, as in adults, has a poor prognosis with high mortality due to bronchiolitis obliterans.

> **Case Study: Part 3**
> The initial treatment of lesional clobetasol cream once a day did not lead to disease control. Therefore, in conjunction with a pediatrician, prednisolone 0.5 mg/kg/day (3 mg) was started, and dosage increased to 1.0 mg/kg/day (5 mg) because of active disease. Topical steroids were maintained. Pain management was optimized, and osteoporosis prophylaxis (vitamin D) and proton pump inhibitor were prescribed during prednisolone treatment, with also regular check-ups of blood glucoses and blood pressure. After 1 month of treatment, prednisolone was tapered to stop in the follow-

ing 2 months. Three months after the initial lesions, she was in complete remission and the topical corticosteroids tapered and ultimately stopped after 4 months, without signs of skin atrophy. No relapse occurred.

Answers

1. b.
2. c.
3. a. and b.
4. a.
5. b

Review Questions

1. What is the most frequent AIBD in children?
   a. BP
   b. LAD
   c. PV
   a. MMP
2. The AIBD with the most favorable clinical course and prognosis is:
   a. MMP
   b. EBA
   c. BP
   d. PV
3. Diagnostics of a child with suspicion of an AIBD should include (more than 1 is right):
   a. DIF biopsy.
   b. Serology for circulating autoantibodies.
   c. Hb, MCV, leucocytes.
   d. Gastroduodenoscopy and colonoscopy.
4. First line therapy of mild infantile BP consists of:
   a. Topical superpotent corticosteroids.
   b. Topical tetracycline cream.
   c. Oral corticosteroids (0.5 mg/kg/day).
   d. Dapsone.
5. Which statement about childhood mechanobullous EBA is incorrect?
   a. Oral mucosa is affected in most of the patients.
   b. It responds well to treatment.
   c. It resembles dystrophic epidermolysis bullosa.
   d. It can be associated with inflammatory bowel disease.

References

1. Hübner F, König IR, Holtsche MM, Zillikens D, Linder R, Schmidt E. Prevalence and age distribution of pemphigus and pemphigoid diseases among paediatric patients in Germany. J Eur Acad Dermatol Venereol. 2020;34(11):2600–5.
2. Welfringer-Morin A, Bekel L, Bellon N, Gantzer A, Boccara O, Hadj-Rabia S, Leclerc-Mercier S, Frassati-Biaggi A, Fraitag S, Bodemer C. Long-term evolving profile of childhood autoimmune blistering diseases: retrospective study on 38 children. J Eur Acad Dermatol Venereol. 2019;33(6):1158–63.
3. Nanda A, Lazarevic V, Rajy JM, Almasry IM, AlSabah H, AlLafi A. Spectrum of autoimmune bullous diseases among children in Kuwait. Pediatr Dermatol. 2021;38(1):50–7.
4. Zhao CY, Chiang YZ, Murrell DF. Neonatal autoimmune blistering disease: a systematic review. Pediatr Dermatol. 2016;33(4):367–74.
5. Fortuna G, Salas-Alanis JC, Guidetti E, Marinkovich MP. A critical reappraisal of the current data on drug-induced linear immunoglobulin A bullous dermatosis: a real and separate nosological entity? J Am Acad Dermatol. 2012;66(6):988–94.
6. Reddy H, Shipman AR, Wojnarowska F. Epidermolysis bullosa acquisita and inflammatory bowel disease: a review of the literature. Clin Exp Dermatol. 2013;38(3):225–9.
7. Marathe K, Lu J, Morel KD. Bullous diseases: kids are not just little people. Clin Dermatol. 2015;33(6):644–56.
8. Schwieger-Briel A, Moellmann C, Mattulat B, Schauer F, Kiritsi D, Schmidt E, Sitaru C, Ott H, Kern JS. Bullous pemphigoid in infants: characteristics, diagnosis and treatment. Orphanet J Rare Dis. 2014;10(9):185.

Wound Care in Autoimmune Bullous Diseases

Josephine C. Duipmans and Maria C. Bolling

Introduction and Aims

Patients with an AIBD suffer from pain, itch and discomfort due to blisters and erosions that may involve large body areas, including the mucosae. The pain they experience brings them stress and influences sleep, altogether hampering recovery. Due to the rarity of the disease, there is often a delay in diagnosis and treatment, leaving patients with multiple, non-healing mucosal and skin erosions. In addition, these wounds can be a porte d'entrée for infections. Despite the differences in the extent and aspect of the skin and mucosal fragility between the different AIBDs, wound and skin care follows the same principles that will be discussed in this chapter.

The aim of this chapter is to learn about factors contributing to wound healing and about the best clinical practices in wound care in AIBDs, in order to optimize comfort and quality of life and facilitate recovery of the patient.

> **Learning Objectives**
> After reading you will be able to list factors that interfere with wound healing in AIBD. You will be able to identify risk factors for hampered wound healing. You will be able to describe goals in skin, wound and blister care in AIBDs. You will be able to set up a plan for proper wound care, create the right conditions for adequate wound care and choose appropriate dressings in order to reduce pain and discomfort and to stimulate optimal wound healing, both in a hospital and a home setting.

> **Case Study: Part 1**
> A previously healthy 41-year-old male attended his general practitioner following a 3-month history of progressive blister formation and erosions on the skin (mainly upper trunk and extremities) and oral mucosa, a sore throat, difficulties in swallowing, and burning eyes. Weight loss was 25 kg in 3 months. The patient was admitted to the dermatology department of a regional hospital. Based on the clinical picture and immunodiagnostic results (perilesional skin biopsy for direct immunofluorescence and serology) a diag-

J. C. Duipmans · M. C. Bolling (✉)
Center for Blistering Diseases, Department of Dermatology, University Medical Center Groningen, University of Groningen,
Groningen, The Netherlands
e-mail: j.c.duipmans@umcg.nl;
m.c.bolling@umcg.nl

nosis of pemphigus vulgaris (PV) was made. Systemic treatment with prednisolone 1 mg/kg/d was initiated and rituximab 1000 mg iv was given. The nursing staff was inexperienced in wound care for blistering skin diseases. The wounds were covered with dry gauze compresses and were changed every day (Fig. 25.1a). By removing the gauzes that were stuck in the wound bed, the wounds started to bleed, and the patient suffered from excruciating pain. Wound healing was hampered by repeatedly damaging the re-epithelializing skin. He suffered from severe pain, anxiety and depressed feelings due to his skin condition.

Didactical Questions

Which factors interfere with wound healing in AIBDs? What are the risks of inadequate wound care? What is the first choice of dressings? Which factors should be optimized before starting a dressing change? How often should wound dressings be changed?

Goals and Challenges in Wound Care in AIBDs

Adequate wound care is essential for recovery of patients with an AIBD as it will stimulate wound healing, reduce pain, itch and stress, prevent infection and unnecessary damage to healing or yet unaffected skin, and it may prevent an unnecessary increase in immunosuppressive treatment (the goals). However, many aspects of an AIBD make proper wound care in these patients challenging. Often large areas of the body are affected, including difficult to dress body sites like groins, axilla and neck. In addition, the extensiveness of wounds and multiple blisters increase the risk of infection and can cause a substantial amount of pain, both during dressing changes and daily activities. Furthermore, these patients have fragile skin with a tendency to develop new blisters. In such circumstances, adhesive dressings and regular tapes are contraindicated and dressings should be held in place with bandages, tubular cotton bandages or soft silicone tape [1]. Finally, the frequently (and sometimes solely) involved mucosae often show poor healing, and it is difficult to protect painful erosions on oral, nasopharyngeal, ocular, and genital sites.

Factors Influencing Wound Healing in AIBDs

Many factors can influence the wound healing process, like medication, ageing, infection, smoking, comorbidities, anemia, malnutrition, immobilization, living alone, stress and lack of sleep. Regarding medication, it is important to consider that the use of the necessary immunosuppressive agents for AIBDs, although neces-

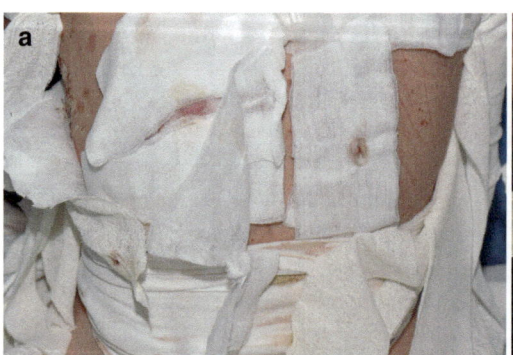
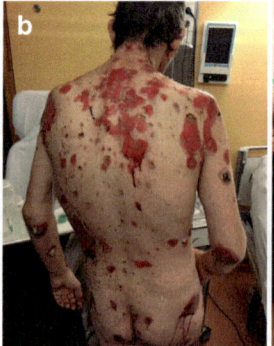
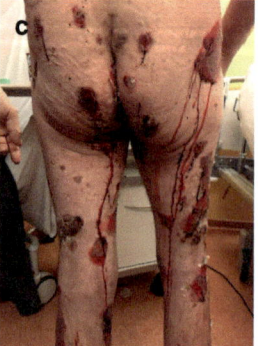

Fig. 25.1 Dry gauzes sticking to the patient's skin erosions and blisters at admission (**a**). Bleeding and de-epithelialized wounds on the back of the patient after careful removal of the dry gauzes (**b** and **c**)

sary, will affect wound healing, increase the risk of infection and may cause anemia. In addition, most AIBD patients are older than 75 years and therefore have slow wound healing. Because of pain, itch and discomfort, sleep may be disturbed, nutrition can be comprised and often mobility is limited. This all influences wound healing in a negative way.

It is important to be aware of these impairing influences on wound healing and manage them if possible.

The 'Mise En Place' for Proper Wound and Skin Care

Severity of the Disease
When more than 30% of the body surface area (BSA) is involved, it is recommended that patients are admitted to a burn care unit, where proper temperature and humidity can be provided. Patients with extensive skin lesions covering less then 30% of the BSA must be hospitalized and isolated, preferably in a low flow room, to prevent infection.

Pain Management
Optimal pain management is vital for patients with AIBDs and includes pharmacological and non-pharmacological interventions. Analgesia, such as paracetamol, NSAID's, and long-acting opioids, may be sufficient to manage pain during the day, while additional opioids and anxiolytics may be necessary for severe pain and anticipatory anxiety before and during dressing changes. Room temperature must be kept on a comfortable temperature. It is important to choose dressings that are pain free on removal. Isotonic salt baths (900 g salt in 100 l water), may reduce pain during bathing.

Infection Prevention
Practicing good hand hygiene and using protective equipment properly is very important to reduce the risk of infection. Hands should be re-washed between removal of used dressings and applying new ones. It is important to be well prepared in advance and make sure all equipment is present and ready to use. Prepare a clean field and spread out all needed materials and ointments for the dressing change. After removal, dirty dressings should be disposed immediately into a disposal bag. The wounds should be cared for using an aseptic or clean technique (an aseptic technique can be challenging when a large area of the body is affected with multiple wounds).

Skin and Mucosal Wound Care in AIBDs

Removal of Dressing and Cleansing of the Wounds

The present dressings should be carefully removed leaving re-epithelializing skin intact and preventing blistering of surrounding skin. If gauzes are stuck into the wound bed, they may be soaked off with water or paraffin/petroleum jelly ointment or a silicon medical adhesive remover (SMAR) can be used. Showering or bathing may help in removing adhesive dressings. If taking off dressings causes too much skin damage, the stuck gauzes should be left in place till they come off like a crust.

All erosions and wounds should be cleansed carefully, for example during showering of bathing if the patient can tolerate this. If not, water or topical products like wound irrigation solution or gel with polyhexamethylene biguanide (PHMB) can be poured onto the wounds. Surrounding wound skin must be cleansed as well.

Blister Management

Blisters in AIBD should be left intact in order to prevent secondary infection. The blister roof provides moist wound healing and is the best natural wound dressing. However, large blisters and blisters that are subject to trauma or on joints, should be lanced using a sterile needle, creating a large hole, preventing the blister from refilling. The roof should be left in place, because deroofing can lead to additional pain. Subsequently, the blister can be covered with a non-adherent dressing.

Wound Care and Dressings

Erosions, blisters and surrounding skin are vulnerable to further damage. Therefore, wounds must be covered with non-adhesive dressings that promote moist wound healing, are comfortable, and are available in large sizes. Silicon or lipido colloïd based foam dressings (Mepilex transfer/lite; urgotul) or hydrofibers (Aquacel) satisfy these demands. As a first wound contact layer soft silicon mesh (Mepitel one) can be applied. This dressing can stay in place up to 5–7 days while topical treatment can be applied on top of the mesh daily. Secondary dressings, on top of the silicon mesh, can be changed every (other) day. If these dressings are not available, a double layer of grease impregnated gauzes can be applied. Great care must be taken to ensure dressings do not slip, which can cause tearing of skin and cause adherence of wounds to clothing or bedding. The use of dry gauzes as a primary wound layer must be avoided.

In case of local infection, topical antibiotics or antiseptics can be used. When application of topicals directly to the skin is too painful, the dressing can be impregnated with the topical product instead and applied. Dry skin and crusts must be kept moist by daily application of emollients.

Frequency of Dressing Changes

Frequent dressing changes can strip the wound of fragile re-epithelialization. It is advised to limit dressing frequency to 3 times a week, unless treatment with daily topical potent corticosteroids is needed, like in bullous pemphigoid, or in case of a wound infection with large amounts of exudate.

> **Case Study: Part 2**
> Because the wound care was so traumatic for the patient, and proper non-adhesive wound dressings were not present, the patient was transferred to the Dutch Center for Blistering Diseases. Prednisolone 1 mg/kg/d was continued, omeprazole and calcium were added. Because of the traumatic experiences, the patient was very anxious about the dressing change. Proper pain medication was given 1 h prior to dressing change. All materials and a clean field were prepared beforehand, and room temperature was set to 24 gr Celsius.
>
> Dry gauzes were removed with great care and bandages stuck in the wound bed were left in place to avoid further skin damage. Skin was cleansed with tap water and eroded areas were carefully treated with a disinfect wound gel (Prontosan wound gel with polyhexanide). All open areas were covered with non-adherent silicon foam dressing (Mepilex transfer) and fixated with tape, that didn't touch the skin (Fig. 25.2a). A shirt, cut out of cotton cloth, was put on top of the dressings and secured with cohesive bandages in a way that shoulders and axillae were covered. For dressing fixation on arms and legs tubular bandages were used. Dressing changes were only needed 3 times a week. Attention was paid to adequate mouth care, and lidocaine 2% gel was started before eating. The patient experienced less pain, no trauma and anxiety, slept well and gained some weight. The combination of the medication with adequate wound care led to fast re-epithelialization of the skin (Fig. 25.2b).

Mucosae

Oral blisters, erosions and ulcerations are very painful, and often heal slowly. Application of local anesthetics (lidocaine 2% gel) may relief pain and promotes food intake. A soft, calory-rich diet and avoidance of spicy and acidic foods are recommended. Adequate oral hygiene, including using diluted antiseptic mouthwashes, and proper periodontal treatment must be supported. Candida and herpes simplex virus infections are common on the mucosae of AIBD patients with oral lesions and/or treated with

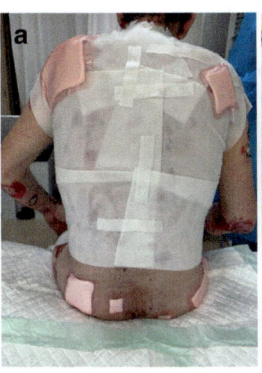 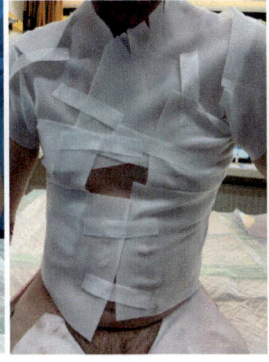 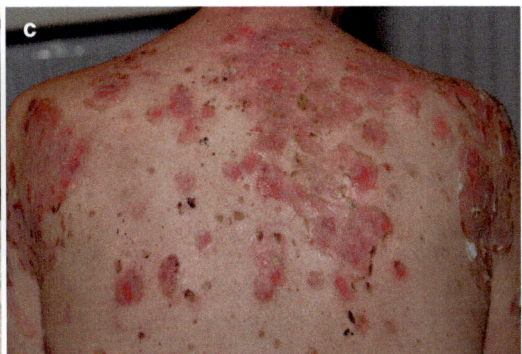

Fig. 25.2 Non-adhesive silicon-based dressings applied to the wounds on the back (**a**) and front (**b**), fixated on the bandages itself. Isolated erosions were covered by silicon based bordered dressings on the buttocks (**a**, pink). Few days later partly re-epithelized skin appeared on the back, and bleeding was absent after removal of the silicon-based bandages (**c**)

immunosuppressants and should be treated timely and appropriately. In case of candida, treat the prosthetics as well if present. Lips can be kept soft with petroleum jelly bidaily or more frequently. Other sites that can be affected include the conjunctival, nasal, pharyngeal, laryngeal, esophageal, genital, and anal mucosa. All affected mucosae should be cleansed daily with water or sterile sodium chloride and, if necessary, an antimicrobial ointment can be applied. Use cotton swabs for eyes and nostrils. Small painful erosions on difficult to dress locations, like labia and nostrils, can be covered with a thin layer of a zinc oxide product.

Wound Care Plan

To ensure well-executed wound care, it is important to make a simple and clear wound care plan and explain and provide it to the patients and immediate caregivers (spouse/children/nurses). The wound care plan is dynamic and should be adjusted, when necessary, based on changes in the skin condition.

Conclusion

Optimal wound care in patients with an AIBD can be challenging. Even though the general principles of wound care also apply to patients with an AIBD, factors like skin fragility, extensive wounds, higher age, use of immunosuppressant medication, wounds on difficult to dress locations, all impact wound care. Therefore, it is important to pay attention to, and individualize skin and mucosal care to the unique needs of AIBD patients from the first visit. Basic principles are pain management, infection prevention, non-adhesive dressings, and paying attention to the general condition of the patient.

Review Questions

1. What is the effect of the immunosuppressive therapy on wound healing in AIBD?
    a. Slowing down wound healing
    b. Increasing the risk of infection
    c. Increasing itch
    d. Reducing wound bleeding
2. What is the general principle for treating blisters in AIBD?
    a. Always pop the blister in order to reduce the risk of infection
    b. Pop the blister only when it is subject to trauma or on joints
    c. Pop blisters when the diameter is >4 cm
    d. Only open blisters on mucosal surfaces
3. What is the first choice of dressings in AIBD?
    a. Impregnated gauzes and hydrocolloid dressings
    b. Hydrofibers, hydrocolloid dressings and silicon- and lipidocolloid based dressings

c. Hydrofibers and silicon- and lipidocolloid-based dressings
d. A good dressing has yet to be invented

Answers

1. a. and b.
2. b.
3. c.

References

1. Nadelmann E, Czernik A. Wound care in immunobullous disease, Chapter 9. In: Gönül M, Cakmak S, editors. Intech open autoimmune bullous diseases; 2018. p. 213–45.
2. Schultz GS, Sibbald RG, Falanga V, Ayello EA, Dowsett C, Harding K, Romanelli M, Stacey MC, Teot L, Vanscheidt W. Wound bed preparation: a systematic approach to wound management. Wound Repair Regen. 2003;11:S1–S28.
3. Denyer J, Pillay E, Clapham J. Practice Guidelines Skin and wound care in Epidermolysis bullosa, an expert working group consensus. Wounds International. 2017. www.woundsinternational.com
4. Armstrong D, Meyr A. Risk factors for impaired wound healing and wound complications. In Berman S, et al (Ed.), UpToDate. Retrieved March 15, 2021, from https://www.uptodate.com/contents/risk-factors-for-impaired-wound-healing-and-wound-complications

Appendix A: Patient Support Groups and International Centers for AIBD

Patients should also be informed about the existence of local or national patient support groups or patients' associations, such as the International Pemphigus and Pemphigoid Foundation (IPPF, www.pemphigus.org) for autoimmune bullous diseases. These associations contribute to promote knowledge of the disease, improve patients' access to information, healthcare and social services and they can help in referring patients to referral centers for AIBD (Table A.1). For example, dermatologists in Europe work together in the Task Force AIBD of the European Academy of Dermatology and Venereology, and in Japan in the Pemphigus Study Group. Referral centers collaborating in the scientific network of RegiSCAR (www.regiscar.org) contribute to the pharmacovigilance of severe cutaneous adverse events.

Table A.1 An overview of national patient support groups and referral centers for AIBD. The provided information may be incomplete

Country	Patient support group	National referral center
Australia	Australasian Blistering Diseases Foundation: http://blisters.org.au	Department of Dermatology at St George Hospital, University of New South Wales, Sydney
Austria		Department of Dermatology, Division of Immunology, Allergy and Infectious Diseases, Medical University of Vienna
Brasil		Department of Dermatology, University of Sao Paulo
Bulgaria		Department of Dermatology, Alexander's University Hospital, Sofia
Canada	Canadian Pemphigus and Pemphigoid Foundation:	Division of Dermatology, Sunnybrook Health Sciences Center, Toronto
Croatia		Department of Dermatology, School of Medicine University of Zagreb, Zagreb, Croatia
Czech Republic		Department of Dermatology, Masaryk University, Brno
Denmark		Department of Dermato-Venereology, Aarhus University
Egypt		Department of Dermatology, Cairo University
Finland		Department of Dermatology, Tampere University Hospital, Tampere
France	Association Pemphigus Pemphigoïde France: www.pemphigus.asso.fr	Groupe Bulle, Dermatology Department, Rouen University Hospital, University of Rouen Groupe Hospitalier Henri-Mondor, Créteil
Germany	Pemphigus und Pemphigoid Selbsthilfegruppe www.pemphigus-pemphigoid-selbsthilfe.de	Department of Dermatology, University of Lubeck Department of Dermatology and Allergology, University Hospital, Philipps-Universität Marburg

(continued)

Table A.1 (continued)

Country	Patient support group	National referral center
Greece		Department of Dermatology, Aristotle University of Thessaloniki, Thessaloniki,
India		Department of Dermatology, Venereology and Leprology, Postgraduate Institute of Medical Education and Research, Chandigarh
		Department of Dermatology and Venereology, All India Institute of Medical Sciences, New Delhi
Indonesia		Department of Dermaotlogy, Gadjah Mada University, Yogyakarta
Iran		Autoimmune Bullous Diseases Research Center, Department of Dermatology, Tehran University of Medical Sciences
Italy	Associazione Nazionale Pemfigo-Pemfigoide Italy, www.pemfigo.it	Istituto Dermopatico dell'Immacolata, IRCCS, Rome
Israel		Department of Dermatology, Tel-Aviv University
Hungary		Department of Dermatology, Semmelweis University Budapest
Japan		Department of Dermatology, Keio University School of Medicine, Tokyo
		Kurume University Institute of Cutaneous Cell Biology, Kurume, Fukuoka
South Korea		Department of Dermatology and Cutaneous Biology Research Institute, Yonsei University College of Medicine, Gangnam Severance Hospital, Seoul
Lebanon		Department of Dermatology, American University of Beirut Medical Center, Riad El Solh/Beirut
Morocco		Service de Dermatologie, CHU Ibn Sina, Université Med V, Souissi, Rabat
Nepal	Blistering Disease Foundation of Nepal	Civil Service Hospital, Naya Baneshwor, Kathmandu
Netherlands	Netwerk voor Blaarziekten www.netwerkblaarziekten.nl	Department of Dermatology, Center for Blistering Diseases, University Medical Center Groningen
Poland		Department of Dermatology, Medical University of Warsaw
Serbia		Clinic of Dermatovenereology, Clinical Center of Serbia, Belgrade
Spain	Asociación Española de Pénfigo, Penfigoide y Otras Enfermedades Vesiculoampollosas, info@aeppeva.org	Department of Dermatology, Hospital Clínic. Universitat de Barcelona
Switzerland		Department of Dermatology, University of Bern, Inselspital,
Tanzania		Regional Dermatology Training Centre at Kilimanjaro Christian Medical University College, Moshi
Tunisia		Department of Dermatology, Charles Nicolle Hospital Tunis
Turkey	www.turkdermatoloji.org.tr	Department of Dermatology, Akdeniz University, Antalya
		Department of Dermatology, Karadeniz Technical University, Trabzon
United Kingdom	http://pemfriends.co.uk http://www.pemphigus.org.uk	Department of Dermatology, Churchill Hospital, Oxford
		St John's Institute of Dermatology, Guy's and St Thomas' Hospital NHS Trust, London

Table A.1 (continued)

Country	Patient support group	National referral center
USA	International Pemphigus Pemphigoid Foundation www.pemphigus.org	Department of Dermatology, University at Buffalo
Department of Dermatology, University of North Carolina at Chapel Hill
Division of Dermatology, Duke Medical Center, Durham
Department of Dermatology, School of Medicine, University of Utah, Salt Lake City
Department of Dermatology, University of Iowa, Iowa City
Department of Dermatology, University of Texas Southwestern Medical Center, Dallas
Department of Dermatology, University of Pennsylvania, Philadelphia
Department of Dermatology, Stanford University
St Joseph Mercy Health System, Department of Dermatology, Ann Arbor
Department of Dermatology, University of California, Irvine
Laboratory for Investigative Dermatology, Rockefeller University, New York
Center for Investigative Dermatology, Division of Dermatology and Cutaneous Sciences, Michigan State University, East Lansing

Index

A

Adaptive immune system, 2, 5, 6
Adult LVP, 126
Agranulocytosis, 163
Anergy, 6
Anti-BP180 IgG antibodies, 55
Anti-epiligrin cicatricial pemphigoid, 126
Antigen-presenting cells, 3
Antigen-specific antibodies, 4
Anti-laminin 332 MMP (anti-LN-332 MMP), 126–129
Anti-p200 pemphigoid, 116, 118, 119
Asboe-Hansen's (or blister spread) sign, 15
Autoimmune blistering diseases, 6, 43, 44
Autoimmune bullous diseases (AIBDs), 192
    clinical presentation, 188–190
    definition, 187, 188
    diagnosis, 190
    differential diagnosis, 190
    patient history, 187, 188
    treatment, 191, 192
    wound care, 197
        disease severity, 195
        factors, 194, 195
        goals and challenges, 194
        infection prevention, 195
        optimal pain management, 195
        patient history, 193, 194
        skin and mucosal wound care, 195–197
Autoimmune disease, 131, 132
Autoimmunity, 6
Auto-reactive B- and T-lymphocytes, 6

B

B- and T-lymphocytes, 4
B cell receptor (BCR), 2
Biopsy
    buccal mucosa, 30
    conjunctiva, 30
    definition, 29
    histopathology, 29–30
    perilesional, 29, 31, 32
    skin, 30
    transport and handling specimens, 32
B-lymphocytes, 6
BP230, 104, 105
BPAG1/type XVII collagen, 105
Brunsting-Perry cicatricial pemphigoid
    clinical symptoms, 114
    definition, 114
    diagnosis, 114, 119
    treatment, 115
Bullous dermatitis artefacta (DA), 185
    blistering, 183
    definition, 181, 182
    diagnosis, 182–185
    epidemiology, 182
    pathogenesis, 182
    treatment, 184, 185
Bullous pemphigoid (BP), 8, 19, 38
    clinical symptoms, 119
    definition, 107–109
    diagnostics, 110, 111
    epidemiology, 108
    follow-up and tapering, 112
    history, 109–111
    initial treatment and therapeutic ladder, 111, 112
    pathogenesis, 109
    physical examination, 109–111
    treatment, 119
180 kDa bullous pemphigoid antigen (BP180), 105
Bullous pemphigoid disease area index (BPDAI), 15, 21
Bullous systemic lupus erythematosus (BSLE), 141
    classification, 138
    clinical presentation, 138
    definition, 137
    diagnosis, 138–140
    epidemiology, 138
    pathogenesis, 138
    treatment, 140

C

Cellular/humoral immune response, 5
Chronic bullous dermatosis of childhood (CBDC), 145
Circulating IgG-dsDNA complexes, 7

Classic subcorneal pustular dermatosis, 95
Clonal deletion or negative selection, 6
Corticosteroids, 73

D
Dapsone, 162, 163
Dapsone hypersensitivity syndrome (DHS), 163
Delayed type hypersensitivity, 7
Deranged cell signaling, 7
Dermatitis herpetiformis (DH), 40, 164
    clinical presentation, 158, 160, 161
    definition, 157, 158
    diagnostics, 160, 162
    epidemiology, 158
    pathogenesis, 158–160
    treatment, 161–163
Desmocollins (Dscs), 63, 64
Desmoglein compensation hypothesis, 68, 69
Desmogleins (Dsgs), 63, 64
Desmoplakin, 63, 64
Desmosomal cadherins, 61
Desmosomes
    cell-cell adhesion structures, 61–63
    isoforms, 63
    proteins, 64
Dipeptidyl peptidase 4 (DPP-4) inhibitors, 152
Direct immunofluorescence (DIF) microscopy, 30, 73, 145, 147, 148, 160
    dermatitis herpetiformis, 40
    laboratory preparation, 35
    pemphigoid, 37, 38
    pemphigus, 36
    porphyria cutanea tarda, 40
    pseudoporphyria, 41
Drug-induced bullous pemphigoid (DIBP), 155
    antigenic properties, 151
    comorbidities, 151
    diagnosis, 152–154
    etiology, 151
    pharmacological groups, 151–153
    treatment, 154
    types, 151
Drug-induced linear IgA disease (DILAD), 154–156
Drug-induced pemphigus
    diagnosis, 101
    non-thiol/non-phenol drugs, 100, 101
    phenol drugs, 100, 101
    thiol-associated drugs, 100, 101
    treatment, 102

E
Efflorescences, 12
Endemic pemphigus foliaceus, 80, 81
Enteropathy associated T-cell lymphoma (EATL), 161
Enzyme-linked immunosorbent assay (ELISA), 56, 57, 73

Epidermal basement membrane, 103, 105, 106
Epidermal basement membrane zone (EBMZ), 121, 151
Epidermolysis bullosa (EB), 49
Epidermolysis bullosa acquisita (EBA), 38, 135, 188
    definition, 131, 132
    diagnosis, 133, 134
    epidemiology, 132
    history, 133
    pathogenesis, 132
    physical examination, 133
    treatment, 134, 135
Epitopes, 55
Erythema exsudativum multiforme (EEM), 165
    characteristics, 174
    classification, 172, 173
    definition, 166, 172
    diagnosis, 174
    differential diagnosis, 173
    epidemiology, 173
    history, 174
    pathogenesis, 173
    treatment, 174, 175
Erythema multiforme, 139
Exfoliation or skin peeling, 12

F
FITC conjugated antibodies, 36
Fluorescent overlay antigen mapping (FOAM), 39
Fogo selvagem ('wildfire'), *see* Endemic pemphigus
Follicle or germinal center, 4

G
Glucose-6-phosphate dehydrogenase (G6 PD) deficiency, 147
Gluten free diet (GFD), 161, 162
Glutens sensitive disease (GSD), 157–158

H
Hemidesmosomes (HDs), 103–105, 107
Hemolysis, 162, 163
Human leucocyte antigens (HLA), 3
Hypersensitivity reactions, 6

I
IgA epidermolysis bullosa acquisita (IgA-EBA), 144, 145
IgA pemphigus (IGAP), 36, 94
    classification, 94
    definition, 93, 94
    epidemiology, 95
    follow-up and tapering, 97
    general diagnostics, 95
    history and physical examination, 95
    initial treatment, 96, 97

pathogenesis, 95
specific diagnostics, 96
Immune system
  adaptive immune system, 2, 5
  innate immune system, 1
Immunoadsorption, 74
Immuno-assays
  ELISA, 56, 57
  immunoblotting, 53–55
  immunoprecipitation, 55, 56
  keratinocyte binding assay, 58
  keratinocyte footprint assay, 58, 59
Immunoblotting, 53–55
Immunofluorescence biopsy, 31
Immunofluorescent techniques, 7
Immunological tolerance, 6
Immunoprecipitation, 55, 56
Immunosuppressive agents, 74
Indirect immunofluorescence (IIF) microscopy, 73, 160
  autoimmune blistering diseases, 43, 44
  circulating antibodies, 43
  human salt split skin, 47, 48
  knock-out skin, 49, 50
  laboratory preparation, 43
  monkey esophagus, 45, 46
  rat bladder, 49
  salt split skin, 48
Infiltrated urticarial plaques, 107
Innate immune system, 1, 2
Integrin α6β4, 105
Intraepidermal neutrophilic IgA dermatosis type (IEN-type), 94
Intravenous immunoglobulin (IVIG), 74, 112, 171
Isotype switching, 4

J
Juvenile/childhood LVP, 126, 129

K
Keratinocyte binding assay, 58
Keratinocyte footprint assay, 58, 59
Knock-out skin, 49, 50

L
Laminins, 105
Lesional peribullous biopsy, 31
Lichen planus pemphigoides (LPP), 115
Linear IgA bullous dermatosis (LABD), 148
  diagnostics, 145, 146, 148
  epidemiology, 144
  history, 145–147
  pathogenesis, 144
  physical examination, 145–147
  treatment, 147, 148
Localized vulvar pemphigoid (LVP)
  clinical symptoms, 126
  definition, 125, 126
  diagnosis, 126
  treatment, 126
Lupus band, 7
Lupus-band phenomenon, 83
Lupus erythematosus (LE), 138

M
Major histocompatibility complex (MHC) molecules, 3
Methemoglobinemia, 163
MMP Disease Area Index (MMPDAI), 123
Monkey esophagus, 45, 46
Mucocutaneous pemphigus vulgaris, 71
Mucosal-dominant pemphigus vulgaris, 70
Mucous membrane pemphigoid (MMP), 38, 152
  definition, 121, 122, 128, 129
  diagnostics, 123, 124
  follow-up and tapering, 124
  history, 122, 123
  initial treatment and treatment ladder, 124
  physical examination, 122, 123
Mucous membrane pemphigoid area index (MMPDAI), 16, 22
Mycoplasma pneumoniae-induced rash and mucositis (MIRM), 173

N
Negative selection/clonal deletion, 5
Neonatal bullous pemphigoid, 191
Nikolsky sign, 108, 109
Nikolsky sign type I procedure, 14
Nonbullous pemphigoid (NBP), 107, 108, 119
  clinical presentation, 113
  definition, 112
  diagnosis, 114
  epidemiology, 113
  pathogenesis, 113
  treatment, 114
16th non-collagenous domain (NC16A), 109
Non-radioactive immunoprecipitation, 56

O
Ocular mucous membrane pemphigoid
  clinical symptoms, 124, 125
  definition, 124
  diagnosis, 125
  treatment, 125

P
p200, 105
Paraneoplastic autoimmune multi-organ syndrome (PAMS), 88

Paraneoplastic pemphigus (PNP), 36, 38, 54
  clinical hallmark, 88
  definition, 87, 88
  diagnosis of, 89
  epidemiology, 88
  history and physical examination, 88, 89
  manifestations of, 87
  pathogenesis, 88
  prognosis, 90
  rat bladder test, 48, 49
  small subset of, 89, 90
  treatment, 90
Pathogen associated molecules, 5
Pemphigoid, 7, 37, 38
Pemphigoid gestationis (PG), 115–117, 119
Pemphigus, 7, 15, 36, 37
Pemphigus disease area index (PDAI), 15, 17
Pemphigus erythematosus (PE), 38, 83, 84
Pemphigus foliaceus (PF), 78, 79
  classification, 78
  definition, 77
  diagnosis of, 79
  epidemiology, 79
  follow-up, 80
  history and physical examination, 79
  initial treatment, 80
  pathogenesis, 79
  tapering, 80
Pemphigus herpetiformis (PH), 81–83
Pemphigus vulgaris
  classification, 67
  corticosteroids, 73
  definition, 67
  direct immunofluorescence microscopy, 73
  enzyme-linked immunosorbent assays, 73
  epidemiology, 67
  follow-up, 75
  general diagnostics, 71
  histopathology, 72
  history and physical examination, 70, 71
  IF findings and clinical symptoms, 66–67
  immunoadsorption, 74
  immunosuppressive agents, 74
  indirect immunofluorescence microscopy, 73
  intravenous immunoglobulin, 74
  pathogenesis, 68
  plasmapheresis, 74
  rituximab, 74
  tapering, 75
  typical features, 66
Perilesional biopsy, 29, 31, 32
Peripheral tolerance, 6
Plakoglobin, 63, 64
Plakophilins (Pkp), 63, 64
Plasmapheresis, 74
Plectin, 104
Polyacrylamide gel electrophoresis (PAGE), 53
Polyhexamethylene biguanide (PHMB), 195
Porphyria cutanea tarda (PCT), 40, 180
  definition, 178
  diagnosis, 179
  epidemiology, 178
  history, 178, 179
  pathogenesis, 178, 179
  patient history, 177, 178
  physical examination, 178, 179
  skin fragility and blistering, 177
  treatment, 179, 180
  triggering factors, 177
Pseudo-Nikolsky's sign, 14, 171
Pseudoporphyria, 41, 179

R
Rat bladder, 49
Regulatory T-cells (Tregs), 6
Reticulocytosis, 162
Rituximab, 74, 112

S
Salt split skin, 48
SCORTEN criteria, 170
Signalling pathways, 68
Silicon medical adhesive remover (SMAR), 195
Skin biopsy, direct immunofluorescence, 96
Sneddon-Wilkinson's disease, 95
Sodium dodecyl sulphate (SDS), 53
Split skin (SSS) substrate, 111
Standard immunoblotting technique, 96
Steric hindrance theory, 7, 68
Stevens Johnson syndrome/Toxic epidermal necrolysis (SJS/TEN), 175
  aetiology, 169
  blisters, 167
  classification, 166, 167
  definition, 166
  diagnosis, 168, 170, 171
  flu-like symptoms, 167
  history, 170
  incidence, 168
  overall mortality rate, 168
  overview, 165
  pathogenesis, 168, 169
  physical examination, 170
  treatment, 171, 172
  visceral involvement (liver), 167
Subacute cutaneous lupus erythematosus (SCLE), 138
Subcorneal pustulosis dermatosis type (SPD-type), 94
Subepidermal autoimmune blistering diseases, 47
Systemic corticosteroids, 73
Systemic lupus erythematosus (SLE), 7

T
Target/iris lesions, 172
T cell receptor (TCR), 2
T-helper cells, 3
Tissue transglutaminase (tTG), 157
T-lymphocytes, 3

Toxic epidermal necrolysis (TEN), 145
Toxic epidermolytic necrolysis (TEN), 139
Type II hypersensitivity, 6
Type IV collagen, 106
Type IV hypersensitivity, 7
Type VII collagen, 105

U
Uroporphyrinogen decarboxylase (UROD), 178

V
Vertical distribution, 158
Vesiculo-bullous diseases
   definition, 12
   physical signs, 13
   symptoms, 12

GPSR Compliance

The European Union's (EU) General Product Safety Regulation (GPSR) is a set of rules that requires consumer products to be safe and our obligations to ensure this.

If you have any concerns about our products, you can contact us on ProductSafety@springernature.com

In case Publisher is established outside the EU, the EU authorized representative is:

Springer Nature Customer Service Center GmbH
Europaplatz 3
69115 Heidelberg, Germany

Batch number: 08823233

Printed by Printforce, the Netherlands